Medical Group Management Association

Physician Compensation and Production Survey

2003 REPORT BASED ON 2002 DATA

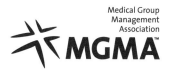

Medical Group
Management
Association

MGMA

www.mgma.com

2002-2003 SURVEY ADVISORY COMMITTEE

John W. Houser, FACMPE, *Chair*
Administrator
Valley Medical Center PLLC
Lewiston, Idaho

Phyllis Brown
Chief Executive Officer
Arkansas Cardiology PA
Little Rock, Arkansas

Sarah H. Patterson, FACMPE
Vice President
Virginia Mason Medical Center
Seattle, Washington

Bruce A. Johnson, JD, MPA
Principal
MGMA Health Care Consulting Group
Medical Group Management Association
Englewood, Colorado

Michael L. Nochomovitz, MD
President and Chief Medical Officer
Univ. of Primary Care Physician Practices
University Hospitals of Cleveland
Cleveland, Ohio

Fred Simmons
Administrator
Clearwater Cardiovascular Consultants
Clearwater, Florida

W. David Holloway, MD
Senior Vice President and Chief Quality Officer
Parkview Health System
Fort Wayne, Indiana

Jeffrey Mossoff, CMPE
Executive Vice President
Univ. Clinical Associates Medical Clinic
Univ. of Mississippi
Jackson, Mississippi

Board Liaison
Christine A. Schon, FACMPE
Sr. Director Physician Operations
Bassett Healthcare
Mary Imogene Bassett Hospital
Cooperstown, New York

Academic Practice Committee Chair
Kathryn A. Mahaffey
Chief Operating Officer
SIU Physicians and Surgeons
Southern Illinois University School of Medicine
Springfield, Illinois

The *Physician Compensation and Production Survey: 2003 Report Based on 2002 Data* was compiled by the Medical Group Management Association (MGMA) Survey Operations Department. MGMA would like to acknowledge Vivian Heggie and Doug Conrad for their assistance with this project. The Survey Operations Department staff members responsible for this and other MGMA surveys are:

Chris A. Adams, Data Specialist
Rochelle V. Cookson, MBA, Senior Analyst
Suman Elizabeth Graeber, MHA, Senior Analyst
Danielle C. Guillen, Data Specialist
Pamela Hart, MA, Senior Analyst
Rusalyn A. Herington, MBA, Production Manager
Heather C. Jones, Department Coordinator
Jan Jordan Krause, MA, CMPE, Project Director

Mariann Lowery, Production Assistant
Lori L. McNeilley, Assistant Analyst
Dean A. Pallozzi, Systems Analyst
Jena M. Pohle, Administrative Assistant
Daniel P. Stech, MBA, Director
Brooke L. Whitten, Assistant Analyst
Jay Y. Whitten, Data Specialist

For further information or questions, please contact Rochelle V. Cookson, MBA, Senior Analyst or Brooke L. Whitten, Assistant Analyst, at 877.ASK.MGMA (275.6462), ext. 895.

ISSN #1064-4563
ISBN #1-56829-051-9

August 2003

Dear Colleague:

Congratulations! You have selected the Medical Group Management Association (MGMA) *Physician Compensation and Production Survey: 2003 Report Based on 2002 Data* as an addition to your collection of practice management resources.

If you received this report due to your participation and submittal of your practice's data, thank you for taking the time to contribute to the advancement of our profession. Part of your reward is this complimentary copy of the report, but take pride in knowing that you have helped to build the best comparative database of medical group practice statistics available anywhere. The other part of your reward is having ready access to reliable information on which to make daily business decisions.

If you were not a contributor but could have been, I encourage you to participate in next year's survey. Participation in the surveys is the one key factor that increases the value of the data. The process is not difficult, and the MGMA Survey Department staff can walk you through it.

The report's contents are sorted to allow you to easily compare your practice's performance and key indicators to that of your peers'. The introductory text and appendices should be reviewed to get the best understanding of the data and most benefit from the report. The observations you can make using the data can have a profound impact on the effectiveness of your organization.

Thanks again for your support of the MGMA surveys and reports. I know you will find them as indispensable as I do.

Sincerely,

John W. Houser, FACMPE
Chair, 2003 MGMA Survey Advisory Committee

TABLE OF CONTENTS

Executive Summary

Demographic Tables and Graphs

Physician Compensation and Benefits

Physician Productivity

Part-Time Physicians

0.7 Clinical FTE

0.4 - 0.6 Clinical FTE

Nonphysician Providers

Compensation

Retirement Benefits

Gross Charges

Ambulatory Encounters

Surgical/Anesthesia Encounters

Appendices

IMPORTANT NOTICE AND DISCLAIMER

The information contained in the *Physician Compensation and Production Survey: 2003 Report Based on 2002 Data* is presented solely for the purpose of informing readers of ranges of compensation reported by Medical Group Management Association member organizations. These data may not be used for the purpose of limiting competition, restraining trade, or reducing or stabilizing salary or benefit levels. Such improper use is prohibited by federal and state antitrust laws and will violate the antitrust compliance program established and enforced by the MGMA Board of Directors.

MGMA publications are intended to provide current and accurate information, and are designed to assist readers in becoming more familiar with the subject matter covered. MGMA published the *Physician Compensation and Production Survey: 2003 Report Based on 2002 Data* for a general audience as well as for MGMA members. Such publications are distributed with the understanding that MGMA does not render any legal, accounting, or professional advice that may be construed as specifically applicable to individual situations. No representations or warranties are made concerning the application of legal or other principles discussed in MGMA publications to any specific factual situation, nor is any prediction made concerning how any particular judge, government official, or other person will interpret or apply such principles. Specific factual situations should be discussed with professional advisors.

EXECUTIVE SUMMARY

INTRODUCTION

Purpose: The Medical Group Management Association (MGMA) *Physician Compensation and Production Survey: 2003 Report Based on 2002 Data* is a census of the MGMA membership designed to assist medical practice executives in evaluating the ranges of compensation and productivity of physicians and nonphysician providers. This report allows users to compare and learn more about the factors affecting compensation and production.

Description: This survey of MGMA member practices has been conducted annually since 1987. Data are reported for 105 physician specialties and 30 nonphysician provider specialties. The report contains sections on physician compensation, benefits, productivity and summary tables for specialties, as well as summary tables for part-time physicians and nonphysician providers. The productivity measures of gross charges, ambulatory encounters, hospital encounters, surgical/anesthesia cases, and total and physician work relative value units (RVUs) are presented.

Four performance ratios – compensation to gross charges ratio, compensation to collections ratio, compensation per total RVU and compensation per physician work RVU – are calculated to illustrate the relationship between compensation and productivity.

MGMA Survey Products: In addition to the *Physician Compensation and Production Survey Report*, the MGMA Survey Operations Department conducts other annual surveys of MGMA member practices.

The *Management Compensation Survey Report* includes compensation, bonus and retirement benefit amounts for physician executives and for middle and upper level manager positions.

The *Cost Survey Report* summarizes the financial performance and productivity of responding medical practices. Significant measures contained in the report are: staffing ratios, medical revenue, staff salary costs, total operating costs, revenue after operating costs, provider costs and net practice income/loss. Accounts receivable, payer mix, collection percentages, financial ratios and balance sheet information are also included.

The Cost Survey is also the basis for additional reports. An in-depth analysis of "better performing" medical group practices is presented in a companion publication, the *Performance and Practices of Successful Medical Groups*. Also, studies have been conducted of various clinical specialties and special interest groups within MGMA. Cost survey reports will be available for orthopedic practices, cardiovascular/thoracic surgery and cardiology practices, and for practices within integrated delivery systems. Additional reports are available for practices in ambulatory surgery centers and management services organizations.

MGMA conducts a parallel survey to this report for the academic sector. *The Academic Practice Compensation and Production Survey for Faculty & Management Report* provides compensation and productivity levels for medical school physician faculty. Clinical science department and practice plan managerial compensation and benefit information is also reported.

The MGMA *Physician Compensation and Production Survey Report* and *Cost Survey Report* are available in both printed format and as an interactive CD-ROM, which includes more comprehensive statistics and additional data not found in the printed report.

A respondent ranking report for *Physician Compensation and Production* data, comparing the respondent's data against the survey medians, is computed and distributed only to respondents to enable them to easily identify measures that might warrant further review and improvement.

Survey Advisory Committee: The MGMA Survey Advisory Committee provided guidance on the format and content of this report as well as the related questionnaire and guide to ensure that the survey addresses current and relevant practice management areas. The committee members are listed on page two.

SURVEY METHODOLOGY

Changes to the Instrument and Report: This year, 39,108 providers are observed in this report versus 33,421 in 2002, which represents a 17.02% increase in published responses. Data were received from 1,831 medical practices in all 50 states and the District of Columbia. Because of the increase in responses, there are additional physician and nonphysician provider specialties included in the report this year. This report includes data on the specialty of sleep medicine and also, includes a table on compensation for part-time physicians categorized as 0.7 FTE.

Another change in this report is reflected by the arrangement of tables. The tables now take the reader from an organizational frame in the beginning of the report down to specific environments relative to medical practice management.

Please note that physician work relative value units are not presented for anesthesiology. Rather, anesthesiology respondents were instructed to provide American Society of Anesthesiologists (ASA) units in the place of Total RVUs for anesthesia. This change was made last year to provide more useful information to anesthesiology practices and was based upon input from members of MGMA's Anesthesia Administrators Assembly.

Data Collection: Survey questionnaires were mailed in February 2003 to MGMA member and non-member organizations. While predominantly medical group practices, the MGMA membership includes many other types of organizations involved in physician practice management. Printed questionnaires were mailed to selected organizations that were, or were presumed to be affiliated with medical practices. Available on the MGMA web site were a downloadable electronic version of the questionnaire, and also a printable version.

Data Editing: A critical aspect of the survey process is the editing phase. Editing identifies reporting errors, mathematical miscalculations, inconsistencies and extreme values for follow-up and resolution. Practices that identified themselves as academic practices, freestanding ambulatory surgery centers, or a nonphysician organization were reclassified as ineligible for inclusion in the survey report.

Guidelines were developed to structure the editing process. The Survey Operations Department staff examined all questionnaires. Data representing outliers were investigated by telephone, e-mail or fax for follow-up and either corrected or suppressed from the database.

Minimum and maximum values were established for compensation and productivity measures to ensure the inclusion of only full-time providers in the report (with the exception of Tables 109-115). An upper limit was imposed on compensation and productivity measures for full-time providers. Data that fell outside these parameters were suppressed from the report. The table below describes the minimum and maximum values used in this report.

Full-time	Minimum	Maximum
Physician		
Compensation		
Primary Care	$60,000	$2,000,000
Specialty Care	$80,000	$2,000,000
Retirement benefits	$2,000	$55,000
Collections	$80,000	n/a
Gross charges	$80,000	$8,000,000
Ambulatory encounters	250	13,500
Hospital encounters	25	3,500
Surgery/anesthesia cases	25	3,500
Total RVUs primary care	3,000	16,000
Total RVUs specialists	3,000	30,000
Physician work RVUs		
primary care	1,500	8,000
Physician work RVUs		
specialists	1,500	15,000
Compensation to gross		
charges ratio	.150	1.00
Compensation to		
Physician work RVUs	10	200
Compensation to		
Total RVUs	10	100

Full-time	Minimum	Maximum
Nonphysician Provider		
Compensation	$25,000	n/a
Gross charges	$40,000	n/a

Part-time	Minimum	Maximum
Physician		
Compensation	$25,000	n/a
Gross charges	$40,000	n/a

Response Rate: A goal of this survey was to obtain as many responses as possible from medical practices. Therefore, organizations that were identified as medical practices, or those with close affiliations with medical practices—consulting practices, accounting firms, etc., were selected from the MGMA constituent database, and survey questionnaires were mailed to member and nonmember individuals associated with one of the previously mentioned organizations. In January 2003, 14,947 organizations were identified in the MGMA constituent database. Of these, 1,075 were determined to be undeliverable. Ultimately, the number of questionnaires actually distributed to organizations identified in the MGMA database was 13,872. Respondents returned 1,831 questionnaires representing 40,089 providers, including 826 surveys in electronic format and 1,005 paper surveys. Of these returned questionnaires, 103 questionnaires were determined to be ineligible or incomplete and were not included in the tables within this report.

In total, data from 1,728 responses were included in this report. Consistent with the goal of increasing the number of responses to the survey, approximately 3,500 additional questionnaires were mailed in this survey cycle than were in the 2002 survey. This increased distribution level tends to lower the overall response rate. The computed gross response rate for this survey was 10.93%. A response rate based on MGMA membership participation was not calculated due to the inability to accurately pinpoint the number of active members at the time of questionnaire distribution. Hospitals, management services organizations that provide or assist in the provision of physician services comprised 461 responses.

Limitations of the Data: It is recommended to use caution in interpreting the data in this report. The report is based on a voluntary response by primarily MGMA member practices and data may not be representative of all providers in medical practices. Providers in the responding organizations may have different compensation and productivity than providers in practices that did not respond to the survey or were not MGMA members. Additionally, note that the respondent sample varies from year to year. Therefore, conclusions about longitudinal trends or year to year fluctuations in summary statistics may not be appropriate.

Confidentiality: The MGMA and MGMA Center for Research Policy on Data Confidentiality states: "All data submitted to MGMA and the MGMA Center for Research will be kept confidential. All submitted data and related materials that identify a specific organization or individual will be safeguarded and will not be published or voluntarily released within the public domain without written permission."

Only summary statistics will be published. A summary statistic will be reported only if there are sufficient responses to be statistically reliable and if the anonymity of those submitting data is protected.

In compliance with the MGMA policy, an asterisk (*) denotes data that have been suppressed to ensure confidentiality.

DATA COMPUTATIONS

Calculations: Some of the values presented in this report are calculated from submitted data. Calculations were performed to convert data into percentages or ratios and were computed individually for each provider. Calculations computed are:

Full-Time Provider:	0.8 - 1.0 clinical FTE
Part-Time Provider:	0.4 - 0.6 clinical FTE
Part-Time Provider:	0.7 clinical FTE (*New*)

Compensation to Gross Charges Ratio: This ratio is computed by dividing compensation by gross charges (excluding technical component and gross charges attributed to nonphysician providers). The formula is:

$$\frac{Compensation}{Gross\ charges}$$

Compensation to Collections Ratio: This ratio is computed by dividing compensation by collections (excluding technical component and gross charges attributed to nonphysician providers). The formula is:

$$\frac{Compensation}{Collections}$$

Compensation per total RVU: This ratio indicates the amount of compensation paid per total RVU of production. RVUs for nonphysician providers are excluded. The formula is:

$$\frac{Compensation}{Total\ RVUs}$$

Compensation per physician work RVU: This ratio indicates the amount of compensation paid per physician work RVU of production. The formula is:

$$\frac{Compensation}{Total\ physician\ work\ RVUs}$$

HOW TO USE THIS REPORT

It is important to understand how the information is collected and defined in the survey. Appendix C and D feature the *2003 Compensation and Production Survey Questionnaire* and *Guide to the Questionnaire* as references for the user.

Report Organization: Data is presented as seven sections within the report. The medical practice and provider demographic tables begin on page 18, followed by physician compensation and benefits (Tables 1-14), physician productivity (Tables 15-63), physician time worked (Tables 64-67), select specialty summary tables (Tables 68-108), part-time physician data (Tables 109-115) and nonphysician provider data (Tables 116-133).

Statistical Interpretation: The median is reported in all tables. In addition to the median, some tables include the 25th, 75th, and 90th percentiles along with the mean and standard deviation, so the reader can better understand the distribution of the data. We strongly encourage the reader to use the median as the measure of central tendency, as the median is not subject to the distortion that may occur in the mean when extremely high or low values are in the data set.

Key Findings: The following results and conclusions were reached by historical and current year trend analyses performed by the MGMA Survey Operations staff. These analyses provide more information on how compensation may change over time as well as factors that influence current compensation and productivity levels. The median is used in the analysis.

The report reflects data submitted for fiscal year 2002 or the medical practice's most recently completed 12-month period. A majority of practices, 81.1%, provided data for calendar year 2002; 9.4% of the respondents reported data for the fiscal year ending June 2002 and another 5.7% of the respondents reported data for the fiscal year ending September 2002, with the remainder reporting data for other fiscal periods.

Note: While gross charges continue to be a prominent measure of productivity within this report and are used throughout the industry, the MGMA Survey Advisory Committee strongly encourages medical practices to adopt relative value units (RVUs) as more precise measures of productivity. MGMA will increasingly support the collection and reporting of RVU data through its survey activities.

Factors Affecting Compensation: The characteristics of the medical practice and individual provider may influence compensation levels. Examples of contributing factors include group type, geographic section and percent of capitation revenue within the practice. Influence of these contributors may differ for primary care and specialty care physicians.

The following sections discuss the association between direct compensation and various practice characteristics. Overall median compensation levels for primary care and specialty care physicians are:

Primary Care	Specialty Care
$153,231	$274,639

Group Type: Group type indicates whether physicians practiced in a single-specialty or multispecialty practice. Median compensation levels for primary care and specialty care physicians in both types of practices are:

Group Type	Primary Care	Specialty Care
Single-Specialty	$157,100	$340,245
Multispecialty	$152,800	$246,866

For primary care physicians, compensation levels increased slightly for those in single-specialty practices. Specialty care physicians' compensation in single-specialty practices experienced a small increase and, in multispecialty practices, the increase was similar.

For specialty care physicians, there continues to be a marked difference between single- and multispecialty practice data. Specialty care physicians continued to earn more in single-specialty groups.

Geographic Section: Differences in compensation may also be reported by geographic section. The figures below present median compensation levels for primary care and specialty care physicians.

Section	Primary Care	Specialty Care
Eastern	$144,996	$247,852
Midwest	$153,832	$299,240
Southern	$161,937	$321,602
Western	$152,907	$246,671

Continuing a trend seen for the last several years, compensation levels were highest in the Southern Section although compensation also increased in the other sections this year. Compensation for primary care physicians was lowest in the Eastern Section and for specialty care physicians it was lowest in the Western Section.

Compensation by Percent of Capitation: The level of capitation within a practice can also affect compensation. Median compensation is reported for four levels of capitation.

% Capitation	Primary Care	Specialty Care
No capitation	$157,702	$315,684
10 % or less	$149,491	$259,548
11% to 50%	$149,531	$239,745
51% to 100%	$154,761	$230,981

As practices increase in percent of capitation revenue, compensation levels tend to exhibit certain patterns. In this year's report, primary care physician's income was lowest at 10% or less capitation. Compensation for primary care is highest at no capitation and at 51% or more capitation. This trend has been observed in past years.

In contrast, specialty care physician income decreased when practices accepted higher levels of capitation contracts.

Multi-Year Compensation and Gross Charges Analyses: Compensation and gross charges were examined for the years 1998 through 2002 for primary care and specialty care physicians. Tables A and B on pages 18-19 report median compensation and gross charges over this five-year period. Because of the more comprehensive specialty list, some specialties were aggregated for the multi-year comparisons and they are denoted with an asterisk. For example, anesthesiology data are separately reported for anesthesiology, anesthesiology: pain management and anesthesiology: pediatric. For purposes of multi-year analysis these three specialties were combined into the specialty of anesthesiology. Other specialties that reflect combined categories in Table A and Table B are cardiology: invasive, dermatology, hematology/oncology, internal medicine, orthopedic surgery, pediatric/adolescent medicine, psychiatry and diagnostic radiology.

Primary Care Multi-Year Compensation and Gross Charges Analyses: The upper portions of Tables A and B focus on the primary care specialties of family practice, internal medicine and pediatrics. Graph 1 on page 20, illustrates the year-to-year changes for primary care physicians since 1992.

Primary Care Compensation

Current Year: Compensation levels for all primary care physicians rose to $153,231 in 2002, a 2.83% increase. Each of the highlighted primary care specialties experienced increases from the previous year with internal medicine having the highest at 3.88%.

Five-Year Trend: The last column in Table A shows the change in compensation levels from 1998 to 2002. Compensation increased for all primary care specialties by 10.04%. Increases ranged from 8.67% for family practice without OB to 13.10% for pediatrics.

The five-year increase of 10.04% for primary care physicians was lower than the increase seen in specialty care physician compensation of 18.38%. The change in nonphysician provider compensation also increased during this five-year period by 13.80%.

Primary Care Gross Charges:

Current Year: Gross charges for all primary care physicians increased by 5.18% in 2002. (Table B on page 17). Within the primary care specialties, gross charges increased 4.13% for internal medicine, 6.78% for family practice and 4.74% for pediatrics.

There was a moderate increase for primary care specialties in gross charges between 2001 and 2002, compared to the previous year. In 2002, median gross charges reported were $439,347 and $417,704 in 2001.

Five-Year Trend: From the period 1998 to 2002, gross charges increased 30.80%. Pediatricians' gross charges increased the most during this period to 35.73%, while family practitioners' and internists' gross charges rose 34.72% and 28.02% respectively.

The year-to-year changes in compensation and gross charges for 1992-2002 for primary care physicians are shown in Graph 1 on page 20. Gross charges continue to outpace increases in compensation for primary care physicians, but this year the ratio difference appears to be leveling off significantly.

Specialty Care Multi-Year Compensation and Gross Charges Analyses: The middle portion of Tables A and B show median compensation and gross charge levels for 17 selected specialties from 1998 to 2002. Graph 2 on page 20, illustrates the year-to-year changes for specialists since 1992.

Specialty Care Compensation

Current Year: Approximately one third of the selected specialties experienced compensation decreases in 2002, cardiology: invasive (-6.17%), noninvasive (-3.90%), ophthalmology (-2.54%), pulmonary medicine (-2.64%), surgery: general (0.80%) and urology (-3.00%). The highest gains occurred in dermatology 25.08%, hematology/oncology: 13.16% and radiology: diagnostic 12.95%.

Five-Year Trend: From 1998 to 2002, compensation levels for specialists increased by 18.38%. Of the selected specialties displayed in Table A, dermatology 39.35%, hematology/oncology: 46.05% and radiology: diagnostic 38.34%, had the most significant gains. Obstetrics/Gynecology experienced the least at 7.75%.

Specialty Care Gross Charges:

Current Year: Increases in specialty care gross charges were moderate but less pronounced in comparison to compensation in 2002 with a 5.50% increase from 2001. Dermatology experienced the largest yearly change in gross charges with an increase of 40.00% offsetting a decline from the prior year. Two specialties, cardiology: invasive (-7.88%) and cardiology: noninvasive (-2.21%) exhibited declines in gross charges.

Five-Year Trend: In examining the change in gross charges since 1998, three of the 17 specialties experienced increases in gross charges of 50% or more:

emergency medicine 61.55%, gastroenterology 59.73% and radiology: diagnostic 51.91%.

Several cautionary caveats are necessary concerning multi-year analyses. Year-to-year differences in response rate, measurement, editing and specialty mix exist that may cause distortion of results. Also, the respondent population was not held constant when analyzing the changes in compensation and gross charges over time.

Nonphysician Providers Analyses: The lower portion of Tables A and B show median compensation and gross charges for six select nonphysician providers. Compensation levels for all nonphysician providers increased by 4.53%. Optometrists experienced the largest compensation increase at 7.22%. This reflects a change from decreases in compensation for optometrists for the previous two years.

Gross Charges for all nonphysician providers increased by 6.73% from 2001 to 2002. Nurse practitioners and CRNA's experienced the greatest increase in gross charges at 10.22% and 10.05% respectively. Gross charges for psychologists dropped (-0.30%) this year following a loss in the previous year.

Five-Year Trend: CRNAs experienced an increase in compensation of 30.03% since 1998. Physician assistants (surgical) reported the lowest change at 3.36%. All the nonphysician providers listed in Table B report an increase in gross charges since 1998, with a range from nurse practitioners reporting 55.24% and psychologists reporting 17.70%.

SUMMARY

Many changes are taking place in the health care sector relative to compensation and productivity. Several demographic and socio-economic factors come into play: the aging population creates new demands in the health care industry and the increase in regulatory issues certainly plays a part. By collecting medical practice data, examining the trends and publishing benchmark reports our members can be confident that they possess a critical tool in medical practice management.

Feedback: If you have questions concerning the survey results or comments on improving this report, survey questionnaire or the guide, please contact the Survey Operations Department toll-free, 877.ASK.MGMA (275.6462), extension 895, or e-mail surveys@mgma.com. Purchasing information for the MGMA survey reports appears on the inside back cover of this report.

NOTES:

MEDICAL GROUP MANAGEMENT ASSOCIATION™

THIS PAGE INTENTIONALLY LEFT BLANK

DEMOGRAPHIC TABLES AND GRAPHS

Table A: Median Compensation for Selected Specialties, 1998-2002

	1998	98-99 change	1999	99-00 change	2000	00-01 change	2001	01-02 change	2002	98-02 change
All Primary Care:	$ 139,244	3.39%	$ 143,970	2.27%	$ 147,232	1.21%	$ 149,009	2.83%	$ 153,231	10.04%
Family Practice (without OB)	$ 138,277	2.33%	$ 141,493	2.56%	$ 145,121	1.02%	$ 146,601	2.50%	$ 150,267	8.67%
Internal Medicine *	$ 141,147	3.01%	$ 145,397	2.55%	$ 149,104	0.41%	$ 149,720	3.88%	$ 155,530	10.19%
Pediatric/Adolescent Medicine*	$ 135,000	5.93%	$ 143,011	-0.93%	$ 141,676	6.03%	$ 150,222	1.64%	$ 152,690	13.10%
All Specialists:	$ 231,993	6.00%	$ 245,910	4.30%	$ 256,494	2.64%	$ 263,254	4.32%	$ 274,639	18.38%
Anesthesiology *	$ 250,200	-2.18%	$ 244,755	14.54%	$ 280,353	1.18%	$ 283,655	8.22%	$ 306,964	22.69%
Cardiology: Invasive *	$ 350,000	-2.85%	$ 340,010	7.61%	$ 365,894	12.14%	$ 410,300	-6.17%	$ 385,000	10.00%
Cardiology: Noninvasive	$ 278,900	-0.07%	$ 278,712	7.66%	$ 300,073	6.68%	$ 320,111	-3.90%	$ 307,618	10.30%
Dermatology *	$ 193,215	8.21%	$ 209,077	2.30%	$ 213,876	0.64%	$ 215,247	25.08%	$ 269,238	39.35%
Emergency Medicine	$ 176,217	5.93%	$ 186,663	6.30%	$ 198,423	6.14%	$ 210,597	0.53%	$ 211,709	20.14%
Gastroenterology	$ 240,278	10.08%	$ 264,500	6.35%	$ 281,308	10.94%	$ 312,074	2.87%	$ 321,023	33.60%
Hematology/Oncology *	$ 212,516	20.07%	$ 255,167	1.27%	$ 258,403	6.14%	$ 274,270	13.16%	$ 310,371	46.05%
Neurology	$ 160,601	10.96%	$ 178,197	-1.71%	$ 175,143	2.96%	$ 180,325	2.96%	$ 185,666	15.61%
Obstetrics/Gynecology	$ 216,307	1.26%	$ 219,022	1.91%	$ 223,207	3.49%	$ 231,000	0.89%	$ 233,061	7.75%
Ophthalmology	$ 213,422	2.96%	$ 219,743	7.56%	$ 236,353	10.43%	$ 261,012	-2.54%	$ 254,376	19.19%
Orthopedic Surgery *	$ 312,356	2.23%	$ 319,315	5.11%	$ 335,646	7.90%	$ 362,173	0.00%	$ 362,181	15.95%
Otorhinolaryngology	$ 229,430	2.84%	$ 235,945	-0.22%	$ 235,415	8.81%	$ 256,160	8.36%	$ 277,585	20.99%
Psychiatry*	$ 142,736	6.42%	$ 151,903	3.02%	$ 156,486	0.65%	$ 157,509	3.58%	$ 163,144	14.30%
Pulmonary Medicine	$ 183,381	4.82%	$ 192,221	1.74%	$ 195,557	10.30%	$ 215,700	-2.64%	$ 210,000	14.52%
Radiology: Diagnostic*	$ 271,828	15.90%	$ 315,048	-5.15%	$ 298,824	11.41%	$ 332,917	12.95%	$ 376,035	38.34%
Surgery: General	$ 225,653	4.84%	$ 236,572	3.79%	$ 245,541	4.87%	$ 257,509	-0.80%	$ 255,438	13.20%
Urology	$ 240,000	12.01%	$ 268,825	12.26%	$ 301,772	0.55%	$ 303,433	-3.00%	$ 294,337	22.64%
All Nonphysician Providers:	$ 60,764	2.30%	$ 62,164	1.41%	$ 63,038	4.95%	$ 66,156	4.53%	$ 69,150	13.80%
Cert. Reg. Nurse Anes.	$ 84,863	9.42%	$ 92,856	2.94%	$ 95,586	14.37%	$ 109,323	0.94%	$ 110,350	30.03%
Nurse Practitioner *	$ 55,433	3.01%	$ 57,100	0.86%	$ 57,593	7.84%	$ 62,111	3.21%	$ 64,105	15.64%
Optometrist	$ 78,000	24.53%	$ 97,133	-6.69%	$ 90,631	-1.22%	$ 89,527	7.22%	$ 95,987	23.06%
Physician Asst. (surgical)	$ 70,950	-0.63%	$ 70,502	2.13%	$ 72,006	-0.61%	$ 71,566	2.47%	$ 73,335	3.36%
Physician Asst. (primary care)	$ 61,411	-2.12%	$ 60,107	7.83%	$ 64,815	1.37%	$ 65,704	5.46%	$ 69,294	12.84%
Psychologist	$ 65,500	7.63%	$ 70,500	-3.63%	$ 67,942	2.04%	$ 69,331	3.69%	$ 71,886	9.75%

* Represents specialties that are combined.

Table B: Median Gross Charges (TC Excluded) for Selected Specialties, 1998-2002

	1998	1999	98-99 change	2000	99-00 change	2001	00-01 change	2002	01-02 change	98-02 change
All Primary Care:	$ 335,890	$ 374,702	11.55%	$ 376,187	0.40%	$ 417,704	11.04%	$ 439,347	5.18%	30.80%
Family Practice (without OB)	$ 320,213	$ 370,832	15.81%	$ 366,892	-1.06%	$ 403,988	10.11%	$ 431,376	6.78%	34.72%
Internal Medicine *	$ 327,280	$ 369,685	12.96%	$ 366,184	-0.95%	$ 402,389	9.89%	$ 418,988	4.13%	28.02%
Pediatric/Adolescent Medicine *	$ 342,927	$ 387,583	13.02%	$ 406,985	5.01%	$ 444,407	9.19%	$ 465,456	4.74%	35.73%
All Specialists:	$ 724,257	$ 785,900	8.51%	$ 823,883	4.83%	$ 866,740	5.20%	$ 914,416	5.50%	26.26%
Anesthesiology *	$ 633,591	$ 643,487	1.56%	$ 698,778	8.59%	$ 691,256	-1.08%	$ 789,169	14.16%	24.55%
Cardiology: Invasive *	$ 1,237,551	$ 1,355,882	9.56%	$ 1,447,063	6.72%	$ 1,648,167	13.90%	$ 1,518,331	-7.88%	22.69%
Cardiology: Noninvasive	$ 907,341	$ 1,029,822	13.50%	$ 1,074,378	4.33%	$ 1,204,105	12.07%	$ 1,177,541	-2.21%	29.78%
Dermatology *	$ 660,009	$ 679,547	2.96%	$ 780,159	14.81%	$ 686,930	-11.95%	$ 961,672	40.00%	45.71%
Emergency Medicine	$ 378,819	$ 462,652	22.13%	$ 455,043	-1.64%	$ 541,700	19.04%	$ 612,001	12.98%	61.55%
Gastroenterology	$ 897,674	$ 1,057,214	17.77%	$ 1,158,324	9.56%	$ 1,261,590	8.92%	$ 1,433,899	13.66%	59.73%
Hematology/Oncology *	$ 467,732	$ 519,083	10.98%	$ 491,946	-5.23%	$ 517,667	5.23%	$ 596,813	15.29%	27.60%
Neurology	$ 475,144	$ 570,370	20.04%	$ 544,380	-4.56%	$ 602,883	10.75%	$ 624,120	3.52%	31.35%
Obstetrics/Gynecology	$ 674,712	$ 755,331	11.95%	$ 744,759	-1.40%	$ 826,626	10.99%	$ 874,092	5.74%	29.55%
Ophthalmology	$ 874,340	$ 930,297	6.40%	$ 1,077,329	15.80%	$ 1,092,642	1.42%	$ 1,150,407	5.29%	31.57%
Orthopedic Surgery *	$ 1,079,330	$ 1,128,647	4.57%	$ 1,178,291	4.40%	$ 1,287,703	9.29%	$ 1,388,129	7.80%	28.61%
Otorhinolaryngology	$ 907,934	$ 995,354	9.63%	$ 988,416	-0.70%	$ 1,106,173	11.91%	$ 1,122,047	1.44%	23.58%
Psychiatry *	$ 275,376	$ 280,793	1.97%	$ 310,471	10.57%	$ 320,599	3.26%	$ 374,539	16.82%	36.01%
Pulmonary Medicine	$ 544,523	$ 544,891	0.07%	$ 613,350	12.56%	$ 673,486	9.80%	$ 707,168	5.00%	29.87%
Radiology: Diagnostic *	$ 946,352	$ 1,100,000	16.24%	$ 1,021,782	-7.11%	$ 1,427,677	39.72%	$ 1,437,575	0.69%	51.91%
Surgery: General	$ 836,555	$ 927,482	10.87%	$ 945,341	1.93%	$ 972,654	2.89%	$ 1,052,897	8.25%	25.86%
Urology	$ 872,966	$ 975,872	11.79%	$ 1,086,174	11.30%	$ 1,257,096	15.74%	$ 1,290,095	2.63%	47.78%
All Nonphysician Providers:	$ 188,126	$ 195,248	3.79%	$ 211,079	8.11%	$ 231,534	9.69%	$ 247,111	6.73%	31.35%
Cert. Reg. Nurse Anes.	$ 255,565	$ 292,896	14.61%	$ 250,944	-14.32%	$ 341,926	36.26%	$ 376,276	10.05%	47.23%
Nurse Practitioner *	$ 151,504	$ 171,739	13.36%	$ 188,443	9.73%	$ 213,387	13.24%	$ 235,196	10.22%	55.24%
Optometrist	$ 254,129	$ 267,011	5.07%	$ 330,507	23.78%	$ 319,000	-3.48%	$ 344,843	8.10%	35.70%
Physician Asst. (surgical)	$ 199,687	$ 215,872	8.11%	$ 272,851	26.39%	$ 270,029	-1.03%	$ 275,450	2.01%	37.94%
Physician Asst. (primary care)	$ 205,254	$ 208,330	1.50%	$ 222,750	6.92%	$ 261,293	17.30%	$ 287,045	9.86%	39.85%
Psychologist	$ 137,091	$ 144,574	5.46%	$ 162,132	12.14%	$ 161,837	-0.18%	$ 161,354	-0.30%	17.70%

* Represents specialties that are combined.

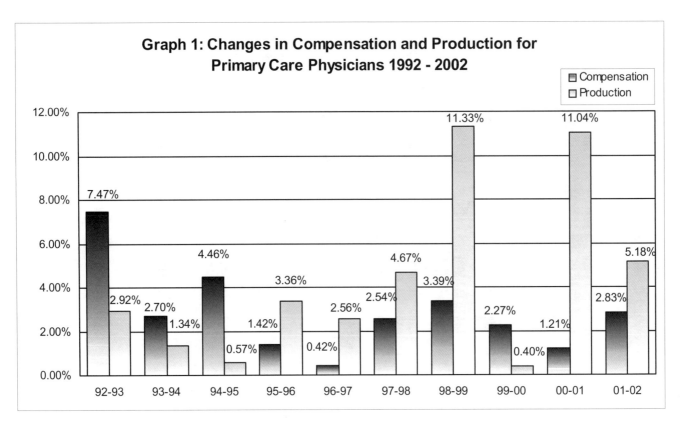

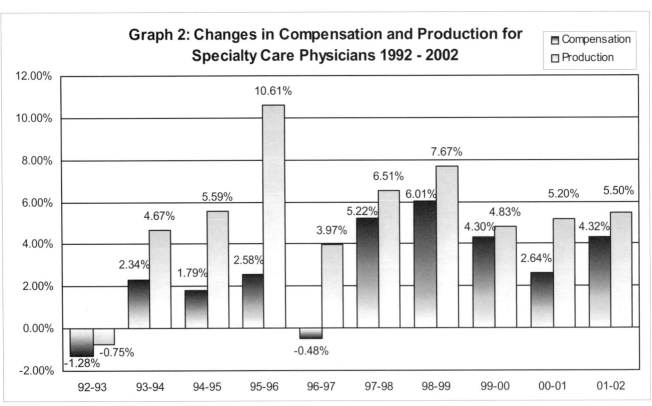

DEMOGRAPHIC TABLES — MEDICAL PRACTICE

1. Responses Received*

	Medical Practices Count	All Providers Count
Questionniares received	1,831	40,089
Ineligible/incomplete cases	103	981
Eligible cases	1,728	39,108

*See page 11 for further explanation.

2. Geographic Section

	Medical Practices		All Providers	
	Count	Percent	Count	Percent
Eastern	383	22.16%	7,491	19.15%
Midwest	535	30.96%	13,473	34.45%
Southern	476	27.55%	7,949	20.33%
Western	334	19.33%	10,195	26.07%
Total	1,728	100.00%	39,108	100.00%

3. Demographic Classification

	Medical Practices		All Providers	
	Count	Percent	Count	Percent
Non-metropolitan (under 50,000)	414	24.30%	5,553	14.40%
Metropolitan (50,000 to 250,000)	550	32.28%	12,442	32.26%
Metropolitan (250,001 to 1,000,000)	478	28.05%	10,137	26.29%
Metropolitan (over 1,000,000)	262	15.38%	10,433	27.05%
Total	1,704	100.00%	38,565	100.00%

MEDICAL GROUP MANAGEMENT ASSOCIATION™

4. State

	Medical Practices		All Providers	
	Count	Percent	Count	Percent
Alabama	21	1.22%	237	.61%
Alaska	7	.41%	47	.12%
Arizona	11	.64%	76	.19%
Arkansas	42	2.43%	479	1.22%
California	63	3.65%	4,363	11.16%
Colorado	47	2.72%	594	1.52%
Connecticut	14	.81%	238	.61%
Delaware	4	.23%	45	.12%
District of Columbia	1	.06%	23	.06%
Florida	63	3.65%	1,028	2.63%
Georgia	54	3.13%	505	1.29%
Hawaii	3	.17%	180	.46%
Idaho	11	.64%	147	.38%
Illinois	69	3.99%	1,874	4.79%
Indiana	58	3.36%	1,035	2.65%
Iowa	40	2.31%	1,093	2.79%
Kansas	28	1.62%	749	1.92%
Kentucky	27	1.56%	512	1.31%
Louisiana	25	1.45%	799	2.04%
Maine	17	.98%	221	.57%
Maryland	15	.87%	165	.42%
Massachusetts	23	1.33%	1,589	4.06%
Michigan	93	5.38%	896	2.29%
Minnesota	54	3.13%	3,153	8.06%
Mississippi	9	.52%	354	.91%
Missouri	21	1.22%	386	.99%
Montana	21	1.22%	488	1.25%
Nebraska	26	1.50%	307	.79%
Nevada	11	.64%	116	.30%
New Hampshire	27	1.56%	216	.55%
New Jersey	16	.93%	169	.43%
New Mexico	4	.23%	151	.39%
New York	54	3.13%	755	1.93%
North Carolina	108	6.25%	1,282	3.28%
North Dakota	10	.58%	912	2.33%
Ohio	119	6.89%	1,622	4.15%
Oklahoma	13	.75%	151	.39%
Oregon	65	3.76%	1,509	3.86%
Pennsylvania	53	3.07%	2,034	5.20%
Rhode Island	3	.17%	52	.13%
South Carolina	24	1.39%	190	.49%
South Dakota	11	.64%	285	.73%
Tennessee	74	4.28%	812	2.08%
Texas	75	4.34%	1,747	4.47%
Utah	15	.87%	586	1.50%
Vermont	3	.17%	16	.04%
Virginia	42	2.43%	674	1.72%
Washington	71	4.11%	1,873	4.79%
West Virginia	3	.17%	12	.03%
Wisconsin	55	3.18%	2,296	5.87%
Wyoming	5	.29%	65	.17%
Total	1,728	100.00%	39,108	100.00%

5. Legal Organization

	Medical Practices		All Providers	
	Count	Percent	Count	Percent
Business corporation	310	17.94%	5,447	13.93%
Limited liability company	135	7.81%	2,387	6.10%
Not-for-profit corporation/foundation	363	21.01%	12,823	32.79%
Partnership	75	4.34%	1,332	3.41%
Professional corporation/association	783	45.31%	16,020	40.96%
Sole proprietorship	19	1.10%	41	.10%
Other	43	2.49%	1,058	2.71%
Total	1,728	100.00%	39,108	100.00%

6. Organization Ownership

	Medical Practices		All Providers	
	Count	Percent	Count	Percent
Government	3	.18%	15	.04%
Hospital/integrated delivery system	415	24.25%	9,279	24.55%
Insurance company or HMO	1	.06%	403	1.07%
MSO or PPMC	28	1.64%	399	1.06%
Physicians	1,208	70.60%	24,245	64.14%
University or medical school	10	.58%	92	.24%
Other	46	2.69%	3,367	8.91%
Total	1,711	100.00%	37,800	100.00%

7. Group Type

	Medical Practices		All Providers	
	Count	Percent	Count	Percent
Single-specialty	1,215	70.31%	10,897	27.86%
Multispecialty	513	29.69%	28,211	72.14%
Total	1,728	100.00%	39,108	100.00%

8. Single-specialty Group Type

	Medical Practices		All Providers	
	Count	Percent	Count	Percent
Allergy/Immunology	11	.91%	65	.60%
Anesthesiology	67	5.51%	1,574	14.44%
Anesthesiology: Pain Management	5	.41%	80	.73%
Cardiology	103	8.48%	1,430	13.12%
Dentistry	2	.16%	16	.15%
Dermatology	12	.99%	48	.44%
Emergency Medicine	10	.82%	231	2.12%
Endocrinology/Metabolism	8	.66%	20	.18%
Family Practice	229	18.85%	1,322	12.13%
Gastroenterology	35	2.88%	334	3.07%
Hematology/Oncology	29	2.39%	188	1.73%
Infectious Disease	8	.66%	42	.39%
Internal Medicine	54	4.44%	339	3.11%
Neonatal Medicine	1	.08%	16	.15%
Nephrology	10	.82%	69	.63%
Neurology	16	1.32%	153	1.40%
Ob/Gyn	91	7.49%	655	6.01%
Ob/Gyn: Gynecological Oncology	2	.16%	14	.13%
Ob/Gyn: Maternal & Fetal Medicine	2	.16%	6	.06%
Ob/Gyn: Reproductive Endocrinology	2	.16%	7	.06%
Occupational Medicine	1	.08%	5	.05%
Ophthalmology	37	3.05%	314	2.88%
Ophthalmology: Retina	6	.49%	34	.31%
Orthopedics (Nonsurgical)	10	.82%	67	.61%
Orthopedic Surgery	133	10.95%	1,189	10.91%
Otorhinolaryngology	21	1.73%	169	1.55%
Pathology	15	1.23%	162	1.49%
Pediatrics	83	6.83%	792	7.27%
Pediatric Cardiology	4	.33%	9	.08%
Pediatric Critical Care/Intensivist	3	.25%	23	.21%
Pediatric Endocrinology	1	.08%	1	.01%
Pediatric Gastroenterology	1	.08%	1	.01%
Pediatric Hematology/Oncology	2	.16%	5	.05%
Pediatric Neurology	1	.08%	1	.01%
Physiatry	7	.58%	25	.23%
Podiatry	1	.08%	8	.07%
Psychiatry	6	.49%	44	.40%
Pulmonary Medicine	14	1.15%	97	.89%
Radiation Oncology	4	.33%	23	.21%
Radiology	35	2.88%	580	5.32%
Rheumatology	3	.25%	11	.10%
Sleep Medicine	3	.25%	7	.06%
Surg: Cardiovasc	14	1.15%	109	1.00%
Surg: Colon and Rectal	2	.16%	9	.08%
Surgery: General	42	3.46%	223	2.05%
Surg: Neurological	17	1.40%	95	.87%
Surg: Oral	2	.16%	10	.09%
Surg: Pediatric	3	.25%	13	.12%
Surg: Plastic & Reconstruction	5	.41%	33	.30%
Surg: Thoracic	1	.08%	17	.16%
Surg: Trauma	2	.16%	5	.05%
Surg: Vascular	4	.33%	18	.17%
Urgent Care	4	.33%	26	.24%
Urology	30	2.47%	162	1.49%
Other Single-specialty	1	.08%	1	.01%
Total	1,215	100.00%	10,897	100.00%

9. Integration Options

	Medical Practices		All Providers	
	Count	Percent	Count	Percent
Hospital Owns Practice				
Yes	415	24.02%	9,279	23.73%
No	1,313	75.98%	29,829	76.27%
Total	1,728	100.00%	39,108	100.00%
Practice Receives Services from a PPMC/MSO				
Yes	272	15.85%	3,978	10.26%
No	1,444	84.15%	34,795	89.74%
Total	1,716	100.00%	38,773	100.00%

10. 2002 Total Medical Revenue

	Medical Practices		All Providers	
	Count	Percent	Count	Percent
$ 2,000,000 or less	377	22.83%	1,223	3.50%
$ 2,000,001 to $ 5,000,000	469	28.41%	3,271	9.35%
$ 5,000,001 to $10,000,000	330	19.99%	4,070	11.63%
$10,000,001 to $20,000,000	222	13.45%	4,706	13.45%
$20,000,001 to $50,000,000	167	10.12%	7,939	22.69%
$50,000,001 or more	86	5.21%	13,779	39.38%
Total	1,651	100.00%	34,988	100.00%

11. 2002 Percent of Capitation Revenue

	Medical Practices		All Providers	
	Count	Percent	Count	Percent
No capitation	1,260	74.56%	19,300	53.20%
10% or less	224	13.25%	7,319	20.18%
11% to 50%	182	10.77%	6,850	18.88%
51% or more	24	1.42%	2,808	7.74%
Total	1,690	100.00%	36,277	100.00%

12. Practice Plans to Change Compensation Methodology

	Medical Practices		All Providers	
	Count	Percent	Count	Percent
Yes	235	14.08%	6,333	16.42%
No	1,434	85.92%	32,226	83.58%
Total	1,669	100.00%	38,559	100.00%

13. Productivity Measures Used in Compensation Methodology

	Medical Practices		All Providers	
	Count	Percent	Count	Percent
Gross Charges				
Yes	205	11.88%	5,736	14.67%
No	1,521	88.12%	33,364	85.33%
Total	1,726	100.00%	39,100	100.00%
Adjusted Charges				
Yes	190	11.01%	5,123	13.10%
No	1,536	88.99%	33,977	86.90%
Total	1,726	100.00%	39,100	100.00%
Collections for Professional Charges				
Yes	553	32.04%	9,711	24.84%
No	1,173	67.96%	29,389	75.16%
Total	1,726	100.00%	39,100	100.00%
Patient Encounters				
Yes	62	3.59%	1,580	4.04%
No	1,664	96.41%	37,520	95.96%
Total	1,726	100.00%	39,100	100.00%
Size of Physician Patient Panel				
Yes	10	.58%	785	2.01%
No	1,716	99.42%	38,315	97.99%
Total	1,726	100.00%	39,100	100.00%
Number of RVUs				
Yes	160	9.27%	6,780	17.34%
No	1,566	90.73%	32,320	82.66%
Total	1,726	100.00%	39,100	100.00%

14. Basis for Incentive/Bonus Used in Compensation Methodology

	Medical Practices		All Providers	
	Count	Percent	Count	Percent
Patient Satisfaction				
Yes	115	6.66%	2,685	6.87%
No	1,611	93.34%	36,415	93.13%
Total	1,726	100.00%	39,100	100.00%
Peer Review				
Yes	26	1.51%	822	2.10%
No	1,700	98.49%	38,278	97.90%
Total	1,726	100.00%	39,100	100.00%
Administrative/Governance Responsibilty				
Yes	157	9.10%	2,949	7.54%
No	1,569	90.90%	36,151	92.46%
Total	1,726	100.00%	39,100	100.00%
Service Quality				
Yes	101	5.85%	1,458	3.73%
No	1,625	94.15%	37,642	96.27%
Total	1,726	100.00%	39,100	100.00%
Seniority in the Medical Practice				
Yes	23	1.33%	664	1.70%
No	1,703	98.67%	38,436	98.30%
Total	1,726	100.00%	39,100	100.00%
Community Outreach				
Yes	33	1.91%	968	2.48%
No	1,693	98.09%	38,132	97.52%
Total	1,726	100.00%	39,100	100.00%

15. Compensation Methodology

	Medical Practices		All Providers	
	Count	Percent	Count	Percent
New Physicians (1 to 2 Years in Specialty)				
Productivity Based	93	7.05%	1,362	3.76%
Guaranteed or Base Salary	536	40.61%	17,871	49.34%
Straight Salary	594	45.00%	14,106	38.94%
Equal Shares	7	.53%	39	.11%
Structured Incentive/Bonus	7	.53%	73	.20%
Other	83	6.29%	2,772	7.65%
Total	1,320	100.00%	36,223	100.00%
Established Primary Care Physicians (More than 2 Years in Specialty)				
Productivity Based	313	34.97%	11,871	39.34%
Guaranteed or Base Salary	240	26.82%	9,290	30.79%
Straight Salary	247	27.60%	4,264	14.13%
Equal Shares	5	.56%	29	.10%
Structured Incentive/Bonus	4	.45%	62	.21%
Other	86	9.61%	4,657	15.43%
Total	895	100.00%	30,173	100.00%
Established Specialist (More than 2 Years in Specialty)				
Productivity Based	439	35.23%	12,345	36.06%
Guaranteed or Base Salary	281	22.55%	8,673	25.33%
Straight Salary	279	22.39%	5,632	16.45%
Equal Shares	90	7.22%	1,087	3.18%
Capitation	2	.16%	14	.04%
Structured Incentive/Bonus	2	.16%	40	.12%
Other	153	12.28%	6,445	18.83%
Total	1,246	100.00%	34,236	100.00%

16. Compensation to Gross Charges (TC/NPP Excluded) Ratio Category

	All Providers	
	Count	Percent
.15 to .19	702	6.41%
.20 to .24	1,446	13.20%
.25 to .29	1,819	16.61%
.30 to .34	1,785	16.30%
.35 to .39	1,769	16.15%
.40 to .44	1,324	12.09%
.45 to .49	806	7.36%
.50 to .54	445	4.06%
.55 to .59	291	2.66%
.60 to .64	194	1.77%
.65 to .69	118	1.08%
.70 to .74	83	.76%
.75 to .79	68	.62%
.80 to .84	35	.32%
.85 to .89	27	.25%
.90 to .94	23	.21%
.95 to 1.00	19	.17%
Total	10,954	100.00%

MEDICAL GROUP MANAGEMENT ASSOCIATION™

17. Physician Specialty

	Physicians	
	Count	Percent
Allergy/Immunology	205	.59%
Anesthesiology	1,802	5.22%
Anesth: Pain Management	94	.27%
Anesth: Pediatric	35	.10%
Cardiology: Electrophysiology	156	.45%
Cardiology: Invasive	630	1.82%
Cardiology: Inv-Intervntnl	754	2.18%
Cardiology: Noninvasive	626	1.81%
Critical Care: Intensivist	64	.19%
Dentistry	58	.17%
Dermatology	379	1.10%
Dermatology: MOHS Surgery	25	.07%
Emergency Medicine	647	1.87%
Endocrinology/Metabolism	232	.67%
Family Practice (w/ OB)	1,462	4.23%
Family Practice (w/o OB)	4,786	13.86%
Family Practice: Sports Med	33	.10%
Gastroenterology	770	2.23%
Gastroenterology: Hepatology	79	.23%
Geriatrics	67	.19%
Hematology/Oncology	419	1.21%
Hema/Oncology: Oncology (only)	106	.31%
Infectious Disease	154	.45%
Internal Medicine: General	4,852	14.05%
Internal Med: Hospitalist	364	1.05%
Internal Med: Ped	114	.33%
Nephrology	281	.81%
Neurology	566	1.64%
OBGYN: General	1,727	5.00%
OBGYN: Gynecology (only)	204	.59%
OBGYN: Gyn Oncology	29	.08%
OBGYN: Maternal & Fetal Med	64	.19%
OBGYN: Repro Endocrinology	40	.12%
Occupational Medicine	167	.48%
Ophthalmology	606	1.75%
Ophthalmology: Pediatric	32	.09%
Ophthalmology: Retina	87	.25%
Orthopedic (Non-surgical)	76	.22%
Orthopedic Surgery: General	934	2.70%
Ortho Surg: Foot & Ankle	57	.17%
Ortho Surg: Hand	142	.41%
Ortho Surg: Hip & Joint	118	.34%
Ortho Surg: Oncology	3	.01%
Ortho Surg: Pediatric	45	.13%
Ortho Surg: Spine	139	.40%
Ortho Surg: Trauma	32	.09%
Ortho Surg: Sports Med	263	.76%
Otorhinolaryngology	465	1.35%
Otorhinolaryngology: Pediatric	18	.05%
Pathology: Anatomic & Clinical	250	.72%
Pathology: Anatomic	61	.18%
Pathology: Clinical	95	.28%

17. Physician Specialty (continued)

	Physicians	
	Count	Percent
Pediatrics: General	2,555	7.40%
Ped: Adolescent Medicine	97	.28%
Ped: Allergy/Immunology	11	.03%
Ped: Cardiology	57	.17%
Ped: Child Development	23	.07%
Ped: Critical Care/Intensivist	69	.20%
Ped: Emergency Medicine	9	.03%
Ped: Endocrinology	25	.07%
Ped: Gastroenterology	28	.08%
Ped: Genetics	20	.06%
Ped: Hematology/Oncology	50	.14%
Ped: Hospitalist	28	.08%
Ped: Infectious Disease	13	.04%
Ped: Neonatal Medicine	107	.31%
Ped: Nephrology	10	.03%
Ped: Neurology	36	.10%
Ped: Pulmonology	21	.06%
Ped: Rheumatology	4	.01%
Ped: Sports Medicine	1	.00%
Physiatry (Physical Med & Re)	201	.58%
Podiatry: General	138	.40%
Podiatry: Surg-Foot & Ankle	94	.27%
Podiatry: Surg-Forefoot Only	16	.05%
Psychiatry: General	431	1.25%
Psychiatry: Child & Adolescent	65	.19%
Psychiatry: Geriatric	14	.04%
Pulmonary Medicine	311	.90%
Pulmonary Medicine: Critical Care	159	.46%
Radiation Oncology	118	.34%
Radiology: Diagnostic-Inv	417	1.21%
Radiology: Diagnostic-Noninv	698	2.02%
Radiology: Nuclear Medicine	62	.18%
Rheumatology	292	.85%
Sleep Medicine	15	.04%
Surgery: General	1,010	2.92%
Surg: Cardiovascular	201	.58%
Surg: Cardiovascular-Pediatric	5	.01%
Surg: Colon and Rectal	46	.13%
Surg: Neurological	210	.61%
Surg: Oncology	10	.03%
Surg: Oral	29	.08%
Surg: Pediatric	23	.07%
Surg: Plastic & Reconstruction	112	.32%
Surg: Plastic & Recon-Hand	18	.05%
Surg: Plastic & Recon-Pediatric	4	.01%
Surg: Thoracic (primary)	57	.17%
Surg: Transplant	16	.05%
Surg: Trauma	24	.07%
Surg: Trauma-Burn	14	.04%
Surg: Vascular (primary)	147	.43%
Urgent Care	481	1.39%
Urology	492	1.42%
Urology: Pediatric	13	.04%
Other physician specialty	12	.03%
Total	34,533	100.00%

18. Physician Years in Specialty

	Physicians	
	Count	Percent
1 to 2 years	2,535	8.53%
3 to 7 years	6,719	22.61%
8 to 12 years	5,934	19.97%
13 to 17 years	5,130	17.26%
18 to 22 years	4,090	13.76%
23 years or more	5,309	17.87%
Total	29,717	100.00%

19. FTE Physicians

	Medical Practices		Physicians	
	Count	Percent	Count	Percent
3 or less	368	22.10%	780	2.30%
4 to 6	404	24.26%	2,007	5.92%
7 to 10	295	17.72%	2,445	7.21%
11 to 25	319	19.16%	4,995	14.73%
26 to 50	141	8.47%	4,919	14.51%
51 to 75	55	3.30%	3,299	9.73%
76 to 100	23	1.38%	1,996	5.89%
101 to 150	26	1.56%	2,998	8.84%
151 or more	34	2.04%	10,463	30.86%
Total	1,665	100.00%	33,902	100.00%

20. Clinical FTE

	Physicians	
	Count	Percent
Less than .39 FTE	408	1.18%
.40 to .60 FTE	1,344	3.89%
.61 to .69 FTE	281	.81%
.70 to .79 FTE	790	2.29%
.80 to .89 FTE	370	1.07%
.90 to .99 FTE	21,118	61.20%
1.00 FTE	10,197	29.55%
Total	34,508	100.00%

21. Gender

	Physicians	
	Count	Percent
Male	25,517	77.24%
Female	7,518	22.76%
Total	33,035	100.00%

22. Reporting Technical Component in Production

	Medical Practices		Physicians	
	Count	Percent	Count	Percent
Professional Gross Charges				
0%	693	49.71%	17,173	65.49%
1-10%	472	33.86%	6,140	23.42%
> 10%	229	16.43%	2,908	11.09%
Total	1,394	100.00%	26,221	100.00%
Total RVUs				
Yes	231	38.89%	5,377	42.08%
No	363	61.11%	7,401	57.92%
Total	594	100.00%	12,778	100.00%

MEDICAL GROUP MANAGEMENT ASSOCIATION™

DEMOGRAPHIC TABLES — PROVIDER

23. Reporting Nonphysician Providers in Production

	Medical Practices		Physicians	
	Count	Percent	Count	Percent
Professional Gross Charges				
Yes	192	14.78%	3,056	12.91%
No	1,107	85.22%	20,607	87.09%
Total	1,299	100.00%	23,663	100.00%
Ambulatory Encounters				
Yes	136	13.17%	2,125	11.65%
No	897	86.83%	16,119	88.35%
Total	1,033	100.00%	18,244	100.00%
Total RVUs				
Yes	57	14.73%	1,389	14.96%
No	330	85.27%	7,894	85.04%
Total	387	100.00%	9,283	100.00%
Work RVUs				
Yes	50	12.66%	1,337	9.32%
No	345	87.34%	13,011	90.68%
Total	395	100.00%	14,348	100.00%

24. Nonphysician Provider (NPP)

	Nonphysician Providers	
	Count	Percent
Audiologist	120	2.62%
Certified Diabetic Educator	11	.24%
Cert Reg Nurse Anesthetist	308	6.73%
Chiropractor	24	.52%
Dietician/Nutritionist	32	.70%
Midwife-Out-/In-patient	138	3.02%
Midwife-Outpatient (primary)	12	.26%
Midwife-Inpatient (primary)	11	.24%
Nurse Practitioner	1,221	26.69%
NP: Adult	11	.24%
NP: Cardiology	19	.42%
NP: Family Practice	78	1.70%
NP: Gerontology/Elder Health	12	.26%
NP: Internal Medicine	43	.94%
NP: Pediatric/Child Health	41	.90%
NP: OBGYN/Women's Health	46	1.01%
Occupational Therapist	43	.94%
Optometrist	288	6.30%
Orthotist/Prosthetist	2	.04%
Perfusionist	6	.13%
Pharmacist	72	1.57%
Physical Therapist	231	5.05%
Physician Asst (surgical)	294	6.43%
Physician Asst (primary care)	775	16.94%
Phys Asst (non-surg./non-prim care)	287	6.27%
Physicist	2	.04%
Psychologist	238	5.20%
Social Worker	124	2.71%
Speech Therapist	15	.33%
Surgeon Assistant	16	.35%
Other nonphysician provider specialty	55	1.20%
Total	4,575	100.00%

25. FTE Nonphysician Providers (NPP)

	Medical Practices		Nonphysician Providers	
	Count	Percent	Count	Percent
1 to 3	20	48.78%	640	14.32%
4 to 9	10	24.39%	1,004	22.46%
10 or more	11	26.83%	2,826	63.22%
Total	41	100.00%	4,470	100.00%

26. Nonphysician Provider (NPP) Clinical FTE

	Nonphysician Providers	
	Count	Percent
Less than .39 FTE	145	3.25%
.40 to .60 FTE	372	8.35%
.61 to .69 FTE	42	.94%
.70 to .79 FTE	156	3.50%
.80 to .89 FTE	110	2.47%
.90 to .99 FTE	2,611	58.58%
1.00 FTE	1,021	22.91%
Total	4,457	100.00%

27. Nonphysician Provider (NPP) Gender

	Nonphysician Providers	
	Count	Percent
Male	1,324	31.13%
Female	2,929	68.87%
Total	4,253	100.00%

THIS PAGE INTENTIONALLY LEFT BLANK

PHYSICIAN COMPENSATION AND BENEFITS

Table 1: Physician Compensation

	Physicians	Medical Practices	Mean	Std. Dev.	25th %tile	Median	75th %tile	90th %tile
Allergy/Immunology	185	94	$300,319	$212,916	$182,988	$235,316	$341,037	$499,421
Anesthesiology	1,702	118	$330,299	$114,693	$250,769	$305,676	$394,371	$485,910
Anesth: Pain Management	84	35	$335,370	$118,392	$247,086	$318,322	$418,361	$496,176
Anesth: Pediatric	35	5	$347,380	$161,522	$224,121	$320,000	$351,946	$647,051
Cardiology: Electrophysiology	148	83	$409,391	$171,321	$289,753	$375,540	$514,015	$610,710
Cardiology: Invasive	601	151	$393,408	$172,447	$286,216	$360,988	$437,260	$608,337
Cardiology: Inv-Intervntnl	720	157	$478,112	$215,985	$351,011	$422,123	$568,144	$749,273
Cardiology: Noninvasive	582	166	$336,094	$144,407	$241,128	$307,618	$391,404	$518,613
Critical Care: Intensivist	62	15	$224,409	$77,205	$180,027	$204,905	$236,708	$295,977
Dentistry	42	9	$160,693	$54,703	$130,182	$145,646	$181,348	$247,393
Dermatology	313	140	$304,158	$154,148	$205,795	$262,782	$367,894	$477,400
Dermatology: MOHS Surgery	22	21	$456,981	$229,183	$288,932	$388,282	$633,141	$854,926
Emergency Medicine	556	49	$224,400	$60,151	$187,351	$211,709	$247,280	$289,470
Endocrinology/Metabolism	207	114	$187,529	$80,820	$141,417	$170,000	$213,878	$273,685
Family Practice (w/ OB)	1,301	219	$167,228	$49,458	$131,429	$156,829	$193,368	$236,076
Family Practice (w/o OB)	4,321	517	$163,151	$57,997	$125,907	$150,267	$185,844	$234,961
Family Practice: Sports Med	28	22	$208,786	$107,546	$140,266	$180,315	$267,533	$348,115
Gastroenterology	720	201	$358,576	$164,116	$250,036	$321,023	$432,604	$559,629
Gastroenterology: Hepatology	75	16	$332,503	$149,752	$238,994	$316,200	$381,576	$482,047
Geriatrics	56	28	$150,215	$46,407	$120,953	$146,016	$166,488	$201,298
Hematology/Oncology	399	124	$394,361	$256,944	$218,052	$299,319	$472,384	$817,611
Hem/Onc: Oncology (only)	95	39	$360,031	$156,197	$238,164	$336,683	$471,481	$547,202
Infectious Disease	146	70	$224,149	$161,429	$140,000	$180,286	$222,954	$409,353
Internal Medicine: General	4,357	438	$165,861	$57,421	$130,229	$154,756	$186,241	$232,886
Internal Med: Hospitalist	350	79	$180,456	$61,303	$147,521	$161,955	$196,036	$248,434
Internal Med: Pediatric	96	35	$160,433	$48,370	$129,813	$141,887	$182,034	$234,840
Nephrology	268	86	$261,919	$136,797	$185,990	$227,385	$302,463	$400,000
Neurology	522	150	$213,082	$97,235	$156,843	$185,666	$236,655	$317,607
OBGYN: General	1,638	284	$257,933	$107,545	$192,370	$233,061	$293,390	$385,521
OBGYN: Gynecology (only)	176	72	$224,273	$109,690	$146,714	$201,420	$270,286	$364,399
OBGYN: Gyn Oncology	26	13	$314,393	$126,179	$228,113	$285,652	$387,008	$507,399
OBGYN: Maternal & Fetal Med	60	19	$358,758	$141,723	$251,534	$337,618	$458,559	$556,652
OBGYN: Repro Endocrinology	36	13	$287,828	$107,007	$216,438	$264,602	$335,492	$427,669
Occupational Medicine	153	55	$197,461	$112,934	$141,282	$164,783	$206,796	$295,765
Ophthalmology	557	155	$301,761	$150,875	$200,000	$254,376	$375,057	$477,124
Ophthalmology: Pediatric	29	20	$316,010	$117,117	$243,592	$284,387	$392,350	$470,613
Ophthalmology: Retina	76	31	$503,859	$254,287	$337,449	$430,834	$623,750	$863,044
Orthopedic (Non-surgical)	51	29	$266,995	$139,572	$152,395	$206,797	$357,964	$457,132
Orthopedic Surgery: General	904	226	$404,263	$186,004	$282,878	$364,060	$482,696	$626,991
Ortho Surg: Foot & Ankle	52	46	$395,985	$151,612	$276,643	$389,487	$476,757	$599,472
Ortho Surg: Hand	140	79	$475,257	$237,377	$288,299	$419,676	$606,250	$774,989
Ortho Surg: Hip & Joint	117	62	$476,283	$229,605	$305,705	$432,531	$632,560	$806,117
Ortho Surg: Oncology	3	3	*	*	*	*	*	*
Ortho Surg: Pediatric	42	28	$333,474	$142,519	$242,546	$294,309	$411,190	$456,138
Ortho Surg: Spine	134	81	$620,380	$332,373	$384,461	$545,412	$806,215	$1,100,000
Ortho Surg: Trauma	30	18	$409,540	$176,683	$265,472	$382,774	$489,928	$636,349
Ortho Surg: Sports Med	260	102	$407,666	$249,561	$234,406	$344,229	$501,908	$717,599
Otorhinolaryngology	424	146	$326,884	$177,842	$220,217	$277,585	$367,484	$545,954
Otorhinolaryngology: Pediatric	17	4	$345,267	$179,717	$202,576	$324,800	$374,310	$687,365
Pathology: Anatomic & Clinical	233	44	$338,344	$173,094	$214,820	$285,087	$445,798	$531,028
Pathology: Anatomic	60	11	$301,352	$110,359	$224,000	$276,687	$394,915	$431,804
Pathology: Clinical	84	18	$207,204	$83,212	$140,838	$196,950	$267,964	$320,810

Table 1: Physician Compensation (continued)

	Physicians	Medical Practices	Mean	Std. Dev.	25th %tile	Median	75th %tile	90th %tile
Pediatrics: General	2,215	321	$164,817	$56,005	$126,862	$153,098	$188,925	$241,844
Ped: Adolescent Medicine	85	14	$154,983	$50,311	$119,406	$145,650	$182,140	$218,718
Ped: Allergy/Immunology	10	8	$186,420	$82,140	$128,143	$153,786	$229,415	$343,186
Ped: Cardiology	53	22	$227,776	$75,124	$178,513	$218,858	$282,360	$338,159
Ped: Child Development	20	11	$128,925	$34,941	$109,152	$122,738	$134,781	$164,116
Ped: Critical Care/Intensivist	67	20	$273,113	$137,429	$182,500	$252,665	$326,368	$382,247
Ped: Emergency Medicine	8	2	*	*	*	*	*	*
Ped: Endocrinology	23	15	$144,706	$25,710	$129,143	$144,311	$163,604	$179,823
Ped: Gastroenterology	28	11	$205,674	$63,907	$167,147	$188,657	$210,965	$284,519
Ped: Genetics	18	7	$191,978	$126,579	$126,500	$162,205	$208,715	$294,504
Ped: Hematology/Oncology	48	20	$193,821	$58,360	$154,501	$181,524	$225,004	$260,879
Ped: Hospitalist	26	12	$155,963	$40,259	$130,056	$151,500	$184,014	$229,648
Ped: Infectious Disease	10	5	$166,744	$35,480	$134,285	$170,829	$199,514	$206,441
Ped: Neonatal Medicine	106	23	$268,765	$137,588	$178,940	$218,522	$296,718	$516,133
Ped: Nephrology	10	7	$174,359	$60,168	$139,011	$161,991	$205,922	$298,796
Ped: Neurology	33	19	$191,626	$75,044	$149,674	$170,004	$213,713	$319,770
Ped: Pulmonology	21	11	$224,278	$87,623	$145,725	$194,723	$297,684	$363,233
Ped: Rheumatology	4	3	*	*	*	*	*	*
Ped: Sports Medicine	1	1	*	*	*	*	*	*
Physiatry (Phys Med & Rehab)	178	81	$234,896	$137,062	$155,434	$192,490	$273,648	$357,265
Podiatry: General	127	72	$162,335	$57,982	$117,574	$151,328	$194,786	$239,272
Podiatry: Surg-Foot & Ankle	92	26	$180,162	$72,098	$144,000	$162,225	$187,513	$249,426
Podiatry: Surg-Forefoot Only	15	6	$154,706	$44,706	$120,000	$150,000	$175,841	$221,234
Psychiatry: General	361	70	$163,906	$42,539	$135,942	$159,444	$184,536	$214,490
Psychiatry: Child & Adolescent	53	19	$180,852	$31,156	$166,265	$180,000	$193,404	$213,976
Psychiatry: Geriatric	13	7	$226,224	$106,929	$135,973	$207,734	$294,083	$425,551
Pulmonary Medicine	295	130	$230,983	$85,034	$175,084	$210,000	$277,140	$331,944
Pulmonary Med: Critical Care	152	45	$254,601	$99,211	$185,421	$234,243	$301,266	$371,766
Radiation Oncology	108	38	$399,597	$138,279	$287,294	$369,424	$490,530	$597,300
Radiology: Diagnostic-Inv	385	59	$412,515	$138,745	$313,604	$377,000	$510,110	$586,751
Radiology: Diagnostic-Noninv	635	94	$367,754	$120,765	$278,822	$348,774	$446,049	$532,497
Radiology: Nuclear Medicine	57	29	$293,682	$110,782	$220,173	$265,000	$377,457	$428,683
Rheumatology	268	131	$222,691	$97,884	$160,480	$193,410	$258,094	$357,635
Sleep Medicine	15	7	$212,877	$99,870	$133,844	$174,400	$256,096	$414,734
Surgery: General	960	252	$286,670	$123,967	$205,782	$255,438	$334,847	$432,072
Surg: Cardiovascular	187	51	$478,315	$210,015	$352,848	$433,353	$552,805	$770,677
Surg: Cardiovascular-Pediatric	5	5	*	*	*	*	*	*
Surg: Colon and Rectal	44	20	$308,064	$119,012	$228,285	$286,200	$383,022	$485,847
Surg: Neurological	201	66	$535,626	$316,926	$337,456	$470,476	$614,020	$855,159
Surg: Oncology	10	6	$377,154	$170,740	$273,140	$359,675	$473,276	$691,314
Surg: Oral	27	13	$270,097	$100,457	$205,798	$228,359	$381,767	$430,767
Surg: Pediatric	22	10	$353,057	$130,800	$252,383	$308,166	$411,532	$626,831
Surg: Plastic & Reconstruction	108	54	$320,552	$164,927	$227,065	$289,561	$338,691	$546,199
Surg: Plastic & Recon-Hand	18	7	$330,994	$181,679	$201,410	$270,500	$472,017	$600,960
Surg: Plastic & Recon-Pediatric	4	2	*	*	*	*	*	*
Surg: Thoracic (primary)	56	16	$388,154	$210,531	$237,780	$288,540	$425,136	$772,900
Surg: Transplant	16	8	$350,965	$69,781	$307,588	$364,246	$393,202	$440,520
Surg: Trauma	24	8	$321,326	$163,463	$197,288	$286,375	$357,739	$675,269
Surg: Trauma-Burn	13	6	$350,032	$145,129	$248,540	$337,667	$483,886	$579,566
Surg: Vascular (primary)	140	53	$325,373	$135,237	$241,988	$303,517	$357,031	$465,179
Urgent Care	405	100	$172,269	$69,754	$131,653	$159,000	$200,779	$240,075
Urology	475	139	$333,712	$159,822	$224,173	$294,337	$401,456	$524,001
Urology: Pediatric	13	4	$201,287	$87,396	$141,153	$149,623	$269,209	$362,850

Medical Group Management Association™

Table 2: Physician Compensation by Group Type

	Single-specialty			Multispecialty		
	Physicians	Medical Practices	Median	Physicians	Medical Practices	Median
Allergy/Immunology	48	11	$340,160	137	83	$214,693
Anesthesiology	1,227	68	$330,823	475	50	$277,647
Anesth: Pain Management	60	20	$329,746	24	15	$273,458
Anesth: Pediatric	20	2	*	15	3	$387,997
Cardiology: Electrophysiology	100	56	$398,119	48	27	$314,251
Cardiology: Invasive	276	69	$372,212	325	82	$350,000
Cardiology: Inv-Intervntnl	461	89	$420,683	259	68	$443,490
Cardiology: Noninvasive	305	76	$355,610	277	90	$284,709
Critical Care: Intensivist	5	2	*	57	13	$202,198
Dentistry	12	2	*	30	7	$145,646
Dermatology	25	10	$392,934	288	130	$256,846
Dermatology: MOHS Surgery	4	4	*	18	17	$375,656
Emergency Medicine	136	10	$240,575	420	39	$208,795
Endocrinology/Metabolism	12	9	$173,508	195	105	$168,239
Family Practice (w/ OB)	282	69	$151,787	1,019	150	$158,711
Family Practice (w/o OB)	714	192	$154,068	3,607	325	$150,000
Family Practice: Sports Med	13	10	$188,818	15	12	$159,244
Gastroenterology	235	31	$337,688	485	170	$309,572
Gastroenterology: Hepatology	57	10	$319,061	18	6	$304,229
Geriatrics	1	1	*	55	27	$146,016
Hematology/Oncology	130	29	$462,386	269	95	$246,299
Hem/Onc: Oncology (only)	38	6	$429,002	57	33	$302,287
Infectious Disease	41	12	$214,544	105	58	$173,939
Internal Medicine: General	295	68	$160,000	4,062	370	$154,469
Internal Med: Hospitalist	6	2	*	344	77	$162,581
Internal Med: Pediatric	4	2	*	92	33	$140,874
Nephrology	68	11	$242,700	200	75	$217,657
Neurology	135	21	$191,459	387	129	$184,576
OBGYN: General	451	88	$238,953	1,187	196	$232,132
OBGYN: Gynecology (only)	47	24	$167,301	129	48	$217,480
OBGYN: Gyn Oncology	1	1	*	25	12	$286,804
OBGYN: Maternal & Fetal Med	11	5	$341,557	49	14	$333,679
OBGYN: Repro Endocrinology	13	5	$323,294	23	8	$251,659
Occupational Medicine	8	3	*	145	52	$164,203
Ophthalmology	179	34	$344,000	378	121	$236,001
Ophthalmology: Pediatric	17	11	$288,993	12	9	$256,936
Ophthalmology: Retina	53	19	$514,246	23	12	$384,348
Orthopedic (Non-surgical)	20	8	$186,770	31	21	$277,942
Orthopedic Surgery: General	403	105	$411,375	501	121	$345,687
Ortho Surg: Foot & Ankle	41	37	$387,854	11	9	$440,696
Ortho Surg: Hand	110	61	$454,517	30	18	$401,339
Ortho Surg: Hip & Joint	91	50	$457,796	26	12	$332,356
Ortho Surg: Oncology	2	2	*	1	1	*
Ortho Surg: Pediatric	27	19	$288,617	15	9	$313,960
Ortho Surg: Spine	97	60	$547,585	37	21	$538,982
Ortho Surg: Trauma	25	16	$439,750	5	2	*
Ortho Surg: Sports Med	158	74	$438,861	102	28	$240,211
Otorhinolaryngology	109	21	$261,685	315	125	$278,307
Otorhinolaryngology: Pediatric	8	2	*	9	2	*
Pathology: Anatomic & Clinical	98	14	$465,150	135	30	$222,923
Pathology: Anatomic	43	6	$349,104	17	5	$226,000
Pathology: Clinical	21	6	$237,044	63	12	$187,635

Table 2: Physician Compensation by Group Type (continued)

	Single-specialty			Multispecialty		
	Physicians	Medical Practices	Median	Physicians	Medical Practices	Median
Pediatrics: General	540	79	$168,244	1,675	242	$150,507
Ped: Adolescent Medicine	4	1	*	81	13	$146,000
Ped: Allergy/Immunology	4	2	*	6	6	*
Ped: Cardiology	22	8	$276,200	31	14	$216,874
Ped: Child Development	*	*	*	20	11	$122,738
Ped: Critical Care/Intensivist	30	7	$279,424	37	13	$243,576
Ped: Emergency Medicine	2	1	*	6	1	*
Ped: Endocrinology	4	3	*	19	12	$137,800
Ped: Gastroenterology	11	4	$198,134	17	7	$185,016
Ped: Genetics	*	*	*	18	7	$162,205
Ped: Hematology/Oncology	14	4	$172,030	34	16	$189,103
Ped: Hospitalist	3	1	*	23	11	$153,000
Ped: Infectious Disease	2	1	*	8	4	*
Ped: Neonatal Medicine	29	4	$301,361	77	19	$202,926
Ped: Nephrology	2	1	*	8	6	*
Ped: Neurology	8	5	*	25	14	$165,578
Ped: Pulmonology	8	3	*	13	8	$165,360
Ped: Rheumatology	1	1	*	3	2	*
Ped: Sports Medicine	*	*	*	1	1	*
Physiatry (Phys Med & Rehab)	49	28	$250,500	129	53	$186,061
Podiatry: General	3	3	*	124	69	$151,638
Podiatry: Surg-Foot & Ankle	14	5	$166,595	78	21	$162,225
Podiatry: Surg-Forefoot Only	1	1	*	14	5	$157,500
Psychiatry: General	10	3	$140,193	351	67	$160,000
Psychiatry: Child & Adolescent	7	3	*	46	16	$181,230
Psychiatry: Geriatric	*	*	*	13	7	$207,734
Pulmonary Medicine	33	11	$196,504	262	119	$218,532
Pulmonary Med: Critical Care	48	8	$231,509	104	37	$235,279
Radiation Oncology	51	12	$471,000	57	26	$358,287
Radiology: Diagnostic-Inv	238	31	$435,000	147	28	$362,500
Radiology: Diagnostic-Noninv	244	28	$392,525	391	66	$324,676
Radiology: Nuclear Medicine	21	11	$374,416	36	18	$231,786
Rheumatology	32	9	$221,281	236	122	$191,670
Sleep Medicine	8	3	*	7	4	*
Surgery: General	187	43	$254,250	773	209	$255,889
Surg: Cardiovascular	88	19	$489,281	99	32	$390,500
Surg: Cardiovascular-Pediatric	3	3	*	2	2	*
Surg: Colon and Rectal	12	6	$235,000	32	14	$291,000
Surg: Neurological	87	20	$510,000	114	46	$443,633
Surg: Oncology	1	1	*	9	5	*
Surg: Oral	13	3	$226,077	14	10	$239,667
Surg: Pediatric	6	2	*	16	8	$294,216
Surg: Plastic & Reconstruction	11	5	$321,309	97	49	$289,062
Surg: Plastic & Recon-Hand	14	4	$221,000	4	3	*
Surg: Plastic & Recon-Pediatric	2	1	*	2	1	*
Surg: Thoracic (primary)	19	2	*	37	14	$281,248
Surg: Transplant	4	1	*	12	7	$364,246
Surg: Trauma	5	2	*	19	6	$271,250
Surg: Trauma-Burn	8	3	*	5	3	*
Surg: Vascular (primary)	33	10	$310,738	107	43	$303,083
Urgent Care	40	5	$131,747	365	95	$161,625
Urology	156	30	$316,151	319	109	$286,230
Urology: Pediatric	2	2	*	11	2	*

MEDICAL GROUP MANAGEMENT ASSOCIATION™

Table 3A: Physician Compensation by Size of Multispecialty Practice (50 or Less FTE Physicians)

	10 FTE or less		11 to 25 FTE		26 to 50 FTE	
	Physicians	Median	Physicians	Median	Physicians	Median
Allergy/Immunology	0	*	2	*	23	$298,503
Anesthesiology	*	*	15	*	40	$315,258
Anesth: Pain Management	1	*	6	*	4	*
Anesth: Pediatric	*	*	1	*	13	*
Cardiology: Electrophysiology	1	*	5	*	8	*
Cardiology: Invasive	*	*	16	$343,791	86	$384,665
Cardiology: Inv-Intervntnl	8	*	33	$359,611	74	$585,162
Cardiology: Noninvasive	2	*	20	$250,150	51	$294,792
Critical Care: Intensivist	1	*	2	*	2	*
Dentistry	0	*	1	*	9	*
Dermatology	*	*	7	*	38	$268,515
Dermatology: MOHS Surgery	*	*	3	*	3	*
Emergency Medicine	8	*	6	*	11	$164,320
Endocrinology/Metabolism	3	*	19	$175,323	20	$146,495
Family Practice (w/ OB)	84	$153,464	153	$156,634	113	$169,999
Family Practice (w/o OB)	218	$149,813	313	$141,919	542	$152,055
Family Practice: Sports Med	4	*	1	*	4	*
Gastroenterology	4	*	41	$358,079	85	$328,043
Gastroenterology: Hepatology	1	*	4	*	3	*
Geriatrics	*	*	6	*	6	*
Hematology/Oncology	4	*	13	$305,000	46	$323,269
Hem/Onc: Oncology (only)	*	*	2	*	9	*
Infectious Disease	2	*	12	$233,922	4	*
Internal Medicine: General	157	$141,180	372	$141,601	575	$160,391
Internal Med: Hospitalist	4	*	21	$161,000	35	$162,318
Internal Med: Pediatric	9	*	21	$166,959	17	$143,147
Nephrology	11	$201,500	6	*	14	$192,197
Neurology	8	*	14	$217,742	34	$201,375
OBGYN: General	31	$275,000	62	$227,662	167	$245,010
OBGYN: Gynecology (only)	1	*	5	*	10	$181,381
OBGYN: Gyn Oncology	0	*	1	*	3	*
OBGYN: Maternal & Fetal Med	2	*	*	*	3	*
OBGYN: Repro Endocrinology	0	*	*	*	7	*
Occupational Medicine	2	*	23	$223,834	8	*
Ophthalmology	4	*	18	$244,791	43	$236,032
Ophthalmology: Pediatric	*	*	4	*	*	*
Ophthalmology: Retina	*	*	2	*	*	*
Orthopedic (Non-surgical)	1	*	1	*	6	*
Orthopedic Surgery: General	5	*	47	$449,661	63	$329,000
Ortho Surg: Foot & Ankle	*	*	1	*	5	*
Ortho Surg: Hand	1	*	3	*	8	*
Ortho Surg: Hip & Joint	1	*	6	*	7	*
Ortho Surg: Oncology	*	*	1	*	*	*
Ortho Surg: Pediatric	*	*	4	*	1	*
Ortho Surg: Spine	8	*	3	*	3	*
Ortho Surg: Sports Med	3	*	5	*	19	$238,019
Otorhinolaryngology	3	*	8	*	74	$298,224
Pathology: Anatomic & Clinical	4	*	4	*	3	*
Pathology: Anatomic	*	*	*	*	4	*
Pathology: Clinical	*	*	*	*	12	$141,445

Table 3A: Physician Compensation by Size of Multispecialty Practice (50 or Less FTE Physicians) (continued)

	10 FTE or less		11 to 25 FTE		26 to 50 FTE	
	Physicians	Median	Physicians	Median	Physicians	Median
Pediatrics: General	41	$148,500	144	$131,474	268	$152,540
Ped: Adolescent Medicine	1	*	3	*	12	$168,805
Ped: Allergy/Immunology	*	*	*	*	1	*
Ped: Cardiology	1	*	0	*	4	*
Ped: Child Development	*	*	4	*	5	*
Ped: Critical Care/Intensivist	*	*	2	*	19	$252,665
Ped: Emergency Medicine	*	*	*	*	6	*
Ped: Endocrinology	*	*	1	*	6	*
Ped: Gastroenterology	*	*	*	*	3	*
Ped: Genetics	*	*	3	*	2	*
Ped: Hematology/Oncology	*	*	5	*	9	*
Ped: Hospitalist	*	*	2	*	2	*
Ped: Infectious Disease	*	*	2	*	*	*
Ped: Neonatal Medicine	*	*	2	*	1	*
Ped: Nephrology	*	*	1	*	*	*
Ped: Neurology	*	*	2	*	3	*
Ped: Pulmonology	*	*	1	*	4	*
Ped: Rheumatology	*	*	*	*	1	*
Physiatry (Phys Med & Rehab)	4	*	13	$160,460	7	*
Podiatry: General	1	*	5	*	11	$183,958
Podiatry: Surg-Foot & Ankle	*	*	1	*	3	*
Podiatry: Surg-Forefoot Only	*	*	*	*	5	*
Psychiatry: General	4	*	5	*	21	$154,253
Psychiatry: Child & Adolescent	*	*	2	*	1	*
Psychiatry: Geriatric	*	*	4	*	7	*
Pulmonary Medicine	5	*	22	$225,526	31	$220,109
Pulmonary Med: Critical Care	2	*	34	$230,128	27	$286,037
Radiation Oncology	*	*	*	*	4	*
Radiology: Diagnostic-Inv	*	*	5	*	9	*
Radiology: Diagnostic-Noninv	*	*	13	$309,222	26	$386,659
Radiology: Nuclear Medicine	1	*	5	*	2	*
Rheumatology	4	*	23	$238,000	30	$256,350
Sleep Medicine	4	*	*	*	*	*
Surgery: General	34	$226,804	47	$246,329	106	$256,984
Surg: Cardiovascular	*	*	*	*	29	$381,294
Surg: Cardiovascular-Pediatric	*	*	*	*	2	*
Surg: Colon and Rectal	2	*	*	*	3	*
Surg: Neurological	13	$531,000	12	$424,761	4	*
Surg: Oncology	2	*	*	*	1	*
Surg: Oral	*	*	*	*	2	*
Surg: Pediatric	2	*	2	*	*	*
Surg: Plastic & Reconstruction	*	*	1	*	7	*
Surg: Plastic & Recon-Hand	*	*	1	*	*	*
Surg: Thoracic (primary)	2	*	4	*	*	*
Surg: Transplant	1	*	*	*	4	*
Surg: Trauma	5	*	*	*	*	*
Surg: Vascular (primary)	12	$289,029	9	*	13	$334,109
Urgent Care	11	$147,502	14	$133,395	61	$150,712
Urology	*	*	10	$294,442	30	$329,226

Table 3B: Physician Compensation by Size of Multispecialty Practice (51 or More FTE Physicians)

	51 to 75 FTE		76 to 150 FTE		151 FTE or more	
	Physicians	Median	Physicians	Median	Physicians	Median
Allergy/Immunology	17	$199,992	32	$214,191	57	$208,842
Anesthesiology	14	$250,528	71	$296,070	320	$280,676
Anesth: Pain Management	1	*	2	*	7	*
Anesth: Pediatric	1	*	*	*	*	*
Cardiology: Electrophysiology	3	*	13	$301,784	18	$303,722
Cardiology: Invasive	40	$334,274	77	$352,445	98	$328,680
Cardiology: Inv-Intervntnl	15	$478,477	56	$367,937	67	$443,490
Cardiology: Noninvasive	28	$234,901	64	$325,775	112	$280,591
Critical Care: Intensivist	1	*	2	*	49	$203,799
Dentistry	*	*	*	*	20	$140,886
Dermatology	47	$291,473	64	$302,606	121	$240,000
Dermatology: MOHS Surgery	1	*	5	*	5	*
Emergency Medicine	12	*	43	$232,119	326	$209,600
Endocrinology/Metabolism	27	$190,688	50	$165,823	74	$175,050
Family Practice (w/ OB)	172	$162,063	158	$157,731	327	$157,385
Family Practice (w/o OB)	544	$155,652	771	$150,028	1,165	$148,346
Family Practice: Sports Med	1	*	3	*	2	*
Gastroenterology	63	$413,309	121	$322,240	163	$266,194
Gastroenterology: Hepatology	5	*	*	*	5	*
Geriatrics	5	*	10	$144,126	24	$150,452
Hematology/Oncology	29	$363,168	64	$274,906	113	$226,205
Hem/Onc: Oncology (only)	10	$290,537	19	$330,321	15	$245,097
Infectious Disease	9	*	28	$178,618	46	$171,065
Internal Medicine: General	510	$158,682	843	$156,200	1,534	$154,358
Internal Med: Hospitalist	25	$165,891	100	$163,937	159	$160,272
Internal Med: Pediatric	13	$125,567	19	$148,500	13	$130,008
Nephrology	28	$227,137	52	$279,485	85	$206,200
Neurology	58	$181,234	85	$202,297	180	$175,564
OBGYN: General	137	$242,619	217	$251,185	550	$223,160
OBGYN: Gynecology (only)	14	$231,712	40	$221,811	59	$220,000
OBGYN: Gyn Oncology	*	*	3	*	18	$294,244
OBGYN: Maternal & Fetal Med	1	*	9	*	34	$365,848
OBGYN: Repro Endocrinology	*	*	2	*	14	$255,926
Occupational Medicine	10	$134,018	25	$190,132	63	$155,000
Ophthalmology	42	$278,172	77	$294,882	186	$225,723
Ophthalmology: Pediatric	0	*	*	*	7	*
Ophthalmology: Retina	2	*	0	*	18	$369,985
Orthopedic (Non-surgical)	6	*	10	$335,801	6	*
Orthopedic Surgery: General	44	$375,925	92	$388,748	230	$328,870
Ortho Surg: Foot & Ankle	*	*	*	*	5	*
Ortho Surg: Hand	1	*	2	*	15	$382,500
Ortho Surg: Hip & Joint	1	*	2	*	9	*
Ortho Surg: Pediatric	*	*	0	*	4	*
Ortho Surg: Spine	4	*	2	*	17	$561,088
Ortho Surg: Trauma	*	*	*	*	5	*
Ortho Surg: Sports Med	6	*	7	*	62	$240,211
Otorhinolaryngology	37	$269,035	74	$274,937	108	$295,569
Otorhinolaryngology: Pediatric	1	*	8	*	*	*
Pathology: Anatomic & Clinical	6	*	15	$284,706	93	$221,191
Pathology: Anatomic	*	*	3	*	10	*
Pathology: Clinical	4	*	15	$229,418	32	$191,262

Table 3B: Physician Compensation by Size of Multispecialty Practice (51 or More FTE Physicians) (continued)

	51 to 75 FTE		76 to 150 FTE		151 FTE or more	
	Physicians	Median	Physicians	Median	Physicians	Median
Pediatrics: General	200	$157,665	328	$151,908	660	$149,851
Ped: Adolescent Medicine	*	*	25	*	40	$141,697
Ped: Allergy/Immunology	*	*	*	*	5	*
Ped: Cardiology	6	*	2	*	17	$210,457
Ped: Child Development	2	*	1	*	8	*
Ped: Critical Care/Intensivist	*	*	1	*	15	$178,583
Ped: Endocrinology	3	*	*	*	9	*
Ped: Gastroenterology	3	*	1	*	10	$184,964
Ped: Genetics	3	*	*	*	10	$170,428
Ped: Hematology/Oncology	4	*	1	*	14	$169,098
Ped: Hospitalist	8	*	1	*	10	$151,500
Ped: Infectious Disease	1	*	*	*	5	*
Ped: Neonatal Medicine	3	*	7	*	64	$203,193
Ped: Nephrology	3	*	*	*	4	*
Ped: Neurology	3	*	3	*	14	$167,641
Ped: Pulmonology	*	*	*	*	8	*
Ped: Rheumatology	2	*	*	*	*	*
Ped: Sports Medicine	*	*	1	*	*	*
Physiatry (Phys Med & Rehab)	8	*	24	$204,274	67	$184,090
Podiatry: General	8	*	40	$160,336	59	$136,050
Podiatry: Surg-Foot & Ankle	6	*	7	*	55	$167,370
Podiatry: Surg-Forefoot Only	*	*	6	*	3	*
Psychiatry: General	19	$166,899	58	$161,288	223	$160,000
Psychiatry: Child & Adolescent	4	*	2	*	33	$183,211
Psychiatry: Geriatric	*	*	1	*	1	*
Pulmonary Medicine	31	$218,298	88	$227,895	78	$201,628
Pulmonary Med: Critical Care	19	$227,497	7	*	11	$235,950
Radiation Oncology	10	$361,457	16	$346,160	27	$370,000
Radiology: Diagnostic-Inv	4	*	34	$508,374	95	$350,000
Radiology: Diagnostic-Noninv	27	$352,845	53	$355,096	245	$318,122
Radiology: Nuclear Medicine	4	*	9	*	14	$242,931
Rheumatology	35	$187,130	58	$202,720	82	$175,924
Sleep Medicine	1	*	2	*	*	*
Surgery: General	88	$258,159	177	$273,428	294	$253,477
Surg: Cardiovascular	1	*	17	$329,669	49	$402,500
Surg: Colon and Rectal	1	*	4	*	21	$295,000
Surg: Neurological	11	$442,180	22	$541,818	45	$412,620
Surg: Oncology	*	*	6	*	*	*
Surg: Oral	*	*	3	*	9	*
Surg: Pediatric	4	*	2	*	6	*
Surg: Plastic & Reconstruction	5	*	22	$304,670	60	$291,480
Surg: Plastic & Recon-Hand	*	*	2	*	1	*
Surg: Plastic & Recon-Pediatric	*	*	2	*	*	*
Surg: Thoracic (primary)	5	*	6	*	19	$239,309
Surg: Transplant	*	*	*	*	7	*
Surg: Trauma	*	*	2	*	12	$309,625
Surg: Trauma-Burn	*	*	1	*	4	*
Surg: Vascular (primary)	4	*	14	$306,171	52	$299,541
Urgent Care	28	$138,434	120	$180,467	123	$163,244
Urology	38	$248,951	82	$314,419	143	$276,860
Urology: Pediatric	11	*	*	*	*	*

MEDICAL GROUP MANAGEMENT ASSOCIATION™

Table 4: Physician Compensation by Hospital Ownership

	Hospital Owned			Non-hospital Owned		
	Physicians	Medical Practices	Median	Physicians	Medical Practices	Median
Allergy/Immunology	18	14	$198,830	162	78	$250,233
Anesthesiology	91	17	$315,000	1,556	98	$306,995
Anesth: Pain Management	8	6	*	73	27	$326,421
Anesth: Pediatric	*	*	*	35	5	$320,000
Cardiology: Electrophysiology	5	3	*	140	79	$377,149
Cardiology: Invasive	38	11	$409,238	552	137	$358,556
Cardiology: Inv-Intervntnl	55	12	$459,518	663	143	$416,382
Cardiology: Noninvasive	55	16	$309,024	511	147	$309,492
Critical Care: Intensivist	13	6	$200,914	47	7	$208,362
Dentistry	3	2	*	28	5	$152,627
Dermatology	53	27	$223,278	246	109	$274,496
Dermatology: MOHS Surgery	7	6	*	14	14	$409,999
Emergency Medicine	161	18	$196,536	369	28	$218,477
Endocrinology/Metabolism	65	35	$162,206	133	76	$177,207
Family Practice (w/ OB)	432	79	$159,984	843	138	$154,962
Family Practice (w/o OB)	1,999	230	$150,000	2,283	282	$151,214
Family Practice: Sports Med	10	8	$214,672	18	14	$166,398
Gastroenterology	81	30	$344,323	614	165	$322,577
Gastroenterology: Hepatology	*	*	*	75	16	$316,200
Geriatrics	22	10	$147,119	34	18	$134,108
Hematology/Oncology	48	18	$241,467	343	102	$320,406
Hem/Onc: Oncology (only)	8	5	*	80	32	$357,625
Infectious Disease	29	21	$176,141	112	47	$182,723
Internal Medicine: General	1,251	151	$154,840	2,974	280	$154,932
Internal Med: Hospitalist	167	32	$162,318	177	45	$162,873
Internal Med: Pediatric	47	17	$140,000	49	18	$145,151
Nephrology	37	14	$203,000	223	69	$230,000
Neurology	68	28	$176,346	434	119	$189,519
OBGYN: General	372	84	$230,055	1,237	197	$235,606
OBGYN: Gynecology (only)	82	20	$223,792	86	50	$175,988
OBGYN: Gyn Oncology	6	4	*	19	8	$301,683
OBGYN: Maternal & Fetal Med	29	8	$401,500	30	10	$304,050
OBGYN: Repro Endocrinology	11	3	$270,000	22	8	$268,849
Occupational Medicine	39	15	$147,568	111	38	$170,820
Ophthalmology	57	23	$250,398	470	127	$262,741
Ophthalmology: Pediatric	1	1	*	27	18	$284,387
Ophthalmology: Retina	2	2	*	73	28	$433,265
Orthopedic (Non-surgical)	10	8	$198,011	40	20	$265,487
Orthopedic Surgery: General	76	30	$360,250	800	192	$372,308
Ortho Surg: Foot & Ankle	*	*	*	51	45	$391,120
Ortho Surg: Hand	3	3	*	133	75	$442,300
Ortho Surg: Hip & Joint	3	1	*	113	60	$429,603
Ortho Surg: Oncology	*	*	*	3	3	*
Ortho Surg: Pediatric	6	3	*	36	25	$278,156
Ortho Surg: Spine	4	3	*	129	77	$548,000
Ortho Surg: Trauma	4	1	*	20	15	$456,085
Ortho Surg: Sports Med	10	7	$260,333	243	93	$347,011
Otorhinolaryngology	65	29	$263,635	343	113	$278,307
Otorhinolaryngology: Pediatric	*	*	*	17	4	$324,800
Pathology: Anatomic & Clinical	28	6	$215,749	200	36	$298,444
Pathology: Anatomic	3	1	*	50	9	$338,848
Pathology: Clinical	14	5	$190,914	65	12	$197,250

Table 4: Physician Compensation by Hospital Ownership (continued)

	Hospital Owned			Non-hospital Owned		
	Physicians	Medical Practices	Median	Physicians	Medical Practices	Median
Pediatrics: General	683	114	$151,754	1,499	203	$154,943
Ped: Adolescent Medicine	27	7	$164,604	57	6	$143,850
Ped: Allergy/Immunology	2	2	*	8	6	*
Ped: Cardiology	7	4	*	46	18	$222,149
Ped: Child Development	8	5	*	9	4	*
Ped: Critical Care/Intensivist	19	6	$252,665	48	14	$248,960
Ped: Emergency Medicine	8	2	*	*	*	*
Ped: Endocrinology	11	7	$137,800	12	8	$144,575
Ped: Gastroenterology	9	5	*	19	6	$200,013
Ped: Genetics	3	2	*	15	5	$163,621
Ped: Hematology/Oncology	20	8	$194,663	28	12	$179,275
Ped: Hospitalist	8	5	*	18	7	$154,016
Ped: Infectious Disease	2	1	*	8	4	*
Ped: Neonatal Medicine	30	8	$246,714	75	14	$213,920
Ped: Nephrology	3	3	*	7	4	*
Ped: Neurology	14	9	$168,200	19	10	$170,004
Ped: Pulmonology	7	4	*	14	7	$213,208
Ped: Rheumatology	*	*	*	4	3	*
Ped: Sports Medicine	*	*	*	1	1	*
Physiatry (Phys Med & Rehab)	38	17	$189,974	138	62	$195,469
Podiatry: General	40	19	$147,101	83	51	$156,918
Podiatry: Surg-Foot & Ankle	7	5	*	85	21	$162,579
Podiatry: Surg-Forefoot Only	5	1	*	10	5	$129,499
Psychiatry: General	114	29	$148,291	221	37	$165,913
Psychiatry: Child & Adolescent	13	9	$172,574	39	9	$181,060
Psychiatry: Geriatric	5	3	*	8	4	*
Pulmonary Medicine	51	23	$231,000	234	105	$206,645
Pulmonary Med: Critical Care	14	8	$219,472	115	35	$233,877
Radiation Oncology	13	7	$303,301	91	30	$393,739
Radiology: Diagnostic-Inv	35	9	$375,000	347	49	$387,438
Radiology: Diagnostic-Noninv	57	14	$318,122	549	78	$355,096
Radiology: Nuclear Medicine	9	4	*	48	25	$287,952
Rheumatology	57	30	$188,916	204	96	$196,239
Sleep Medicine	1	1	*	9	5	*
Surgery: General	172	58	$258,380	762	190	$254,250
Surg: Cardiovascular	20	9	$457,500	163	40	$431,245
Surg: Cardiovascular-Pediatric	2	2	*	3	3	*
Surg: Colon and Rectal	0	*	*	38	19	$283,935
Surg: Neurological	21	12	$440,500	174	52	$473,867
Surg: Oncology	*	*	*	10	6	$359,675
Surg: Oral	3	2	*	23	10	$246,263
Surg: Pediatric	11	6	$263,203	11	4	$407,505
Surg: Plastic & Reconstruction	16	10	$325,362	88	42	$287,690
Surg: Plastic & Recon-Hand	1	1	*	17	6	$244,000
Surg: Plastic & Recon-Pediatric	*	*	*	4	2	*
Surg: Thoracic (primary)	3	3	*	53	13	$283,155
Surg: Transplant	8	4	*	8	4	*
Surg: Trauma	16	5	$238,821	8	3	*
Surg: Trauma-Burn	1	1	*	12	5	$325,411
Surg: Vascular (primary)	14	9	$285,625	124	43	$306,555
Urgent Care	100	29	$148,797	296	69	$163,048
Urology	50	22	$286,480	412	114	$292,564
Urology: Pediatric	9	1	*	4	3	*

MEDICAL GROUP MANAGEMENT ASSOCIATION™

Table 5A: Physician Compensation by Geographic Section for All Practices

	Eastern		Midwest		Southern		Western	
	Physicians	Median	Physicians	Median	Physicians	Median	Physicians	Median
Allergy/Immunology	26	$305,845	52	$239,487	58	$305,208	49	$197,263
Anesthesiology	264	$270,000	450	$380,758	511	$346,000	477	$261,514
Anesth: Pain Management	25	$310,000	17	$315,236	36	$361,439	6	*
Anesth: Pediatric	*	*	1	*	29	$330,487	5	*
Cardiology: Electrophysiology	28	$372,673	46	$372,466	51	$406,407	23	$344,329
Cardiology: Invasive	96	$353,849	177	$383,000	188	$378,270	140	$315,885
Cardiology: Inv-Intervntnl	95	$385,000	228	$426,210	275	$447,984	122	$368,949
Cardiology: Noninvasive	227	$296,800	144	$308,451	135	$350,114	76	$278,831
Critical Care: Intensivist	9	*	8	*	4	*	41	$206,010
Dentistry	27	$149,000	*	*	5	*	10	*
Dermatology	48	$226,037	103	$273,665	50	$275,839	112	$262,791
Dermatology: MOHS Surgery	3	*	6	*	8	*	5	*
Emergency Medicine	157	$194,230	141	$223,162	59	$270,820	199	$210,385
Endocrinology/Metabolism	42	$150,034	59	$175,828	50	$182,706	56	$162,758
Family Practice (w/ OB)	105	$135,784	743	$162,450	187	$154,999	266	$148,717
Family Practice (w/o OB)	758	$142,018	1,660	$148,281	938	$167,314	965	$149,397
Family Practice: Sports Med	1	*	12	$190,659	5	*	10	$212,686
Gastroenterology	143	$302,467	233	$339,397	153	$352,659	191	$291,963
Gastroenterology: Hepatology	22	$312,750	17	*	29	$281,000	7	*
Geriatrics	20	$132,379	18	$147,184	4	*	14	$146,016
Hematology/Oncology	73	$250,000	139	$379,872	87	$327,723	100	$243,174
Hem/Onc: Oncology (only)	36	$348,710	28	$264,984	10	$354,963	21	$388,321
Infectious Disease	35	$171,591	39	$181,095	27	$190,602	45	$178,539
Internal Medicine: General	864	$147,377	1,313	$153,856	796	$163,199	1,384	$154,619
Internal Med: Hospitalist	47	$151,052	134	$165,000	96	$169,007	73	$157,140
Internal Med: Pediatric	6	*	60	$142,971	20	$142,960	10	$139,992
Nephrology	63	$226,362	67	$216,745	71	$267,500	67	$213,633
Neurology	137	$185,200	189	$201,071	88	$184,892	108	$178,937
OBGYN: General	282	$204,736	543	$258,904	298	$255,778	515	$221,800
OBGYN: Gynecology (only)	34	$180,008	76	$233,704	46	$182,922	20	$184,369
OBGYN: Gyn Oncology	5	*	6	*	7	*	8	*
OBGYN: Maternal & Fetal Med	10	$253,068	31	$401,500	5	*	14	$299,669
OBGYN: Repro Endocrinology	7	*	14	$282,940	1	*	14	$248,348
Occupational Medicine	13	$137,767	62	$158,567	16	$237,326	62	$168,753
Ophthalmology	90	$291,504	189	$296,461	108	$267,134	170	$234,704
Ophthalmology: Pediatric	9	*	8	*	4	*	8	*
Ophthalmology: Retina	14	$384,147	26	$480,156	20	$473,436	16	$395,912
Orthopedic (Non-surgical)	7	*	16	$186,727	10	$175,064	18	$335,801
Orthopedic Surgery: General	156	$370,732	307	$389,650	193	$403,053	248	$329,643
Ortho Surg: Foot & Ankle	10	$316,168	17	$391,120	16	$415,390	9	*
Ortho Surg: Hand	28	$334,122	41	$462,523	46	$433,967	25	$442,300
Ortho Surg: Hip & Joint	33	$389,237	39	$457,984	20	$456,098	25	$381,147
Ortho Surg: Oncology	1	*	*	*	2	*	*	*
Ortho Surg: Pediatric	8	*	14	$340,459	12	$327,468	8	*
Ortho Surg: Spine	38	$545,412	48	$590,223	20	$536,250	28	$505,828
Ortho Surg: Trauma	12	$443,760	4	*	7	*	7	*
Ortho Surg: Sports Med	33	$473,000	63	$403,753	72	$364,246	92	$252,655
Otorhinolaryngology	91	$261,820	134	$301,647	118	$288,926	81	$243,671
Otorhinolaryngology: Pediatric	8	*	8	*	1	*	*	*
Pathology: Anatomic & Clinical	28	$226,730	73	$333,958	47	$349,210	85	$226,715
Pathology: Anatomic	7	*	3	*	27	$349,104	23	$312,116
Pathology: Clinical	34	$151,922	23	$228,168	12	$219,067	15	$215,275

Table 5A: Physician Compensation by Geographic Section for All Practices (continued)

	Eastern		Midwest		Southern		Western	
	Physicians	Median	Physicians	Median	Physicians	Median	Physicians	Median
Pediatrics: General	387	$148,226	736	$155,758	411	$150,046	681	$154,656
Ped: Adolescent Medicine	2	*	48	$154,766	35	$131,850	0	*
Ped: Allergy/Immunology	1	*	4	*	1	*	4	*
Ped: Cardiology	10	$208,563	11	$219,017	11	$215,184	21	$218,858
Ped: Child Development	5	*	10	$123,812	2	*	3	*
Ped: Critical Care/Intensivist	4	*	30	$252,665	20	$270,673	13	$255,481
Ped: Emergency Medicine	2	*	6	*	*	*	*	*
Ped: Endocrinology	1	*	10	$141,250	3	*	9	*
Ped: Gastroenterology	3	*	11	$180,000	1	*	13	$203,606
Ped: Genetics	3	*	3	*	1	*	11	$173,531
Ped: Hematology/Oncology	4	*	18	$203,408	5	*	21	$180,746
Ped: Hospitalist	2	*	5	*	7	*	12	$155,296
Ped: Infectious Disease	*	*	0	*	3	*	7	*
Ped: Neonatal Medicine	20	$175,000	29	$246,714	22	$395,120	35	$213,111
Ped: Nephrology	1	*	3	*	*	*	6	*
Ped: Neurology	4	*	19	$175,139	2	*	8	*
Ped: Pulmonology	3	*	11	$187,211	1	*	6	*
Ped: Rheumatology	1	*	*	*	*	*	3	*
Ped: Sports Medicine	1	*	*	*	*	*	*	*
Physiatry (Phys Med & Rehab)	25	$176,425	68	$220,246	25	$210,244	60	$169,278
Podiatry: General	14	$130,881	62	$161,013	22	$135,720	29	$151,948
Podiatry: Surg-Foot & Ankle	5	*	19	$153,632	4	*	64	$162,225
Podiatry: Surg-Forefoot Only	5	*	3	*	5	*	2	*
Psychiatry: General	86	$144,999	128	$155,563	20	$145,804	127	$171,351
Psychiatry: Child & Adolescent	3	*	13	$180,000	10	$169,680	27	*
Psychiatry: Geriatric	4	*	2	*	4	*	3	*
Pulmonary Medicine	53	$192,000	113	$230,000	64	$219,204	65	$204,244
Pulmonary Med: Critical Care	39	$223,873	36	$251,030	41	$250,990	36	$200,972
Radiation Oncology	9	*	32	$396,980	39	$471,000	28	$348,073
Radiology: Diagnostic-Inv	43	$317,053	108	$506,893	108	$456,093	126	$341,264
Radiology: Diagnostic-Noninv	83	$300,000	168	$422,283	166	$380,977	218	$305,559
Radiology: Nuclear Medicine	13	$225,858	11	$362,700	5	*	28	$329,051
Rheumatology	46	$177,244	87	$201,823	63	$215,172	72	$178,606
Sleep Medicine	9	*	3	*	2	*	1	*
Surgery: General	151	$213,211	354	$287,776	198	$286,887	257	$247,170
Surg: Cardiovascular	30	$447,466	44	$405,577	74	$430,140	39	$460,000
Surg: Cardiovascular-Pediatric	*	*	2	*	2	*	1	*
Surg: Colon and Rectal	18	$240,000	11	$394,000	4	*	11	$231,532
Surg: Neurological	49	$440,500	72	$531,292	43	$528,324	37	$411,078
Surg: Oncology	2	*	7	*	*	*	1	*
Surg: Oral	9	*	7	*	5	*	6	*
Surg: Pediatric	5	*	2	*	7	*	8	*
Surg: Plastic & Reconstruction	16	$259,115	27	$301,135	21	$300,000	44	$272,386
Surg: Plastic & Recon-Hand	14	$221,000	3	*	1	*	*	*
Surg: Plastic & Recon-Pediatric	2	*	*	*	2	*	*	*
Surg: Thoracic (primary)	4	*	33	$362,617	0	*	19	$281,479
Surg: Transplant	4	*	1	*	10	$379,959	1	*
Surg: Trauma	3	*	13	$320,141	8	*	*	*
Surg: Trauma-Burn	2	*	4	*	6	*	1	*
Surg: Vascular (primary)	33	$301,250	33	$328,670	29	$353,905	45	$270,000
Urgent Care	35	$140,000	160	$161,350	63	$170,255	147	$157,162
Urology	76	$298,678	139	$332,888	112	$334,971	148	$255,779
Urology: Pediatric	*	*	9	*	1	*	3	*

Table 5B: Physician Compensation by Geographic Section for Single-specialty Practices

	Eastern		Midwest		Southern		Western	
	Physicians	Median	Physicians	Median	Physicians	Median	Physicians	Median
Allergy/Immunology	10	$378,919	*	*	31	$339,029	7	*
Anesthesiology	175	$270,000	336	$386,481	445	$353,468	271	$257,228
Anesth: Pain Management	14	$402,650	11	$293,313	32	$361,439	3	*
Anesth: Pediatric	*	*	*	*	15	*	5	*
Cardiology: Electrophysiology	19	$414,080	29	$406,984	39	$417,991	13	$359,125
Cardiology: Invasive	54	$374,854	85	$393,051	107	$369,905	30	$296,726
Cardiology: Inv-Intervntnl	54	$410,734	119	$420,218	214	$431,593	74	$371,344
Cardiology: Noninvasive	150	$355,591	53	$363,991	89	$353,000	13	$337,707
Critical Care: Intensivist	1	*	*	*	4	*	*	*
Dentistry	2	*	*	*	*	*	10	*
Dermatology	8	*	2	*	2	*	13	$358,700
Dermatology: MOHS Surgery	1	*	2	*	1	*	*	*
Emergency Medicine	44	*	*	*	45	$289,529	47	$239,690
Endocrinology/Metabolism	4	*	4	*	4	*	*	*
Family Practice (w/ OB)	35	$143,985	127	$158,906	38	$154,988	82	$133,498
Family Practice (w/o OB)	166	$160,523	199	$143,927	251	$166,752	98	$137,211
Family Practice: Sports Med	0	*	9	*	2	*	2	*
Gastroenterology	58	$328,844	83	$329,828	58	$396,647	36	$303,821
Gastroenterology: Hepatology	17	$328,800	17	*	21	$263,966	2	*
Geriatrics	*	*	*	*	*	*	1	*
Hematology/Oncology	32	$341,924	51	$796,894	31	$439,295	16	$403,670
Hem/Onc: Oncology (only)	24	$371,479	3	*	*	*	11	*
Infectious Disease	16	$204,640	6	*	10	$209,475	9	*
Internal Medicine: General	90	$158,992	87	$167,630	62	$173,601	56	$146,093
Internal Med: Hospitalist	*	*	*	*	4	*	2	*
Internal Med: Pediatric	*	*	4	*	*	*	*	*
Nephrology	37	$242,700	2	*	24	$186,716	5	*
Neurology	40	$191,480	54	$211,844	24	$164,863	17	$231,000
OBGYN: General	97	$204,472	132	$259,115	127	$262,524	95	$233,000
OBGYN: Gynecology (only)	15	$140,000	4	*	25	$176,538	3	*
OBGYN: Gyn Oncology	1	*	*	*	*	*	*	*
OBGYN: Maternal & Fetal Med	2	*	3	*	3	*	3	*
OBGYN: Repro Endocrinology	*	*	6	*	1	*	6	*
Occupational Medicine	0	*	3	*	5	*	*	*
Ophthalmology	45	$388,177	46	$362,840	49	$278,023	39	$327,036
Ophthalmology: Pediatric	8	*	4	*	1	*	4	*
Ophthalmology: Retina	12	$461,051	21	$470,954	15	$520,000	5	*
Orthopedic (Non-surgical)	6	*	3	*	4	*	7	*
Orthopedic Surgery: General	96	$422,589	119	$394,361	113	$402,894	75	$399,199
Ortho Surg: Foot & Ankle	9	*	10	$338,393	13	$458,314	9	*
Ortho Surg: Hand	23	$381,979	24	$452,075	42	$462,129	21	$442,300
Ortho Surg: Hip & Joint	33	$389,237	23	$578,800	17	$457,952	18	$370,307
Ortho Surg: Oncology	1	*	*	*	1	*	*	*
Ortho Surg: Pediatric	5	*	9	*	11	$354,936	2	*
Ortho Surg: Spine	29	$595,914	33	$534,104	19	$580,733	16	$501,923
Ortho Surg: Trauma	8	*	3	*	7	*	7	*
Ortho Surg: Sports Med	30	$473,861	43	$403,753	52	$444,737	33	$434,257
Otorhinolaryngology	18	$252,962	20	*	55	$287,432	16	$231,112
Otorhinolaryngology: Pediatric	*	*	7	*	1	*	*	*
Pathology: Anatomic & Clinical	8	*	37	$472,000	28	$511,177	25	$413,379
Pathology: Anatomic	*	*	*	*	22	$372,450	21	$312,116
Pathology: Clinical	*	*	5	*	2	*	14	$226,160

Table 5B: Physician Compensation by Geographic Section for Single-specialty Practices (continued)

	Eastern		Midwest		Southern		Western	
	Physicians	Median	Physicians	Median	Physicians	Median	Physicians	Median
Pediatrics: General	145	$169,637	192	$164,827	95	$176,100	108	$170,345
Ped: Adolescent Medicine	*	*	*	*	4	*	0	*
Ped: Allergy/Immunology	*	*	*	*	*	*	4	*
Ped: Cardiology	5	*	5	*	7	*	5	*
Ped: Critical Care/Intensivist	*	*	11	*	7	*	12	*
Ped: Emergency Medicine	2	*	*	*	*	*	*	*
Ped: Endocrinology	*	*	*	*	1	*	3	*
Ped: Gastroenterology	*	*	5	*	1	*	5	*
Ped: Hematology/Oncology	*	*	2	*	3	*	9	*
Ped: Hospitalist	*	*	*	*	*	*	3	*
Ped: Infectious Disease	*	*	*	*	*	*	2	*
Ped: Neonatal Medicine	*	*	*	*	16	*	13	*
Ped: Nephrology	*	*	*	*	*	*	2	*
Ped: Neurology	1	*	4	*	1	*	2	*
Ped: Pulmonology	*	*	5	*	*	*	3	*
Ped: Rheumatology	*	*	*	*	*	*	1	*
Physiatry (Phys Med & Rehab)	7	*	13	$280,000	13	$300,000	16	$207,430
Podiatry: General	*	*	1	*	2	*	*	*
Podiatry: Surg-Foot & Ankle	1	*	12	$166,595	*	*	1	*
Podiatry: Surg-Forefoot Only	*	*	*	*	*	*	1	*
Psychiatry: General	4	*	6	*	*	*	*	*
Psychiatry: Child & Adolescent	1	*	*	*	6	*	*	*
Pulmonary Medicine	16	$174,912	9	*	3	*	5	*
Pulmonary Med: Critical Care	19	*	3	*	14	*	12	$174,242
Radiation Oncology	2	*	8	*	29	$547,776	12	*
Radiology: Diagnostic-Inv	22	$340,201	57	$510,391	89	$450,000	70	$356,076
Radiology: Diagnostic-Noninv	26	$441,783	49	$484,715	102	$447,264	67	$361,484
Radiology: Nuclear Medicine	1	*	4	*	2	*	14	$373,448
Rheumatology	8	*	2	*	14	*	8	*
Sleep Medicine	5	*	2	*	1	*	*	*
Surgery: General	43	$191,501	39	$240,281	83	$286,816	22	$280,955
Surg: Cardiovascular	18	$470,156	14	$600,487	36	$519,617	20	$552,221
Surg: Cardiovascular-Pediatric	*	*	*	*	2	*	1	*
Surg: Colon and Rectal	9	*	1	*	*	*	2	*
Surg: Neurological	26	$510,000	32	$496,943	23	$531,126	6	*
Surg: Oncology	*	*	1	*	*	*	*	*
Surg: Oral	6	*	*	*	3	*	4	*
Surg: Pediatric	*	*	2	*	4	*	0	*
Surg: Plastic & Reconstruction	*	*	*	*	7	*	4	*
Surg: Plastic & Recon-Hand	13	$221,000	*	*	1	*	*	*
Surg: Plastic & Recon-Pediatric	*	*	*	*	2	*	*	*
Surg: Thoracic (primary)	2	*	17	*	0	*	*	*
Surg: Transplant	*	*	*	*	4	*	*	*
Surg: Trauma	*	*	2	*	3	*	*	*
Surg: Trauma-Burn	*	*	1	*	6	*	1	*
Surg: Vascular (primary)	12	$268,102	1	*	11	*	9	*
Urgent Care	15	*	4	*	19	*	2	*
Urology	35	$313,397	28	$363,211	52	$327,528	41	$290,986
Urology: Pediatric	*	*	*	*	1	*	1	*

Table 5C: Physician Compensation by Geographic Section for Multispecialty Practices

	Eastern		Midwest		Southern		Western	
	Physicians	Median	Physicians	Median	Physicians	Median	Physicians	Median
Allergy/Immunology	16	$208,751	52	$239,487	27	$246,800	42	$194,739
Anesthesiology	89	$260,010	114	$339,415	66	$296,252	206	$265,614
Anesth: Pain Management	11	$246,115	6	*	4	*	3	*
Anesth: Pediatric	*	*	1	*	14	*	*	*
Cardiology: Electrophysiology	9	*	17	$318,503	12	$342,270	10	$336,110
Cardiology: Invasive	42	$305,548	92	$378,152	81	$389,920	110	$317,498
Cardiology: Inv-Intervntnl	41	$339,000	109	$457,056	61	$621,411	48	$366,940
Cardiology: Noninvasive	77	$260,416	91	$293,265	46	$339,989	63	$276,925
Critical Care: Intensivist	8	*	8	*	*	*	41	$206,010
Dentistry	25	$151,239	*	*	5	*	0	*
Dermatology	40	$218,193	101	$269,329	48	$272,588	99	$254,537
Dermatology: MOHS Surgery	2	*	4	*	7	*	5	*
Emergency Medicine	113	$192,767	141	$223,162	14	$249,112	152	$205,386
Endocrinology/Metabolism	38	$149,994	55	$177,792	46	$182,706	56	$162,758
Family Practice (w/ OB)	70	$133,012	616	$163,069	149	$154,999	184	$153,990
Family Practice (w/o OB)	592	$138,300	1,461	$148,778	687	$167,607	867	$150,852
Family Practice: Sports Med	1	*	3	*	3	*	8	*
Gastroenterology	85	$278,000	150	$344,323	95	$339,706	155	$285,000
Gastroenterology: Hepatology	5	*	*	*	8	*	5	*
Geriatrics	20	$132,379	18	$147,184	4		13	$146,016
Hematology/Oncology	41	$224,718	88	$317,607	56	$263,641	84	$227,879
Hem/Onc: Oncology (only)	12	$200,800	25	$262,552	10	$354,963	10	$324,920
Infectious Disease	19	$139,280	33	$167,240	17	$187,226	36	$177,193
Internal Medicine: General	774	$145,890	1,226	$153,378	734	$162,608	1,328	$154,881
Internal Med: Hospitalist	47	$151,052	134	$165,000	92	$171,979	71	$157,357
Internal Med: Pediatric	6	*	56	$141,887	20	$142,960	10	$139,992
Nephrology	26	$180,156	65	$216,745	47	$308,946	62	$213,605
Neurology	97	$179,110	135	$200,900	64	$195,463	91	$178,000
OBGYN: General	185	$205,000	411	$258,904	171	$255,130	420	$220,954
OBGYN: Gynecology (only)	19	$197,810	72	$235,540	21	$218,499	17	$197,747
OBGYN: Gyn Oncology	4	*	6	*	7	*	8	*
OBGYN: Maternal & Fetal Med	8	*	28	$392,463	2	*	11	*
OBGYN: Repro Endocrinology	7	*	8	*	*	*	8	*
Occupational Medicine	13	$137,767	59	$161,553	11	$137,451	62	$168,753
Ophthalmology	45	$220,000	143	$280,868	59	$263,798	131	$230,181
Ophthalmology: Pediatric	1	*	4	*	3	*	4	*
Ophthalmology: Retina	2	*	5	*	5	*	11	$379,531
Orthopedic (Non-surgical)	1	*	13	$206,797	6	*	11	$322,249
Orthopedic Surgery: General	60	$300,000	188	$388,025	80	$403,183	173	$316,313
Ortho Surg: Foot & Ankle	1	*	7	*	3	*	*	*
Ortho Surg: Hand	5	*	17	$462,523	4	*	4	*
Ortho Surg: Hip & Joint	*	*	16	$318,636	3	*	7	*
Ortho Surg: Oncology	*	*	*	*	1	*	*	*
Ortho Surg: Pediatric	3	*	5	*	1	*	6	*
Ortho Surg: Spine	9	*	15	$633,972	1	*	12	$536,564
Ortho Surg: Trauma	4	*	1	*	*	*	0	*
Ortho Surg: Sports Med	3	*	20	$400,975	20	$203,901	59	$240,009
Otorhinolaryngology	73	$269,035	114	$308,907	63	$303,793	65	$243,671
Otorhinolaryngology: Pediatric	8	*	1	*	*	*	*	*
Pathology: Anatomic & Clinical	20	$214,934	36	$275,725	19	$264,992	60	$221,017
Pathology: Anatomic	7	*	3	*	5	*	2	*
Pathology: Clinical	34	$151,922	18	$211,667	10	$219,067	1	*

Table 5C: Physician Compensation by Geographic Section for Multispecialty Practices (continued)

	Eastern		Midwest		Southern		Western	
	Physicians	Median	Physicians	Median	Physicians	Median	Physicians	Median
Pediatrics: General	242	$139,767	544	$153,460	316	$144,606	573	$152,659
Ped: Adolescent Medicine	2	*	48	$154,766	31	$139,544	*	*
Ped: Allergy/Immunology	1	*	4	*	1	*	*	*
Ped: Cardiology	5	*	6	*	4	*	16	$234,444
Ped: Child Development	5	*	10	$123,812	2	*	3	*
Ped: Critical Care/Intensivist	4	*	19	$252,665	13	$200,160	1	*
Ped: Emergency Medicine	*	*	6	*	*	*	*	*
Ped: Endocrinology	1	*	10	$141,250	2	*	6	*
Ped: Gastroenterology	3	*	6	*	*	*	8	*
Ped: Genetics	3	*	3	*	1	*	11	$173,531
Ped: Hematology/Oncology	4	*	16	$212,351	2	*	12	$186,754
Ped: Hospitalist	2	*	5	*	7	*	9	*
Ped: Infectious Disease	*	*	0	*	3	*	5	*
Ped: Neonatal Medicine	20	$175,000	29	$246,714	6	*	22	*
Ped: Nephrology	1	*	3	*	*	*	4	*
Ped: Neurology	3	*	15	$170,004	1	*	6	*
Ped: Pulmonology	3	*	6	*	1	*	3	*
Ped: Rheumatology	1	*	*	*	*	*	2	*
Ped: Sports Medicine	1	*	*	*	*	*	*	*
Physiatry (Phys Med & Rehab)	18	$168,979	55	$215,576	12	$193,090	44	$162,135
Podiatry: General	14	$130,881	61	$161,796	20	$135,720	29	$151,948
Podiatry: Surg-Foot & Ankle	4	*	7	*	4	*	63	$161,871
Podiatry: Surg-Forefoot Only	5	*	3	*	5	*	1	*
Psychiatry: General	82	$145,725	122	$156,912	20	$145,804	127	$171,351
Psychiatry: Child & Adolescent	2	*	13	$180,000	4	*	27	*
Psychiatry: Geriatric	4	*	2	*	4	*	3	*
Pulmonary Medicine	37	$210,320	104	$232,395	61	$220,109	60	$199,735
Pulmonary Med: Critical Care	20	$213,314	33	$246,851	27	$277,569	24	$210,679
Radiation Oncology	7	*	24	$386,677	10	$367,674	16	$314,131
Radiology: Diagnostic-Inv	21	$295,100	51	$486,109	19	$529,769	56	$337,550
Radiology: Diagnostic-Noninv	57	$272,656	119	$421,448	64	$358,074	151	$291,748
Radiology: Nuclear Medicine	12	$215,894	7	*	3	*	14	$242,931
Rheumatology	38	$172,429	85	$204,950	49	$212,205	64	$176,434
Sleep Medicine	4	*	1	*	1	*	1	*
Surgery: General	108	$226,510	315	$292,655	115	$287,117	235	$244,544
Surg: Cardiovascular	12	$423,966	30	$365,917	38	$358,169	19	$460,000
Surg: Cardiovascular-Pediatric	*	*	2	*	*	*	*	*
Surg: Colon and Rectal	9	*	10	$434,514	4	*	9	*
Surg: Neurological	23	$356,130	40	$535,609	20	$522,904	31	$412,620
Surg: Oncology	2	*	6	*	*	*	1	*
Surg: Oral	3	*	7	*	2	*	2	*
Surg: Pediatric	5	*	*	*	3	*	8	*
Surg: Plastic & Reconstruction	16	$259,115	27	$301,135	14	$268,158	40	$284,985
Surg: Plastic & Recon-Hand	1	*	3	*	*	*	*	*
Surg: Plastic & Recon-Pediatric	2	*	*	*	*	*	*	*
Surg: Thoracic (primary)	2	*	16	$279,929	*	*	19	$281,479
Surg: Transplant	4	*	1	*	6	*	1	*
Surg: Trauma	3	*	11	$347,207	5	*	*	*
Surg: Trauma-Burn	2	*	3	*	*	*	*	*
Surg: Vascular (primary)	21	$301,250	32	$326,712	18	$335,470	36	$280,153
Urgent Care	20	$131,546	156	$162,940	44	$203,223	145	$156,687
Urology	41	$286,730	111	$331,722	60	$345,411	107	$245,333
Urology: Pediatric	*	*	9	*	*	*	2	*

Table 6: Physician Compensation by Demographic Classification

	Non-metropolitan (under 50,000)		Metropolitan (50,000 to 250,000)		Metropolitan (250,001 to 1,000,000)		Metropolitan (over 1,000,000)	
	Physicians	Median	Physicians	Median	Physicians	Median	Physicians	Median
Allergy/Immunology	12	$205,789	63	$229,401	49	$323,752	61	$199,561
Anesthesiology	98	$263,090	482	$340,348	480	$300,435	613	$295,238
Anesth: Pain Management	10	$246,115	32	$324,545	20	$398,450	21	$310,000
Anesth: Pediatric	*	*	2	*	20	*	13	*
Cardiology: Electrophysiology	6	*	24	$389,915	69	$406,984	45	$369,040
Cardiology: Invasive	47	$318,847	168	$389,503	200	$350,104	179	$365,801
Cardiology: Inv-Intervntnl	30	$375,522	192	$466,211	314	$420,723	168	$416,143
Cardiology: Noninvasive	43	$262,923	150	$350,266	232	$299,999	148	$322,043
Critical Care: Intensivist	8	*	5	*	4	*	45	$208,362
Dentistry	7	*	0	*	24	$147,837	10	*
Dermatology	41	$272,847	120	$304,356	61	$273,665	86	$231,525
Dermatology: MOHS Surgery	2	*	11	$522,460	4	*	5	*
Emergency Medicine	48	$172,732	130	$228,162	131	$209,568	212	$210,770
Endocrinology/Metabolism	24	$161,599	74	$165,787	52	$172,806	54	$175,050
Family Practice (w/ OB)	440	$158,153	497	$160,000	176	$147,537	160	$151,238
Family Practice (w/o OB)	950	$142,976	1,501	$154,105	1,046	$148,312	759	$156,603
Family Practice: Sports Med	6	*	13	$197,096	4	*	5	*
Gastroenterology	67	$310,832	255	$344,323	135	$320,636	243	$285,751
Gastroenterology: Hepatology	2	*	22	$263,878	11	$280,992	39	$343,391
Geriatrics	13	$151,516	11	$140,031	24	$134,108	6	*
Hematology/Oncology	41	$231,320	145	$362,488	110	$344,154	98	$227,879
Hem/Onc: Oncology (only)	6	*	43	$359,566	14	$326,674	31	$331,214
Infectious Disease	12	$139,640	52	$168,963	36	$209,804	43	$180,204
Internal Medicine: General	609	$145,384	1,207	$159,948	940	$151,109	1,545	$156,900
Internal Med: Hospitalist	23	$152,122	154	$165,000	85	$159,431	85	$161,193
Internal Med: Pediatric	16	$139,992	26	$140,000	37	$159,094	17	$130,008
Nephrology	33	$195,000	101	$281,481	46	$197,784	88	$211,040
Neurology	86	$199,854	171	$194,879	109	$188,911	150	$177,774
OBGYN: General	245	$228,995	466	$254,836	372	$237,991	539	$221,479
OBGYN: Gynecology (only)	23	$197,870	53	$194,149	73	$206,569	25	$210,614
OBGYN: Gyn Oncology	0	*	8	*	7	*	11	$286,804
OBGYN: Maternal & Fetal Med	2	*	23	$346,157	20	$497,436	14	$299,669
OBGYN: Repro Endocrinology	0	*	5	*	16	$246,324	15	$308,549
Occupational Medicine	16	$141,172	49	$183,110	32	$153,013	55	$164,783
Ophthalmology	82	$222,773	171	$300,000	108	$343,796	193	$230,802
Ophthalmology: Pediatric	4	*	8	*	8	*	9	*
Ophthalmology: Retina	7	*	18	$452,545	15	$426,872	36	$395,912
Orthopedic (Non-surgical)	7	*	29	$277,942	2	*	12	$176,828
Orthopedic Surgery: General	180	$341,126	307	$420,334	197	$390,000	216	$329,201
Ortho Surg: Foot & Ankle	1	*	17	$377,992	19	$350,000	15	$452,788
Ortho Surg: Hand	4	*	40	$492,833	54	$449,200	42	$341,116
Ortho Surg: Hip & Joint	2	*	38	$360,937	47	$421,201	30	$460,476
Ortho Surg: Oncology	*	*	1	*	1	*	1	*
Ortho Surg: Pediatric	3	*	8	*	15	$347,483	16	$266,294
Ortho Surg: Spine	8	*	42	$726,332	44	$462,200	40	$557,877
Ortho Surg: Trauma	8	*	6	*	8	*	8	*
Ortho Surg: Sports Med	15	$347,000	79	$373,870	61	$497,003	104	$252,422
Otorhinolaryngology	56	$257,929	180	$296,106	107	$251,513	71	$277,455
Otorhinolaryngology: Pediatric	*	*	15	*	1	*	1	*
Pathology: Anatomic & Clinical	29	$226,730	53	$413,660	58	$414,315	93	$221,687
Pathology: Anatomic	3	*	6	*	7	*	44	$314,757
Pathology: Clinical	25	$142,659	32	$220,413	11	$226,000	16	$217,638

Table 6: Physician Compensation by Demographic Classification (continued)

	Non-metropolitan (under 50,000)		Metropolitan (50,000 to 250,000)		Metropolitan (250,001 to 1,000,000)		Metropolitan (over 1,000,000)	
	Physicians	Median	Physicians	Median	Physicians	Median	Physicians	Median
Pediatrics: General	290	$143,369	622	$159,247	566	$153,114	709	$153,039
Ped: Adolescent Medicine	10	$132,906	45	$159,434	2	*	28	*
Ped: Allergy/Immunology	2	*	2	*	4	*	2	*
Ped: Cardiology	5	*	10	$214,869	18	$298,000	20	$217,021
Ped: Child Development	1	*	4	*	10	$123,812	3	*
Ped: Critical Care/Intensivist	2	*	15	$220,000	21	$252,665	29	$261,543
Ped: Emergency Medicine	*	*	*	*	8	*	*	*
Ped: Endocrinology	1	*	1	*	11	$144,699	10	$144,575
Ped: Gastroenterology	3	*	2	*	6	*	17	$200,013
Ped: Genetics	3	*	3	*	2	*	10	$165,473
Ped: Hematology/Oncology	1	*	6	*	18	$203,408	23	$177,803
Ped: Hospitalist	*	*	2	*	8	*	15	$154,000
Ped: Infectious Disease	*	*	*	*	2	*	8	*
Ped: Neonatal Medicine	16	$157,653	24	$227,352	15	$276,629	51	$238,857
Ped: Nephrology	1	*	1	*	2	*	6	*
Ped: Neurology	2	*	12	$163,639	7	*	12	$179,951
Ped: Pulmonology	2	*	1	*	8	*	10	$246,990
Ped: Rheumatology	*	*	*	*	1	*	3	*
Ped: Sports Medicine	*	*	1	*	*	*	*	*
Physiatry (Phys Med & Rehab)	23	$186,061	49	$209,936	44	$242,046	62	$169,476
Podiatry: General	25	$156,918	44	$160,336	25	$153,513	32	$135,585
Podiatry: Surg-Foot & Ankle	4	*	19	$153,632	12	$130,364	57	$162,579
Podiatry: Surg-Forefoot Only	*	*	14	$157,500	*	*	1	*
Psychiatry: General	39	$149,277	84	$166,338	95	$145,000	134	$168,156
Psychiatry: Child & Adolescent	2	*	10	$176,287	12	$167,013	29	$181,400
Psychiatry: Geriatric	3	*	9	*	1	*	*	*
Pulmonary Medicine	33	$192,000	151	$223,878	58	$209,000	50	$198,366
Pulmonary Med: Critical Care	9	*	56	$234,889	50	$237,562	34	$234,913
Radiation Oncology	9	*	25	$368,847	35	$379,394	39	$393,739
Radiology: Diagnostic-Inv	24	$325,697	118	$435,309	139	$388,606	102	$359,966
Radiology: Diagnostic-Noninv	65	$313,917	177	$428,435	103	$384,078	281	$306,502
Radiology: Nuclear Medicine	5	*	12	$339,118	20	$360,149	20	$246,137
Rheumatology	36	$195,352	107	$195,619	60	$217,321	59	$176,116
Sleep Medicine	2	*	3	*	1	*	5	*
Surgery: General	202	$235,713	330	$291,983	186	$261,343	231	$242,304
Surg: Cardiovascular	15	$439,932	40	$431,194	82	$479,543	50	$379,727
Surg: Cardiovascular-Pediatric	1	*	1	*	3	*	*	*
Surg: Colon and Rectal	2	*	11	$282,319	6	*	25	$285,550
Surg: Neurological	28	$393,989	42	$472,131	69	$555,934	61	$422,911
Surg: Oncology	2	*	5	*	2	*	1	*
Surg: Oral	4	*	9	*	8	*	6	*
Surg: Pediatric	2	*	4	*	3	*	13	$400,153
Surg: Plastic & Reconstruction	8	*	32	$248,516	24	$296,856	43	$301,135
Surg: Plastic & Recon-Hand	2	*	10	$297,321	5	*	1	*
Surg: Plastic & Recon-Pediatric	*	*	2	*	*	*	2	*
Surg: Thoracic (primary)	2	*	26	$420,924	6	*	22	$264,518
Surg: Transplant	1	*	9	*	2	*	4	*
Surg: Trauma	*	*	4	*	8	*	12	$203,413
Surg: Trauma-Burn	1	*	7	*	2	*	3	*
Surg: Vascular (primary)	11	$226,423	25	$345,501	49	$336,337	54	$290,415
Urgent Care	31	$164,914	191	$167,713	99	$157,562	83	$141,424
Urology	57	$286,230	154	$342,067	99	$327,688	163	$260,230
Urology: Pediatric	*	*	*	*	10	*	3	*

MEDICAL GROUP MANAGEMENT ASSOCIATION™

Table 7A: Physician Compensation by Percent of Capitation Revenue for All Practices

	No capitation		10% or less		11% to 50%		51% or more	
	Physicians	Median	Physicians	Median	Physicians	Median	Physicians	Median
Allergy/Immunology	78	$268,830	49	$300,306	30	$227,656	18	$208,919
Anesthesiology	1,232	$330,823	136	$336,543	162	$261,550	30	$265,596
Anesth: Pain Management	68	$345,558	2	*	11	$246,115	3	*
Anesth: Pediatric	17	$319,812	*	*	5	*	*	*
Cardiology: Electrophysiology	105	$382,052	33	$368,275	9	*	1	*
Cardiology: Invasive	386	$381,108	128	$338,762	31	$330,430	18	$296,952
Cardiology: Inv-Intervntnl	510	$434,333	159	$372,196	27	$365,000	8	*
Cardiology: Noninvasive	336	$344,329	126	$327,571	75	$275,000	21	$296,321
Critical Care: Intensivist	7	*	7	*	9	*	3	*
Dentistry	12	*	4	*	15	$153,382	10	*
Dermatology	124	$329,894	63	$243,990	64	$239,299	37	$244,695
Dermatology: MOHS Surgery	10	$476,731	8	*	2	*	1	*
Emergency Medicine	221	$228,753	84	$216,706	112	$196,319	18	*
Endocrinology/Metabolism	81	$172,813	59	$162,136	42	$149,994	10	$172,016
Family Practice (w/ OB)	546	$160,119	344	$161,712	341	$154,962	54	*
Family Practice (w/o OB)	1,982	$154,516	990	$144,076	934	$145,945	242	$160,966
Family Practice: Sports Med	13	$149,470	10	$198,744	4	*	*	*
Gastroenterology	436	$348,255	105	$315,788	97	$296,951	33	$284,000
Gastroenterology: Hepatology	63	$319,061	4	*	3	*	5	*
Geriatrics	7	*	26	$146,016	19	$148,222	4	*
Hematology/Oncology	206	$400,321	78	$267,495	52	$234,472	14	$221,737
Hem/Onc: Oncology (only)	70	$373,195	5	*	16	$240,074	4	*
Infectious Disease	70	$201,376	25	$184,780	29	$157,400	7	*
Internal Medicine: General	1,608	$157,935	885	$151,972	883	$150,140	387	$158,789
Internal Med: Hospitalist	169	$165,000	77	$160,690	46	$150,160	47	$168,112
Internal Med: Pediatric	37	$143,181	35	$140,000	22	$144,725	1	*
Nephrology	138	$242,700	41	$216,250	51	$200,932	8	*
Neurology	254	$198,593	102	$176,880	107	$177,692	32	$178,570
OBGYN: General	777	$247,649	240	$230,471	285	$233,385	140	$220,471
OBGYN: Gynecology (only)	113	$210,496	34	$183,644	19	$202,840	10	$178,049
OBGYN: Gyn Oncology	8	*	6	*	5	*	*	*
OBGYN: Maternal & Fetal Med	33	$360,996	6	*	12	$284,178	*	*
OBGYN: Repro Endocrinology	17	$323,294	8	*	3	*	2	*
Occupational Medicine	58	$158,091	20	$180,774	26	$157,813	21	$168,264
Ophthalmology	280	$310,071	90	$267,928	76	$235,877	46	$231,694
Ophthalmology: Pediatric	22	$304,628	1	*	2	*	1	*
Ophthalmology: Retina	55	$514,246	5	*	5	*	2	*
Orthopedic (Non-surgical)	34	$193,382	5	*	2	*	9	*
Orthopedic Surgery: General	578	$409,527	89	$318,762	99	$350,147	45	$328,480
Ortho Surg: Foot & Ankle	42	$389,487	3	*	6	*	*	*
Ortho Surg: Hand	112	$462,579	11	$377,654	15	$378,604	1	*
Ortho Surg: Hip & Joint	106	$441,946	5	*	4	*	1	*
Ortho Surg: Oncology	3	*	*	*	*	*	*	*
Ortho Surg: Pediatric	26	$341,143	5	*	3	*	6	*
Ortho Surg: Spine	110	$497,220	3	*	9	*	2	*
Ortho Surg: Trauma	25	$439,750	*	*	5	*	*	*
Ortho Surg: Sports Med	178	$405,181	12	$268,225	11	$428,493	7	*
Otorhinolaryngology	244	$286,645	67	$263,421	79	$275,255	34	$233,924
Otorhinolaryngology: Pediatric	17	$324,800	*	*	*	*	*	*
Pathology: Anatomic & Clinical	115	$415,251	45	$304,912	20	$224,185	17	$205,774
Pathology: Anatomic	34	$372,450	16	*	10	*	*	*
Pathology: Clinical	31	$212,134	21	$270,427	31	$160,000	*	*

Table 7A: Physician Compensation by Percent of Capitation Revenue for All Practices (continued)

	No capitation		10% or less		11% to 50%		51% or more	
	Physicians	Median	Physicians	Median	Physicians	Median	Physicians	Median
Pediatrics: General	921	$165,011	347	$148,258	498	$147,239	203	$146,687
Ped: Adolescent Medicine	31	$164,604	31	$129,650	19	$151,104	*	*
Ped: Allergy/Immunology	1	*	3	*	6	*	*	*
Ped: Cardiology	17	$225,280	22	$225,659	7	*	1	*
Ped: Child Development	2	*	9	*	9	*	*	*
Ped: Critical Care/Intensivist	23	$300,867	16	$200,060	19	$252,665	*	*
Ped: Emergency Medicine	8	*	*	*	*	*	*	*
Ped: Endocrinology	6	*	6	*	8	*	*	*
Ped: Gastroenterology	7	*	9	*	7	*	*	*
Ped: Genetics	3	*	9	*	*	*	*	*
Ped: Hematology/Oncology	11	$178,340	18	$171,162	11	$225,011	1	*
Ped: Hospitalist	3	*	14	$148,375	5	*	3	*
Ped: Infectious Disease	*	*	6	*	*	*	*	*
Ped: Neonatal Medicine	20	$246,714	44	$291,641	21	$175,000	1	*
Ped: Nephrology	1	*	6	*	2	*	*	*
Ped: Neurology	14	$185,328	9	*	7	*	*	*
Ped: Pulmonology	6	*	3	*	9	*	*	*
Ped: Rheumatology	*	*	3	*	1	*	*	*
Ped: Sports Medicine	1	*	*	*	*	*	*	*
Physiatry (Phys Med & Rehab)	99	$207,430	21	$215,576	27	$201,668	7	*
Podiatry: General	55	$160,229	26	$137,394	27	$167,205	18	$123,840
Podiatry: Surg-Foot & Ankle	21	$179,557	9	*	6	*	13	$138,916
Podiatry: Surg-Forefoot Only	11	$165,000	3	*	*	*	1	*
Psychiatry: General	68	$164,469	82	$140,169	94	$150,671	40	$165,345
Psychiatry: Child & Adolescent	12	$171,287	8	*	5	*	5	*
Psychiatry: Geriatric	8	*	3	*	1	*	*	*
Pulmonary Medicine	145	$223,419	72	$219,438	56	$193,486	18	$193,216
Pulmonary Med: Critical Care	115	$237,531	22	$227,295	11	$273,521	4	*
Radiation Oncology	70	$385,707	10	$354,721	26	$360,807	1	*
Radiology: Diagnostic-Inv	205	$375,000	80	$350,000	66	$510,595	6	*
Radiology: Diagnostic-Noninv	325	$392,000	79	$349,291	90	$320,000	56	$321,159
Radiology: Nuclear Medicine	30	$373,448	6	*	7	*	2	*
Rheumatology	132	$212,205	66	$197,031	34	$168,537	14	$178,299
Sleep Medicine	10	$169,700	4	*	1	*	*	*
Surgery: General	502	$274,900	187	$241,877	132	$252,880	58	$252,297
Surg: Cardiovascular	125	$439,919	23	$473,441	29	$417,440	2	*
Surg: Cardiovascular-Pediatric	3	*	1	*	1	*	*	*
Surg: Colon and Rectal	16	$235,000	5	*	14	$301,000	1	*
Surg: Neurological	127	$510,000	28	$356,245	29	$375,000	4	*
Surg: Oncology	4	*	*	*	6	*	*	*
Surg: Oral	18	$225,322	2	*	4	*	1	*
Surg: Pediatric	4	*	7	*	9	*	*	*
Surg: Plastic & Reconstruction	33	$289,062	26	$284,231	28	$299,818	2	*
Surg: Plastic & Recon-Hand	16	$232,500	*	*	2	*	*	*
Surg: Plastic & Recon-Pediatric	2	*	2	*	*	*	*	*
Surg: Thoracic (primary)	35	$362,617	3	*	1	*	4	*
Surg: Transplant	10	$379,959	3	*	3	*	*	*
Surg: Trauma	12	$213,640	3	*	9	*	*	*
Surg: Trauma-Burn	8	*	1	*	4	*	*	*
Surg: Vascular (primary)	73	$309,260	16	$320,007	23	$311,250	4	*
Urgent Care	209	$163,244	72	$143,953	77	$157,562	45	$180,317
Urology	253	$329,251	78	$302,857	66	$300,000	34	$272,297
Urology: Pediatric	2	*	2	*	9	*	*	*

MEDICAL GROUP MANAGEMENT ASSOCIATION™

Table 7B: Physician Compensation by Percent of Capitation Revenue for Single-specialty Practices

	No capitation		10% or less		11% to 50%		51% or more	
	Physicians	Median	Physicians	Median	Physicians	Median	Physicians	Median
Allergy/Immunology	24	$365,323	22	$323,247	2	*	*	*
Anesthesiology	1,100	$329,973	64	*	63	*	*	*
Anesth: Pain Management	60	$329,746	*	*	*	*	*	*
Anesth: Pediatric	15	*	*	*	5	*	*	*
Cardiology: Electrophysiology	86	$385,025	13	$440,541	1	*	*	*
Cardiology: Invasive	235	$377,373	40	$341,018	1	*	*	*
Cardiology: Inv-Intervntnl	373	$429,263	80	$371,051	8	*	*	*
Cardiology: Noninvasive	250	$347,677	51	$457,056	4	*	*	*
Critical Care: Intensivist	5	*	*	*	*	*	*	*
Dentistry	12	*	*	*	*	*	*	*
Dermatology	19	$402,206	*	*	6	*	*	*
Dermatology: MOHS Surgery	4	*	*	*	*	*	*	*
Emergency Medicine	135	$241,200	1	*	*	*	*	*
Endocrinology/Metabolism	10	$183,877	2	*	*	*	*	*
Family Practice (w/ OB)	145	$155,000	62	$150,953	64	$148,515	*	*
Family Practice (w/o OB)	408	$158,304	123	$144,985	144	$151,634	4	*
Family Practice: Sports Med	6	*	5	*	1	*	*	*
Gastroenterology	225	$334,644	4	*	6	*	*	*
Gastroenterology: Hepatology	54	$315,350	*	*	3	*	*	*
Geriatrics	*	*	1	*	*	*	*	*
Hematology/Oncology	119	$490,063	4	*	*	*	*	*
Hem/Onc: Oncology (only)	38	$429,002	*	*	*	*	*	*
Infectious Disease	32	$215,584	9	*	*	*	*	*
Internal Medicine: General	216	$161,749	40	$149,401	32	$162,755	*	*
Internal Med: Hospitalist	*	*	*	*	2	*	*	*
Internal Med: Pediatric	*	*	1	*	3	*	*	*
Nephrology	50	$242,700	*	*	16	$249,857	*	*
Neurology	113	$193,773	22	*	*	*	*	*
OBGYN: General	408	$238,977	12	*	29	$264,795	2	*
OBGYN: Gynecology (only)	40	$174,159	5	*	2	*	*	*
OBGYN: Gyn Oncology	1	*	*	*	*	*	*	*
OBGYN: Maternal & Fetal Med	9	*	*	*	2	*	*	*
OBGYN: Repro Endocrinology	13	$323,294	*	*	*	*	*	*
Occupational Medicine	8	*	*	*	*	*	*	*
Ophthalmology	154	$353,453	19	$278,023	3	*	3	*
Ophthalmology: Pediatric	17	$288,993	*	*	*	*	*	*
Ophthalmology: Retina	50	$506,299	3	*	*	*	*	*
Orthopedic (Non-surgical)	20	$186,770	*	*	*	*	*	*
Orthopedic Surgery: General	374	$409,954	15	*	7	*	1	*
Ortho Surg: Foot & Ankle	37	$387,854	1	*	2	*	*	*
Ortho Surg: Hand	98	$474,893	6	*	5	*	*	*
Ortho Surg: Hip & Joint	88	$457,874	*	*	2	*	*	*
Ortho Surg: Oncology	2	*	*	*	*	*	*	*
Ortho Surg: Pediatric	23	$300,000	1	*	1	*	*	*
Ortho Surg: Spine	91	$534,104	2	*	1	*	*	*
Ortho Surg: Trauma	25	$439,750	*	*	*	*	*	*
Ortho Surg: Sports Med	151	$443,098	2	*	4	*	*	*
Otorhinolaryngology	93	$261,685	*	*	16	*	*	*
Otorhinolaryngology: Pediatric	8	*	*	*	*	*	*	*
Pathology: Anatomic & Clinical	82	$463,299	16	*	*	*	*	*
Pathology: Anatomic	27	$393,596	16	*	*	*	*	*
Pathology: Clinical	14	$206,263	5	*	2	*	*	*

Table 7B: Physician Compensation by Percent of Capitation Revenue for Single-specialty Practices (continued)

	No capitation		10% or less		11% to 50%		51% or more	
	Physicians	Median	Physicians	Median	Physicians	Median	Physicians	Median
Pediatrics: General	375	$177,840	35	$155,259	110	$151,046	11	*
Ped: Adolescent Medicine	*	*	0	*	*	*	*	*
Ped: Allergy/Immunology	*	*	2	*	2	*	*	*
Ped: Cardiology	10	$276,200	12	$255,105	*	*	*	*
Ped: Critical Care/Intensivist	17	$304,677	8	*	5	*	*	*
Ped: Emergency Medicine	2	*	*	*	*	*	*	*
Ped: Endocrinology	1	*	2	*	1	*	*	*
Ped: Gastroenterology	6	*	5	*	*	*	*	*
Ped: Hematology/Oncology	5	*	7	*	2	*	*	*
Ped: Hospitalist	*	*	3	*	*	*	*	*
Ped: Infectious Disease	*	*	2	*	*	*	*	*
Ped: Neonatal Medicine	1	*	28	$298,373	*	*	*	*
Ped: Nephrology	*	*	2	*	*	*	*	*
Ped: Neurology	6	*	2	*	*	*	*	*
Ped: Pulmonology	5	*	2	*	1	*	*	*
Ped: Rheumatology	*	*	1	*	*	*	*	*
Physiatry (Phys Med & Rehab)	45	$280,000	1	*	3	*	*	*
Podiatry: General	3	*	*	*	*	*	*	*
Podiatry: Surg-Foot & Ankle	14	$166,595	*	*	*	*	*	*
Podiatry: Surg-Forefoot Only	1	*	*	*	*	*	*	*
Psychiatry: General	3	*	4	*	3	*	*	*
Psychiatry: Child & Adolescent	6	*	1	*	*	*	*	*
Pulmonary Medicine	27	$179,141	6	*	*	*	*	*
Pulmonary Med: Critical Care	48	$231,509	*	*	*	*	*	*
Radiation Oncology	41	$472,930	*	*	10	*	*	*
Radiology: Diagnostic-Inv	161	$372,919	48	*	29	*	*	*
Radiology: Diagnostic-Noninv	232	$417,824	12	*	*	*	*	*
Radiology: Nuclear Medicine	19	$377,837	2	*	*	*	*	*
Rheumatology	28	$256,324	4	*	*	*	*	*
Sleep Medicine	8	*	*	*	*	*	*	*
Surgery: General	164	$268,875	22	$177,565	*	*	*	*
Surg: Cardiovascular	73	$528,501	10	*	5	*	*	*
Surg: Cardiovascular-Pediatric	2	*	1	*	*	*	*	*
Surg: Colon and Rectal	12	$235,000	*	*	*	*	*	*
Surg: Neurological	72	$510,000	6	*	9	*	*	*
Surg: Oncology	1	*	*	*	*	*	*	*
Surg: Oral	13	$226,077	*	*	*	*	*	*
Surg: Pediatric	2	*	0	*	4	*	*	*
Surg: Plastic & Reconstruction	4	*	7	*	*	*	*	*
Surg: Plastic & Recon-Hand	14	$221,000	*	*	*	*	*	*
Surg: Plastic & Recon-Pediatric	*	*	2	*	*	*	*	*
Surg: Thoracic (primary)	19	*	*	*	*	*	*	*
Surg: Transplant	4	*	*	*	*	*	*	*
Surg: Trauma	5	*	*	*	*	*	*	*
Surg: Trauma-Burn	7	*	1	*	*	*	*	*
Surg: Vascular (primary)	31	$350,651	2	*	*	*	*	*
Urgent Care	40	$131,747	*	*	*	*	*	*
Urology	128	$316,789	9	*	19	$320,530	*	*
Urology: Pediatric	2	*	*	*	*	*	*	*

MEDICAL GROUP MANAGEMENT ASSOCIATION™

Table 7C: Physician Compensation by Percent of Capitation Revenue for Multispecialty Practices

	No capitation		10% or less		11% to 50%		51% or more	
	Physicians	Median	Physicians	Median	Physicians	Median	Physicians	Median
Allergy/Immunology	54	$229,636	27	$214,704	28	$227,656	18	$208,919
Anesthesiology	132	$334,716	72	$276,155	99	$263,699	30	$265,596
Anesth: Pain Management	8	*	2	*	11	$246,115	3	*
Anesth: Pediatric	2	*	*	*	*	*	*	*
Cardiology: Electrophysiology	19	$375,000	20	$327,903	8	*	1	*
Cardiology: Invasive	151	$393,323	88	$337,321	30	$327,503	18	$296,952
Cardiology: Inv-Intervntnl	137	$511,868	79	$375,605	19	$450,000	8	*
Cardiology: Noninvasive	86	$341,031	75	$279,712	71	$263,898	21	$296,321
Critical Care: Intensivist	2	*	7	*	9	*	3	*
Dentistry	0	*	4	*	15	$153,382	10	*
Dermatology	105	$301,103	63	$243,990	58	$231,533	37	$244,695
Dermatology: MOHS Surgery	6	*	8	*	2	*	1	*
Emergency Medicine	86	$219,275	83	$217,319	112	$196,319	18	*
Endocrinology/Metabolism	71	$171,612	57	$162,136	42	$149,994	10	$172,016
Family Practice (w/ OB)	401	$162,839	282	$166,062	277	$156,634	54	*
Family Practice (w/o OB)	1,574	$153,508	867	$144,022	790	$145,000	238	$161,029
Family Practice: Sports Med	7	*	5	*	3	*	*	*
Gastroenterology	211	$369,369	101	$315,788	91	$285,806	33	$284,000
Gastroenterology: Hepatology	9	*	4	*	*	*	5	*
Geriatrics	7	*	25	$146,016	19	$148,222	4	*
Hematology/Oncology	87	$376,420	74	$263,904	52	$234,472	14	$221,737
Hem/Onc: Oncology (only)	32	$344,483	5	*	16	$240,074	4	*
Infectious Disease	38	$169,653	16	$174,349	29	$157,400	7	*
Internal Medicine: General	1,392	$157,097	845	$152,380	851	$149,311	387	$158,789
Internal Med: Hospitalist	169	$165,000	77	$160,690	44	$150,000	47	$168,112
Internal Med: Pediatric	37	$143,181	34	$140,142	19	$142,795	1	*
Nephrology	88	$258,927	41	$216,250	35	$192,596	8	*
Neurology	141	$201,405	80	$173,135	107	$177,692	32	$178,570
OBGYN: General	369	$258,904	228	$235,204	256	$228,772	138	$221,863
OBGYN: Gynecology (only)	73	$225,285	29	$197,870	17	$209,000	10	$178,049
OBGYN: Gyn Oncology	7	*	6	*	5	*	*	*
OBGYN: Maternal & Fetal Med	24	$375,600	6	*	10	$258,568	*	*
OBGYN: Repro Endocrinology	4	*	8	*	3	*	2	*
Occupational Medicine	50	$152,381	20	$180,774	26	$157,813	21	$168,264
Ophthalmology	126	$264,118	71	$265,268	73	$238,754	43	$230,976
Ophthalmology: Pediatric	5	*	1	*	2	*	1	*
Ophthalmology: Retina	5	*	2	*	5	*	2	*
Orthopedic (Non-surgical)	14	$242,370	5	*	2	*	9	*
Orthopedic Surgery: General	204	$403,944	74	$293,247	92	$350,000	44	$330,857
Ortho Surg: Foot & Ankle	5	*	2	*	4	*	*	*
Ortho Surg: Hand	14	$408,492	5	*	10	$357,957	1	*
Ortho Surg: Hip & Joint	18	$318,636	5	*	2	*	1	*
Ortho Surg: Oncology	1	*	*	*	*	*	*	*
Ortho Surg: Pediatric	3	*	4	*	2	*	6	*
Ortho Surg: Spine	19	$403,846	1	*	8	*	2	*
Ortho Surg: Trauma	0	*	*	*	5	*	*	*
Ortho Surg: Sports Med	27	$265,982	10	$258,162	7	*	7	*
Otorhinolaryngology	151	$308,620	67	$263,421	63	$275,255	34	$233,924
Otorhinolaryngology: Pediatric	9	*	*	*	*	*	*	*
Pathology: Anatomic & Clinical	33	$285,087	29	$267,912	20	$224,185	17	$205,774
Pathology: Anatomic	7	*	*	*	10	*	*	*
Pathology: Clinical	17	$212,134	16	$211,667	29	$151,922	*	*

Table 7C: Physician Compensation by Percent of Capitation Revenue for Multispecialty Practices (continued)

	No capitation		10% or less		11% to 50%		51% or more	
	Physicians	Median	Physicians	Median	Physicians	Median	Physicians	Median
Pediatrics: General	546	$157,057	312	$147,695	388	$146,289	192	$146,320
Ped: Adolescent Medicine	31	$164,604	31	$129,650	19	$151,104	*	*
Ped: Allergy/Immunology	1	*	1	*	4	*	*	*
Ped: Cardiology	7	*	10	$225,659	7	*	1	*
Ped: Child Development	2	*	9	*	9	*	*	*
Ped: Critical Care/Intensivist	6	*	8	*	14	$252,665	*	*
Ped: Emergency Medicine	6	*	*	*	*	*	*	*
Ped: Endocrinology	5	*	4	*	7	*	*	*
Ped: Gastroenterology	1	*	4	*	7	*	*	*
Ped: Genetics	3	*	9	*	*	*	*	*
Ped: Hematology/Oncology	6	*	11	$173,264	9	*	1	*
Ped: Hospitalist	3	*	11	$154,031	5	*	3	*
Ped: Infectious Disease	*	*	4	*	*	*	*	*
Ped: Neonatal Medicine	19	$246,714	16	$282,263	21	$175,000	1	*
Ped: Nephrology	1	*	4	*	2	*	*	*
Ped: Neurology	8	*	7	*	7	*	*	*
Ped: Pulmonology	1	*	1	*	8	*	*	*
Ped: Rheumatology	*	*	2	*	1	*	*	*
Ped: Sports Medicine	1	*	*	*	*	*	*	*
Physiatry (Phys Med & Rehab)	54	$190,213	20	$210,529	24	$194,588	7	*
Podiatry: General	52	$160,655	26	$137,394	27	$167,205	18	$123,840
Podiatry: Surg-Foot & Ankle	7	*	9	*	6	*	13	$138,916
Podiatry: Surg-Forefoot Only	10	*	3	*	*	*	1	*
Psychiatry: General	65	$165,913	78	$140,708	91	$150,966	40	$165,345
Psychiatry: Child & Adolescent	6	*	7	*	5	*	5	*
Psychiatry: Geriatric	8	*	3	*	1	*	*	*
Pulmonary Medicine	118	$240,534	66	$219,438	56	$193,486	18	$193,216
Pulmonary Med: Critical Care	67	$244,770	22	$227,295	11	$273,521	4	*
Radiation Oncology	29	$354,066	10	$354,721	16	$370,492	1	*
Radiology: Diagnostic-Inv	44	$375,000	32	$343,879	37	$497,000	6	*
Radiology: Diagnostic-Noninv	93	$381,553	67	$355,000	90	$320,000	56	$321,159
Radiology: Nuclear Medicine	11	$234,504	4	*	7	*	2	*
Rheumatology	104	$208,762	62	$198,500	34	$168,537	14	$178,299
Sleep Medicine	2	*	4	*	1	*	*	*
Surgery: General	338	$276,222	165	$256,010	132	$252,880	58	$252,297
Surg: Cardiovascular	52	$379,147	13	$385,176	24	$412,720	2	*
Surg: Cardiovascular-Pediatric	1	*	*	*	1	*	*	*
Surg: Colon and Rectal	4	*	5	*	14	$301,000	1	*
Surg: Neurological	55	$513,000	22	$335,811	20	$399,291	4	*
Surg: Oncology	3	*	*	*	6	*	*	*
Surg: Oral	5	*	2	*	4	*	1	*
Surg: Pediatric	2	*	7	*	5	*	*	*
Surg: Plastic & Reconstruction	29	$291,364	19	$238,171	28	$299,818	2	*
Surg: Plastic & Recon-Hand	2	*	*	*	2	*	*	*
Surg: Plastic & Recon-Pediatric	2	*	*	*	*	*	*	*
Surg: Thoracic (primary)	16	$283,525	3	*	1	*	4	*
Surg: Transplant	6	*	3	*	3	*	*	*
Surg: Trauma	7	*	3	*	9	*	*	*
Surg: Trauma-Burn	1	*	*	*	4	*	*	*
Surg: Vascular (primary)	42	$309,230	14	$333,053	23	$311,250	4	*
Urgent Care	169	$171,650	72	$143,953	77	$157,562	45	$180,317
Urology	125	$339,913	69	$310,928	47	$300,000	34	$272,297
Urology: Pediatric	*	*	2	*	9	*	*	*

MEDICAL GROUP MANAGEMENT ASSOCIATION™

Table 8A: Physician Compensation by Method of Compensation (1-2 Years in Specialty)

	Productivity Based		Guaranteed or Base Salary		Straight Salary	
	Physicians	Median	Physicians	Median	Physicians	Median
Allergy/Immunology	*	*	5	*	3	*
Anesthesiology	7	*	17	$220,696	116	$257,474
Anesth: Pain Management	*	*	1	*	5	*
Anesth: Pediatric	*	*	2	*	*	*
Cardiology: Electrophysiology	*	*	2	*	4	*
Cardiology: Invasive	*	*	6	*	18	$236,721
Cardiology: Inv-Intervntnl	*	*	12	$253,500	13	$268,336
Cardiology: Noninvasive	*	*	2	*	12	$227,414
Critical Care: Intensivist	*	*	*	*	8	*
Dermatology	1	*	7	*	7	*
Dermatology: MOHS Surgery	*	*	*	*	1	*
Emergency Medicine	2	*	17	$175,645	41	$184,251
Endocrinology/Metabolism	*	*	4	*	3	*
Family Practice (w/ OB)	1	*	52	$136,836	48	$130,391
Family Practice (w/o OB)	12	$163,023	166	$125,066	80	$129,069
Family Practice: Sports Med	*	*	1	*	2	*
Gastroenterology	*	*	15	$291,727	21	$211,117
Gastroenterology: Hepatology	*	*	1	*	*	*
Geriatrics	1	*	1	*	*	*
Hematology/Oncology	0	*	9	*	13	$189,213
Infectious Disease	*	*	6	*	4	*
Internal Medicine: General	2	*	117	$124,052	248	$129,441
Internal Med: Hospitalist	3	*	33	$152,500	14	$143,408
Internal Med: Pediatric	*	*	13	$130,008	3	*
Nephrology	1	*	8	*	14	$189,328
Neurology	*	*	10	$195,565	17	$150,000
OBGYN: General	4	*	42	$179,564	64	$184,961
OBGYN: Gynecology (only)	*	*	1	*	2	*
OBGYN: Gyn Oncology	*	*	*	*	1	*
OBGYN: Maternal & Fetal Med	1	*	1	*	1	*
OBGYN: Repro Endocrinology	*	*	*	*	3	*
Occupational Medicine	*	*	3	*	12	*
Ophthalmology	*	*	9	*	18	$164,437
Ophthalmology: Retina	*	*	*	*	3	*
Orthopedic (Non-surgical)	*	*	*	*	1	*
Orthopedic Surgery: General	4	*	13	$390,000	31	$270,261
Ortho Surg: Foot & Ankle	*	*	2	*	4	*
Ortho Surg: Hand	1	*	2	*	1	*
Ortho Surg: Hip & Joint	*	*	3	*	1	*
Ortho Surg: Oncology	*	*	*	*	1	*
Ortho Surg: Pediatric	*	*	*	*	2	*
Ortho Surg: Spine	2	*	1	*	8	*
Ortho Surg: Trauma	*	*	*	*	1	*
Ortho Surg: Sports Med	1	*	4	*	21	$193,300
Otorhinolaryngology	0	*	11	$279,869	4	*
Pathology: Anatomic & Clinical	*	*	3	*	13	$173,715
Pathology: Clinical	*	*	2	*	3	*

Table 8A: Physician Compensation by Method of Compensation (1-2 Years in Specialty) (continued)

	Productivity Based		Guaranteed or Base Salary		Straight Salary	
	Physicians	Median	Physicians	Median	Physicians	Median
Pediatrics: General	3	*	62	$120,000	80	$119,962
Ped: Adolescent Medicine	*	*	1	*	3	*
Ped: Cardiology	*	*	2	*	*	*
Ped: Critical Care/Intensivist	1	*	1	*	3	*
Ped: Endocrinology	*	*	3	*	2	*
Ped: Gastroenterology	*	*	1	*	1	*
Ped: Genetics	*	*	*	*	1	*
Ped: Hematology/Oncology	*	*	*	*	2	*
Ped: Hospitalist	*	*	2	*	*	*
Ped: Neonatal Medicine	*	*	*	*	3	*
Ped: Neurology	*	*	3	*	*	*
Ped: Pulmonology	*	*	1	*	*	*
Physiatry (Phys Med & Rehab)	*	*	7	*	9	*
Podiatry: General	0	*	5	*	3	*
Podiatry: Surg-Foot & Ankle	*	*	*	*	5	*
Psychiatry: General	*	*	10	$143,131	21	$147,173
Psychiatry: Child & Adolescent	*	*	1	*	4	*
Pulmonary Medicine	*	*	4	*	5	*
Pulmonary Med: Critical Care	2	*	3	*	2	*
Radiation Oncology	*	*	1	*	3	*
Radiology: Diagnostic-Inv	*	*	6	*	21	$238,469
Radiology: Diagnostic-Noninv	*	*	11	$250,000	27	$240,234
Radiology: Nuclear Medicine	*	*	1	*	2	*
Rheumatology	*	*	3	*	3	*
Sleep Medicine	*	*	*	*	1	*
Surgery: General	2	*	26	$214,320	34	$209,736
Surg: Cardiovascular	*	*	2	*	6	*
Surg: Cardiovascular-Pediatric	*	*	*	*	1	*
Surg: Colon and Rectal	*	*	*	*	2	*
Surg: Neurological	*	*	4	*	7	*
Surg: Pediatric	*	*	3	*	*	*
Surg: Plastic & Reconstruction	*	*	4	*	6	*
Surg: Thoracic (primary)	*	*	*	*	3	*
Surg: Transplant	*	*	2	*	1	*
Surg: Trauma	*	*	2	*	*	*
Surg: Trauma-Burn	*	*	*	*	1	*
Surg: Vascular (primary)	*	*	1	*	10	$258,525
Urgent Care	*	*	11	$165,084	5	*
Urology	*	*	8	*	19	$198,462

Table 8B: Physician Compensation by Method of Compensation (More than 2 Years in Specialty)

	Productivity Based		Guaranteed or Base Salary		Straight Salary	
	Physicians	Median	Physicians	Median	Physicians	Median
Allergy/Immunology	63	$270,832	40	$257,840	7	*
Anesthesiology	237	$320,020	47	$350,002	143	$285,000
Anesth: Pain Management	14	$312,798	2	*	9	*
Anesth: Pediatric	*	*	1	*	*	*
Cardiology: Electrophysiology	23	$537,820	19	$390,000	26	$343,074
Cardiology: Invasive	114	$377,305	76	$351,764	70	$347,289
Cardiology: Inv-Intervntnl	172	$489,760	95	$407,769	64	$362,366
Cardiology: Noninvasive	97	$300,000	74	$288,577	89	$292,050
Critical Care: Intensivist	2	*	10	$195,228	3	*
Dentistry	15	$140,395	3	*	0	*
Dermatology	98	$277,219	51	$327,536	16	$195,539
Dermatology: MOHS Surgery	5	*	6	*	2	*
Emergency Medicine	51	$232,283	73	$199,814	38	$218,996
Endocrinology/Metabolism	59	$175,828	32	$137,309	15	$156,000
Family Practice (w/ OB)	434	$161,661	238	$158,457	48	$151,787
Family Practice (w/o OB)	1,498	$152,974	561	$151,557	183	$144,957
Family Practice: Sports Med	9	*	4	*	3	*
Gastroenterology	226	$381,029	73	$311,193	47	$212,592
Gastroenterology: Hepatology	29	$357,512	13	*	*	*
Geriatrics	18	$136,661	11	$150,904	1	*
Hematology/Oncology	101	$327,723	53	$329,035	18	$230,631
Hem/Onc: Oncology (only)	26	$348,189	10	$549,288	24	$307,165
Infectious Disease	49	$207,240	19	$163,192	8	*
Internal Medicine: General	1,329	$159,005	584	$157,745	265	$147,782
Internal Med: Hospitalist	87	$165,000	37	$162,318	16	$165,723
Internal Med: Pediatric	14	$141,975	5	*	4	*
Nephrology	51	$226,362	36	$242,700	15	$180,000
Neurology	169	$197,000	49	$179,951	25	$172,000
OBGYN: General	413	$257,784	222	$249,203	94	$221,800
OBGYN: Gynecology (only)	94	$207,346	16	$182,365	13	$195,000
OBGYN: Gyn Oncology	3	*	7	*	*	*
OBGYN: Maternal & Fetal Med	23	$346,157	9	*	2	*
OBGYN: Repro Endocrinology	13	$339,558	2	*	3	*
Occupational Medicine	43	$201,896	17	$176,505	2	*
Ophthalmology	186	$293,295	76	$278,172	32	$212,500
Ophthalmology: Pediatric	11	$320,262	1	*	*	*
Ophthalmology: Retina	17	$433,265	2	*	7	*
Orthopedic (Non-surgical)	22	$264,206	9	*	1	*
Orthopedic Surgery: General	349	$398,302	109	$350,180	35	$350,000
Ortho Surg: Foot & Ankle	22	$405,867	5	*	3	*
Ortho Surg: Hand	65	$493,443	11	$462,523	7	*
Ortho Surg: Hip & Joint	43	$337,790	12	$566,366	7	*
Ortho Surg: Oncology	1	*	1	*	*	*
Ortho Surg: Pediatric	14	$276,499	1	*	6	*
Ortho Surg: Spine	56	$644,788	12	$788,934	2	*
Ortho Surg: Trauma	7	*	4	*	2	*
Ortho Surg: Sports Med	82	$428,287	28	$374,419	8	*
Otorhinolaryngology	196	$299,739	60	$248,107	18	$278,750
Otorhinolaryngology: Pediatric	*	*	1	*	7	*
Pathology: Anatomic & Clinical	30	$322,765	29	$297,831	30	$376,703
Pathology: Anatomic	7	*	*	*	11	*
Pathology: Clinical	24	$151,922	5	*	5	*

Table 8B: Physician Compensation by Method of Compensation (More than 2 Years in Specialty) (continued)

	Productivity Based		Guaranteed or Base Salary		Straight Salary	
	Physicians	Median	Physicians	Median	Physicians	Median
Pediatrics: General	671	$167,500	318	$153,796	134	$145,218
Ped: Adolescent Medicine	1	*	26	$153,325	11	$115,342
Ped: Allergy/Immunology	3	*	1	*	2	*
Ped: Cardiology	8	*	*	*	11	$234,444
Ped: Child Development	1	*	0	*	2	*
Ped: Critical Care/Intensivist	7	*	3	*	24	$252,665
Ped: Emergency Medicine	*	*	6	*	2	*
Ped: Endocrinology	1	*	1	*	8	*
Ped: Gastroenterology	2	*	*	*	10	$192,515
Ped: Genetics	2	*	2	*	3	*
Ped: Hematology/Oncology	4	*	3	*	22	$187,998
Ped: Hospitalist	1	*	2	*	11	*
Ped: Infectious Disease	*	*	0	*	3	*
Ped: Neonatal Medicine	23	$281,500	15	$276,629	13	*
Ped: Nephrology	*	*	2	*	4	*
Ped: Neurology	6	*	6	*	5	*
Ped: Pulmonology	2	*	2	*	4	*
Ped: Rheumatology	1	*	*	*	3	*
Physiatry (Phys Med & Rehab)	52	$222,040	20	$218,033	17	$185,603
Podiatry: General	43	$137,069	26	$166,467	8	*
Podiatry: Surg-Foot & Ankle	6	*	21	$150,303	0	*
Podiatry: Surg-Forefoot Only	7	*	*	*	1	*
Psychiatry: General	53	$155,426	40	$161,956	28	$153,843
Psychiatry: Child & Adolescent	7	*	2	*	*	*
Psychiatry: Geriatric	9	*	1	*	*	*
Pulmonary Medicine	93	$224,000	48	$202,805	19	$197,500
Pulmonary Med: Critical Care	45	$236,955	21	$248,953	6	*
Radiation Oncology	18	$374,697	5	*	14	$372,086
Radiology: Diagnostic-Inv	40	$362,422	33	$435,000	101	$383,261
Radiology: Diagnostic-Noninv	88	$370,925	69	$446,814	60	$320,000
Radiology: Nuclear Medicine	7	*	2	*	14	$376,127
Rheumatology	90	$204,318	30	$167,738	10	$161,078
Sleep Medicine	7	*	*	*	*	*
Surgery: General	278	$277,899	133	$275,952	63	$234,000
Surg: Cardiovascular	46	$406,292	29	$527,793	15	$439,932
Surg: Cardiovascular-Pediatric	1	*	1	*	1	*
Surg: Colon and Rectal	8	*	5	*	11	*
Surg: Neurological	45	$445,085	13	$442,180	11	$325,000
Surg: Oncology	1	*	2	*	*	*
Surg: Oral	6	*	2	*	7	*
Surg: Pediatric	1	*	3	*	6	*
Surg: Plastic & Reconstruction	33	$321,309	18	$224,996	3	*
Surg: Plastic & Recon-Hand	8	*	2	*	4	*
Surg: Plastic & Recon-Pediatric	2	*	*	*	*	*
Surg: Thoracic (primary)	2	*	3	*	4	*
Surg: Transplant	8	*	2	*	*	*
Surg: Trauma	*	*	11	$262,642	5	*
Surg: Trauma-Burn	6	*	1	*	*	*
Surg: Vascular (primary)	23	$329,275	23	$303,950	8	*
Urgent Care	127	$173,558	83	$154,400	27	$119,676
Urology	99	$304,940	72	$290,646	41	$291,704
Urology: Pediatric	*	*	2	*	2	*

Table 9A: Physician Compensation by Years in Specialty

	1 to 2 years		3 to 7 years		8 to 17 years		18 years or more	
	Physicians	Median	Physicians	Median	Physicians	Median	Physicians	Median
Allergy/Immunology	8	*	23	$186,180	65	$253,598	71	$274,279
Anesthesiology	155	$249,823	275	$299,479	627	$319,167	330	$310,712
Anesth: Pain Management	7	*	19	$281,991	33	$323,000	15	$331,000
Anesth: Pediatric	2	*	7	*	15	$333,160	6	*
Cardiology: Electrophysiology	6	*	34	$388,999	65	$369,040	24	$425,545
Cardiology: Invasive	29	$238,586	143	$350,451	202	$374,194	153	$360,000
Cardiology: Inv-Intervntnl	26	$259,500	111	$413,850	271	$439,575	228	$435,673
Cardiology: Noninvasive	16	$227,414	83	$311,669	140	$327,282	237	$294,792
Critical Care: Intensivist	8	*	11	$176,586	26	$208,689	13	$220,000
Dentistry	1	*	1	*	9	*	12	$144,698
Dermatology	16	$202,476	53	$276,352	102	$259,503	104	$275,302
Dermatology: MOHS Surgery	2	*	8	*	5	*	6	*
Emergency Medicine	76	$184,376	140	$206,686	175	$216,607	116	$225,752
Endocrinology/Metabolism	9	*	29	$149,747	73	$177,464	61	$171,612
Family Practice (w/ OB)	107	$136,320	346	$148,421	401	$166,333	287	$167,230
Family Practice (w/o OB)	290	$129,069	833	$142,839	1,255	$153,695	1,227	$158,076
Family Practice: Sports Med	3	*	5	*	12	$180,315	5	*
Gastroenterology	44	$232,846	105	$306,591	265	$321,767	211	$323,197
Gastroenterology: Hepatology	3	*	8	*	29	$341,000	35	$328,800
Geriatrics	3	*	4	*	23	$146,016	14	$150,452
Hematology/Oncology	24	$192,310	65	$240,000	122	$311,684	141	$328,323
Hem/Onc: Oncology (only)	0	*	10	$225,967	32	$371,253	36	$346,048
Infectious Disease	11	$140,000	29	$146,697	49	$186,443	38	$213,578
Internal Medicine: General	410	$129,029	974	$149,430	1,233	$162,872	1,070	$165,351
Internal Med: Hospitalist	59	$149,999	118	$165,000	95	$169,933	38	$173,749
Internal Med: Pediatric	17	$130,008	38	$142,971	20	$156,890	5	*
Nephrology	24	$175,943	44	$203,375	74	$227,413	84	$266,773
Neurology	30	$154,843	108	$171,608	170	$198,961	142	$187,229
OBGYN: General	116	$181,709	352	$224,109	546	$248,495	364	$240,811
OBGYN: Gynecology (only)	3	*	11	$275,028	44	$241,315	104	$181,557
OBGYN: Gyn Oncology	3	*	5	*	9	*	5	*
OBGYN: Maternal & Fetal Med	3	*	13	$311,365	23	$354,367	14	$371,066
OBGYN: Repro Endocrinology	4	*	5	*	14	$290,010	6	*
Occupational Medicine	15	$151,916	31	$159,043	57	$179,261	38	$159,038
Ophthalmology	31	$163,874	112	$228,876	207	$287,000	151	$281,931
Ophthalmology: Pediatric	*	*	7	*	15	$283,147	4	*
Ophthalmology: Retina	3	*	20	$319,414	35	$587,714	16	$411,962
Orthopedic (Non-surgical)	2	*	11	$172,246	14	$356,177	20	$199,304
Orthopedic Surgery: General	58	$286,192	148	$351,133	290	$387,783	334	$365,310
Ortho Surg: Foot & Ankle	8	*	18	$406,514	20	$449,490	5	*
Ortho Surg: Hand	4	*	39	$373,464	49	$492,222	45	$426,945
Ortho Surg: Hip & Joint	4	*	14	$439,133	51	$457,796	44	$371,878
Ortho Surg: Oncology	1	*	*	*	1	*	1	*
Ortho Surg: Pediatric	2	*	14	$280,446	16	$412,626	9	*
Ortho Surg: Spine	12	$495,517	27	$534,146	58	$590,223	34	$425,947
Ortho Surg: Trauma	1	*	13	$336,899	9	*	6	*
Ortho Surg: Sports Med	30	$201,041	56	$351,710	121	$376,000	48	$298,743
Otorhinolaryngology	19	$226,877	75	$245,107	117	$288,307	163	$277,670
Otorhinolaryngology: Pediatric	1	*	2	*	7	*	6	*
Pathology: Anatomic & Clinical	16	$172,595	38	$219,645	82	$307,956	85	$319,740
Pathology: Anatomic	*	*	10	$215,535	19	$298,924	28	$346,098
Pathology: Clinical	5	*	14	$182,552	25	$197,922	32	$217,638

Table 9A: Physician Compensation by Years in Specialty (continued)

	1 to 2 years		3 to 7 years		8 to 17 years		18 years or more	
	Physicians	Median	Physicians	Median	Physicians	Median	Physicians	Median
Pediatrics: General	158	$119,907	459	$140,404	631	$161,326	639	$166,955
Ped: Adolescent Medicine	4	*	19	$121,000	28	$148,218	29	$145,650
Ped: Allergy/Immunology	*	*	1	*	3	*	6	*
Ped: Cardiology	2	*	14	$184,828	17	$215,184	16	$236,811
Ped: Child Development	1	*	4	*	2	*	3	*
Ped: Critical Care/Intensivist	5	*	13	$237,980	42	$253,505	6	*
Ped: Emergency Medicine	*	*	1	*	5	*	2	*
Ped: Endocrinology	5	*	5	*	5	*	5	*
Ped: Gastroenterology	2	*	9	*	8	*	7	*
Ped: Genetics	1	*	6	*	6	*	4	*
Ped: Hematology/Oncology	2	*	12	$165,000	17	$197,587	14	$193,701
Ped: Hospitalist	3	*	8	*	5	*	5	*
Ped: Infectious Disease	1	*	1	*	6	*	2	*
Ped: Neonatal Medicine	3	*	14	$222,666	42	$210,636	26	$218,522
Ped: Nephrology	*	*	1	*	5	*	3	*
Ped: Neurology	3	*	10	$164,042	11	$190,019	7	*
Ped: Pulmonology	1	*	7	*	10	$190,967	3	*
Ped: Rheumatology	*	*	2	*	2	*	*	*
Ped: Sports Medicine	*	*	*	*	1	*	*	*
Physiatry (Phys Med & Rehab)	18	$145,222	50	$188,977	74	$209,715	20	$184,628
Podiatry: General	10	$118,000	26	$137,537	41	$134,372	27	$153,106
Podiatry: Surg-Foot & Ankle	5	*	20	$138,976	42	$164,783	21	$182,886
Podiatry: Surg-Forefoot Only	1	*	2	*	7	*	4	*
Psychiatry: General	36	$146,232	73	$156,391	126	$156,646	81	$171,170
Psychiatry: Child & Adolescent	6	*	15	$175,012	20	$182,035	5	*
Psychiatry: Geriatric	*	*	1	*	5	*	7	*
Pulmonary Medicine	9	*	30	$215,905	100	$209,927	94	$195,246
Pulmonary Med: Critical Care	10	$182,506	27	$230,124	62	$241,722	39	$246,851
Radiation Oncology	4	*	23	$354,066	39	$387,923	22	$411,694
Radiology: Diagnostic-Inv	29	$238,469	65	$344,933	153	$422,548	100	$373,960
Radiology: Diagnostic-Noninv	42	$243,432	106	$308,998	216	$355,712	195	$355,717
Radiology: Nuclear Medicine	4	*	8	*	18	$254,064	24	$317,237
Rheumatology	10	$159,088	31	$180,841	77	$192,672	106	$200,504
Sleep Medicine	2	*	3	*	3	*	6	*
Surgery: General	66	$209,736	169	$253,043	308	$264,800	285	$253,971
Surg: Cardiovascular	11	$233,613	40	$445,585	75	$473,441	38	$430,140
Surg: Cardiovascular-Pediatric	1	*	1	*	3	*	*	*
Surg: Colon and Rectal	2	*	9	*	16	$280,155	12	$337,625
Surg: Neurological	13	$388,075	45	$470,476	61	$525,114	56	$450,144
Surg: Oncology	*	*	1	*	3	*	*	*
Surg: Oral	1	*	3	*	10	$246,668	11	$232,261
Surg: Pediatric	3	*	8	*	4	*	7	*
Surg: Plastic & Reconstruction	10	$230,601	27	$280,907	33	$306,000	26	$270,496
Surg: Plastic & Recon-Hand	*	*	2	*	8	*	5	*
Surg: Plastic & Recon-Pediatric	*	*	2	*	2	*	*	*
Surg: Thoracic (primary)	4	*	12	$352,205	23	$293,186	11	$239,309
Surg: Transplant	3	*	2	*	8	*	3	*
Surg: Trauma	2	*	5	*	12	$312,260	3	*
Surg: Trauma-Burn	2	*	1	*	2	*	7	*
Surg: Vascular (primary)	13	$256,770	29	$284,637	51	$324,223	32	$308,167
Urgent Care	17	$155,000	83	$154,043	137	$161,625	102	$156,737
Urology	30	$197,679	83	$250,000	156	$327,466	158	$287,856
Urology: Pediatric	*	*	2	*	2	*	*	*

MEDICAL GROUP MANAGEMENT ASSOCIATION™

Table 9B: Physician Compensation for 1-2 Years in Specialty

	Physicians	Medical Practices	Mean	Std. Dev.	25th %tile	Median	75th %tile	90th %tile
Allergy/Immunology	8	7	*	*	*	*	*	*
Anesthesiology	155	35	$265,039	$74,276	$216,849	$249,823	$321,842	$367,969
Anesth: Pain Management	7	6	*	*	*	*	*	*
Anesth: Pediatric	2	1	*	*	*	*	*	*
Cardiology: Electrophysiology	6	6	*	*	*	*	*	*
Cardiology: Invasive	29	21	$246,373	$69,765	$197,103	$238,586	$297,794	$350,000
Cardiology: Inv-Intervntnl	26	24	$285,874	$110,905	$216,892	$259,500	$328,554	$437,914
Cardiology: Noninvasive	16	12	$245,326	$73,294	$204,492	$227,414	$259,838	$387,451
Critical Care: Intensivist	8	1	*	*	*	*	*	*
Dentistry	1	1	*	*	*	*	*	*
Dermatology	16	13	$208,813	$82,355	$140,979	$202,476	$283,848	$341,316
Dermatology: MOHS Surgery	2	2	*	*	*	*	*	*
Emergency Medicine	76	19	$190,237	$35,774	$175,694	$184,376	$198,663	$232,389
Endocrinology/Metabolism	9	9	*	*	*	*	*	*
Family Practice (w/ OB)	107	61	$137,704	$30,528	$115,141	$136,320	$155,305	$173,299
Family Practice (w/o OB)	290	128	$132,989	$33,759	$114,945	$129,069	$141,916	$167,051
Family Practice: Sports Med	3	3	*	*	*	*	*	*
Gastroenterology	44	29	$291,945	$173,445	$190,744	$232,846	$297,144	$533,075
Gastroenterology: Hepatology	3	2	*	*	*	*	*	*
Geriatrics	3	3	*	*	*	*	*	*
Hematology/Oncology	24	14	$238,660	$109,444	$177,651	$192,310	$244,634	$457,420
Hem/Onc: Oncology (only)	0	*	*	*	*	*	*	*
Infectious Disease	11	9	$150,385	$32,437	$131,500	$140,000	$160,000	$214,590
Internal Medicine: General	410	121	$134,856	$30,532	$120,289	$129,029	$140,132	$161,118
Internal Med: Hospitalist	59	31	$152,052	$25,485	$139,908	$149,999	$161,629	$183,333
Internal Med: Pediatric	17	12	$138,995	$34,058	$122,209	$130,008	$144,250	$206,724
Nephrology	24	13	$177,977	$45,948	$149,898	$175,943	$202,691	$219,872
Neurology	30	22	$163,443	$43,384	$134,966	$154,843	$195,239	$238,732
OBGYN: General	116	57	$186,950	$41,305	$164,017	$181,709	$203,219	$230,796
OBGYN: Gynecology (only)	3	3	*	*	*	*	*	*
OBGYN: Gyn Oncology	3	2	*	*	*	*	*	*
OBGYN: Maternal & Fetal Med	3	3	*	*	*	*	*	*
OBGYN: Repro Endocrinology	4	3	*	*	*	*	*	*
Occupational Medicine	15	3	$156,907	$25,532	$144,478	$151,916	$164,203	$204,227
Ophthalmology	31	17	$169,721	$26,061	$157,000	$163,874	$183,710	$197,242
Ophthalmology: Retina	3	3	*	*	*	*	*	*
Orthopedic (Non-surgical)	2	2	*	*	*	*	*	*
Orthopedic Surgery: General	58	36	$326,025	$139,321	$245,989	$286,192	$390,248	$541,551
Ortho Surg: Foot & Ankle	8	8	*	*	*	*	*	*
Ortho Surg: Hand	4	4	*	*	*	*	*	*
Ortho Surg: Hip & Joint	4	4	*	*	*	*	*	*
Ortho Surg: Oncology	1	1	*	*	*	*	*	*
Ortho Surg: Pediatric	2	2	*	*	*	*	*	*
Ortho Surg: Spine	12	10	$481,296	$167,610	$340,778	$495,517	$587,884	$726,349
Ortho Surg: Trauma	1	1	*	*	*	*	*	*
Ortho Surg: Sports Med	30	19	$272,694	$169,120	$176,842	$201,041	$326,226	$514,274
Otorhinolaryngology	19	16	$237,962	$88,076	$176,000	$226,877	$280,918	$399,696
Otorhinolaryngology: Pediatric	1	1	*	*	*	*	*	*
Pathology: Anatomic & Clinical	16	7	$190,347	$37,084	$164,443	$172,595	$224,987	$255,448
Pathology: Clinical	5	4	*	*	*	*	*	*

Table 9B: Physician Compensation for 1-2 Years in Specialty (continued)

	Physicians	Medical Practices	Mean	Std. Dev.	25th %tile	Median	75th %tile	90th %tile
Pediatrics: General	158	76	$120,500	$22,267	$110,000	$119,907	$130,060	$146,332
Ped: Adolescent Medicine	4	4	*	*	*	*	*	*
Ped: Cardiology	2	1	*	*	*	*	*	*
Ped: Child Development	1	1	*	*	*	*	*	*
Ped: Critical Care/Intensivist	5	5	*	*	*	*	*	*
Ped: Endocrinology	5	4	*	*	*	*	*	*
Ped: Gastroenterology	2	2	*	*	*	*	*	*
Ped: Genetics	1	1	*	*	*	*	*	*
Ped: Hematology/Oncology	2	1	*	*	*	*	*	*
Ped: Hospitalist	3	3	*	*	*	*	*	*
Ped: Infectious Disease	1	1	*	*	*	*	*	*
Ped: Neonatal Medicine	3	2	*	*	*	*	*	*
Ped: Neurology	3	3	*	*	*	*	*	*
Ped: Pulmonology	1	1	*	*	*	*	*	*
Physiatry (Phys Med & Rehab)	18	11	$156,128	$67,241	$115,001	$145,222	$159,193	$303,026
Podiatry: General	10	9	$130,610	$36,820	$103,328	$118,000	$172,614	$192,749
Podiatry: Surg-Foot & Ankle	5	1	*	*	*	*	*	*
Podiatry: Surg-Forefoot Only	1	1	*	*	*	*	*	*
Psychiatry: General	36	18	$152,499	$30,184	$135,512	$146,232	$159,476	$190,579
Psychiatry: Child & Adolescent	6	3	*	*	*	*	*	*
Pulmonary Medicine	9	8	*	*	*	*	*	*
Pulmonary Med: Critical Care	10	9	$196,660	$64,292	$155,096	$182,506	$216,514	$341,650
Radiation Oncology	4	3	*	*	*	*	*	*
Radiology: Diagnostic-Inv	29	17	$248,564	$74,158	$197,160	$238,469	$301,403	$364,874
Radiology: Diagnostic-Noninv	42	19	$266,834	$73,613	$228,399	$243,432	$275,098	$355,737
Radiology: Nuclear Medicine	4	3	*	*	*	*	*	*
Rheumatology	10	8	$182,093	$62,544	$146,780	$159,088	$208,349	$298,858
Sleep Medicine	2	2	*	*	*	*	*	*
Surgery: General	66	41	$224,364	$71,687	$181,510	$209,736	$246,001	$310,869
Surg: Cardiovascular	11	8	$248,874	$93,803	$200,000	$233,613	$352,374	$375,818
Surg: Cardiovascular-Pediatric	1	1	*	*	*	*	*	*
Surg: Colon and Rectal	2	2	*	*	*	*	*	*
Surg: Neurological	13	11	$379,353	$117,321	$300,000	$388,075	$416,216	$597,186
Surg: Oral	1	1	*	*	*	*	*	*
Surg: Pediatric	3	3	*	*	*	*	*	*
Surg: Plastic & Reconstruction	10	6	$231,207	$50,180	$183,369	$230,601	$270,498	$302,907
Surg: Thoracic (primary)	4	2	*	*	*	*	*	*
Surg: Transplant	3	3	*	*	*	*	*	*
Surg: Trauma	2	2	*	*	*	*	*	*
Surg: Trauma-Burn	2	2	*	*	*	*	*	*
Surg: Vascular (primary)	13	6	$262,532	$91,795	$223,555	$256,770	$283,588	$438,253
Urgent Care	17	9	$151,507	$44,951	$128,242	$155,000	$179,977	$223,914
Urology	30	20	$202,905	$67,080	$169,007	$197,679	$213,307	$311,734

　　　MEDICAL GROUP MANAGEMENT ASSOCIATION™

Table 10: Physician Compensation by Gender

	Male			Female		
	Physicians	Medical Practices	Median	Physicians	Medical Practices	Median
Allergy/Immunology	144	79	$254,299	31	21	$190,983
Anesthesiology	1,361	111	$322,543	220	73	$258,253
Anesth: Pain Management	68	30	$324,711	12	8	$191,374
Anesth: Pediatric	25	5	$330,487	10	3	$259,999
Cardiology: Electrophysiology	131	79	$377,951	13	11	$344,329
Cardiology: Invasive	542	147	$369,905	45	31	$286,178
Cardiology: Inv-Intervntnl	673	152	$424,820	22	21	$344,785
Cardiology: Noninvasive	515	158	$323,093	59	40	$261,124
Critical Care: Intensivist	53	13	$202,198	6	3	*
Dentistry	31	8	$151,872	11	7	$134,939
Dermatology	213	113	$277,757	80	55	$223,874
Dermatology: MOHS Surgery	16	15	$418,906	5	5	*
Emergency Medicine	436	43	$213,793	75	27	$191,883
Endocrinology/Metabolism	149	92	$178,539	43	38	$148,008
Family Practice (w/ OB)	898	185	$165,092	353	149	$136,346
Family Practice (w/o OB)	3,234	491	$156,998	844	308	$131,016
Family Practice: Sports Med	23	18	$197,096	5	5	*
Gastroenterology	628	190	$328,779	64	47	$275,974
Gastroenterology: Hepatology	70	16	$320,617	5	4	*
Geriatrics	42	23	$149,111	13	8	$126,022
Hematology/Oncology	326	115	$317,935	60	42	$238,495
Hem/Onc: Oncology (only)	70	34	$339,150	17	10	$331,214
Infectious Disease	108	58	$195,631	29	18	$143,528
Internal Medicine: General	3,201	418	$161,696	994	269	$135,960
Internal Med: Hospitalist	227	71	$164,914	84	46	$154,931
Internal Med: Pediatric	63	28	$154,686	33	20	$132,674
Nephrology	217	80	$241,417	39	25	$178,387
Neurology	392	133	$193,179	103	61	$160,000
OBGYN: General	953	260	$247,601	661	208	$216,012
OBGYN: Gynecology (only)	92	58	$187,561	34	24	$204,212
OBGYN: Gyn Oncology	19	10	$318,447	6	5	*
OBGYN: Maternal & Fetal Med	37	15	$341,557	16	9	$305,831
OBGYN: Repro Endocrinology	23	12	$270,203	12	7	$250,287
Occupational Medicine	118	45	$169,274	25	17	$147,840
Ophthalmology	449	139	$276,614	85	54	$224,570
Ophthalmology: Pediatric	25	17	$288,993	3	3	*
Ophthalmology: Retina	70	29	$452,545	4	4	*
Orthopedic (Non-surgical)	43	27	$293,000	7	5	*
Orthopedic Surgery: General	841	217	$371,162	18	7	$279,151
Ortho Surg: Foot & Ankle	46	40	$422,894	4	4	*
Ortho Surg: Hand	127	72	$456,100	6	6	*
Ortho Surg: Hip & Joint	115	61	$429,603	*	*	*
Ortho Surg: Oncology	3	3	*	*	*	*
Ortho Surg: Pediatric	37	26	$313,960	5	4	*
Ortho Surg: Spine	133	80	$547,585	*	*	*
Ortho Surg: Trauma	25	17	$439,750	5	3	*
Ortho Surg: Sports Med	236	97	$350,044	15	6	$202,081
Otorhinolaryngology	366	137	$277,835	35	25	$275,044
Otorhinolaryngology: Pediatric	14	4	$290,835	3	2	*
Pathology: Anatomic & Clinical	169	41	$299,057	58	24	$226,677
Pathology: Anatomic	39	10	$365,195	14	3	$244,780
Pathology: Clinical	51	16	$200,000	28	12	$170,043

Table 10: Physician Compensation by Gender (continued)

	Male			Female		
	Physicians	Medical Practices	Median	Physicians	Medical Practices	Median
Pediatrics: General	1,255	276	$167,242	907	267	$136,642
Ped: Adolescent Medicine	44	11	$151,247	27	8	$124,394
Ped: Allergy/Immunology	8	6	*	1	1	*
Ped: Cardiology	47	22	$219,017	6	5	*
Ped: Child Development	11	8	$125,749	9	7	*
Ped: Critical Care/Intensivist	50	20	$253,505	17	11	$176,822
Ped: Emergency Medicine	6	2	*	2	1	*
Ped: Endocrinology	14	11	$137,800	9	7	*
Ped: Gastroenterology	23	11	$198,134	5	3	*
Ped: Genetics	8	4	*	10	5	$150,000
Ped: Hematology/Oncology	35	18	$190,500	13	9	$175,000
Ped: Hospitalist	16	9	$155,870	10	6	$131,885
Ped: Infectious Disease	8	3	*	2	2	*
Ped: Neonatal Medicine	70	18	$246,714	34	16	$182,649
Ped: Nephrology	6	4	*	3	2	*
Ped: Neurology	24	16	$175,381	6	6	*
Ped: Pulmonology	18	9	$206,420	2	2	*
Ped: Rheumatology	3	2	*	1	1	*
Ped: Sports Medicine	*	*	*	1	1	*
Physiatry (Phys Med & Rehab)	122	62	$194,604	44	30	$174,041
Podiatry: General	103	63	$153,106	15	14	$111,092
Podiatry: Surg-Foot & Ankle	88	25	$163,541	4	3	*
Podiatry: Surg-Forefoot Only	12	5	$168,497	3	3	*
Psychiatry: General	248	62	$162,527	86	31	$149,218
Psychiatry: Child & Adolescent	31	14	$172,574	21	7	$181,400
Psychiatry: Geriatric	11	7	$217,843	2	1	*
Pulmonary Medicine	253	117	$211,691	21	18	$210,320
Pulmonary Med: Critical Care	134	43	$236,314	14	11	$212,886
Radiation Oncology	84	33	$389,925	14	12	$339,544
Radiology: Diagnostic-Inv	324	54	$385,290	43	17	$304,427
Radiology: Diagnostic-Noninv	485	82	$361,484	113	47	$283,613
Radiology: Nuclear Medicine	46	25	$261,922	11	9	$274,300
Rheumatology	217	115	$197,000	42	31	$159,725
Sleep Medicine	13	7	$210,575	2	2	*
Surgery: General	839	242	$257,249	83	54	$212,030
Surg: Cardiovascular	170	46	$433,850	6	5	*
Surg: Cardiovascular-Pediatric	5	5	*	*	*	*
Surg: Colon and Rectal	32	15	$283,935	4	4	*
Surg: Neurological	173	60	$487,000	15	10	$337,031
Surg: Oncology	7	5	*	3	2	*
Surg: Oral	23	12	$224,567	2	2	*
Surg: Pediatric	20	10	$317,972	2	2	*
Surg: Plastic & Reconstruction	87	46	$298,500	16	13	$272,320
Surg: Plastic & Recon-Hand	14	6	$232,500	1	1	*
Surg: Plastic & Recon-Pediatric	4	2	*	*	*	*
Surg: Thoracic (primary)	55	16	$283,894	1	1	*
Surg: Transplant	16	8	$364,246	*	*	*
Surg: Trauma	20	7	$286,375	2	2	*
Surg: Trauma-Burn	13	6	$337,667	0	*	*
Surg: Vascular (primary)	126	50	$309,230	10	6	$261,090
Urgent Care	312	91	$162,940	80	49	$147,192
Urology	437	131	$294,337	15	13	$196,896
Urology: Pediatric	12	4	$161,824	1	1	*

Table 11: Physician Compensation by Hours Worked per Week

	Less than 40 hours		40 hours or more	
	Physicians	Median	Physicians	Median
Allergy/Immunology	35	$306,478	86	$258,536
Anesthesiology	77	$250,294	1,229	$326,051
Anesth: Pain Management	3	*	71	$315,591
Anesth: Pediatric	2	*	32	$327,462
Cardiology: Electrophysiology	6	*	116	$380,002
Cardiology: Invasive	44	$309,164	416	$370,000
Cardiology: Inv-Intervntnl	46	$450,000	548	$426,277
Cardiology: Noninvasive	76	$273,006	337	$325,405
Critical Care: Intensivist	3	*	17	$210,624
Dentistry	10	*	29	$140,395
Dermatology	64	$274,506	129	$272,847
Dermatology: MOHS Surgery	3	*	12	$374,371
Emergency Medicine	162	$209,801	142	$196,260
Endocrinology/Metabolism	42	$156,946	93	$175,000
Family Practice (w/ OB)	201	$146,746	734	$156,893
Family Practice (w/o OB)	1,077	$149,397	2,382	$150,024
Family Practice: Sports Med	8	*	15	$160,985
Gastroenterology	63	$285,751	429	$349,000
Gastroenterology: Hepatology	0	*	57	$281,000
Geriatrics	12	$134,187	31	$146,016
Hematology/Oncology	44	$290,074	239	$340,216
Hem/Onc: Oncology (only)	4	*	59	$350,361
Infectious Disease	19	$163,192	79	$180,079
Internal Medicine: General	763	$150,963	2,201	$155,530
Internal Med: Hospitalist	91	$166,999	170	$161,549
Internal Med: Pediatric	25	$140,978	60	$146,826
Nephrology	20	$187,398	147	$226,362
Neurology	56	$181,695	311	$190,365
OBGYN: General	256	$221,253	815	$241,224
OBGYN: Gynecology (only)	74	$201,282	76	$222,978
OBGYN: Gyn Oncology	2	*	9	*
OBGYN: Maternal & Fetal Med	10	$530,442	31	$319,102
OBGYN: Repro Endocrinology	1	*	28	$265,854
Occupational Medicine	27	$147,568	56	$190,918
Ophthalmology	110	$233,868	263	$325,584
Ophthalmology: Pediatric	6	*	18	$304,207
Ophthalmology: Retina	9	*	51	$498,351
Orthopedic (Non-surgical)	15	$203,976	26	$199,464
Orthopedic Surgery: General	79	$287,000	524	$401,343
Ortho Surg: Foot & Ankle	5	*	42	$370,419
Ortho Surg: Hand	10	$417,548	112	$404,210
Ortho Surg: Hip & Joint	13	$454,400	92	$431,067
Ortho Surg: Oncology	1	*	2	*
Ortho Surg: Pediatric	3	*	25	$323,909
Ortho Surg: Spine	7	*	99	$580,958
Ortho Surg: Trauma	4	*	24	$421,545
Ortho Surg: Sports Med	16	$415,279	183	$400,000
Otorhinolaryngology	66	$271,389	238	$283,355
Otorhinolaryngology: Pediatric	1	*	13	$300,000
Pathology: Anatomic & Clinical	22	$188,347	126	$414,315
Pathology: Anatomic	*	*	57	$312,116
Pathology: Clinical	16	$168,399	53	$193,000

Table 11: Physician Compensation by Hours Worked per Week (continued)

	Less than 40 hours		40 hours or more	
	Physicians	Median	Physicians	Median
Pediatrics: General	481	$146,640	1,129	$157,000
Ped: Adolescent Medicine	2	*	30	$160,957
Ped: Allergy/Immunology	*	*	7	*
Ped: Cardiology	2	*	32	$215,613
Ped: Child Development	0	*	12	$126,800
Ped: Critical Care/Intensivist	7	*	46	$252,665
Ped: Emergency Medicine	2	*	5	*
Ped: Endocrinology	2	*	15	$144,839
Ped: Gastroenterology	3	*	19	$185,016
Ped: Genetics	2	*	8	*
Ped: Hematology/Oncology	4	*	33	$187,000
Ped: Hospitalist	1	*	20	$151,500
Ped: Infectious Disease	0	*	5	*
Ped: Neonatal Medicine	3	*	50	$265,530
Ped: Nephrology	1	*	7	*
Ped: Neurology	1	*	21	$175,139
Ped: Pulmonology	*	*	15	$187,211
Ped: Rheumatology	1	*	3	*
Ped: Sports Medicine	*	*	1	*
Physiatry (Phys Med & Rehab)	15	$224,995	96	$207,430
Podiatry: General	34	$142,231	50	$147,679
Podiatry: Surg-Foot & Ankle	8	*	29	$179,557
Podiatry: Surg-Forefoot Only	7	*	6	*
Psychiatry: General	57	$143,925	144	$154,007
Psychiatry: Child & Adolescent	3	*	15	$172,574
Psychiatry: Geriatric	*	*	13	$207,734
Pulmonary Medicine	26	$180,919	162	$208,768
Pulmonary Med: Critical Care	7	*	107	$237,531
Radiation Oncology	10	$308,519	68	$385,707
Radiology: Diagnostic-Inv	19	$337,500	265	$431,769
Radiology: Diagnostic-Noninv	55	$328,841	361	$373,593
Radiology: Nuclear Medicine	5	*	32	$371,786
Rheumatology	38	$177,115	142	$205,642
Sleep Medicine	2	*	12	$192,488
Surgery: General	95	$238,971	534	$260,000
Surg: Cardiovascular	4	*	115	$439,919
Surg: Cardiovascular-Pediatric	*	*	5	*
Surg: Colon and Rectal	3	*	22	$240,000
Surg: Neurological	8	*	123	$487,000
Surg: Oncology	*	*	1	*
Surg: Oral	6	*	15	$226,077
Surg: Pediatric	2	*	17	$300,380
Surg: Plastic & Reconstruction	5	*	50	$307,264
Surg: Plastic & Recon-Hand	*	*	15	$221,000
Surg: Plastic & Recon-Pediatric	*	*	4	*
Surg: Thoracic (primary)	3	*	27	$398,992
Surg: Transplant	4	*	9	*
Surg: Trauma	1	*	16	$266,946
Surg: Trauma-Burn	1	*	12	$325,411
Surg: Vascular (primary)	6	*	78	$318,850
Urgent Care	76	$128,988	170	$164,013
Urology	44	$298,136	266	$316,151
Urology: Pediatric	*	*	4	*

Table 12: Physician Compensation by Weeks Worked per Year

	Less than 46 weeks		46 weeks or more	
	Physicians	Median	Physicians	Median
Allergy/Immunology	24	$201,963	109	$285,683
Anesthesiology	933	$330,823	391	$302,863
Anesth: Pain Management	42	$322,835	33	$303,168
Anesth: Pediatric	21	*	13	$276,352
Cardiology: Electrophysiology	61	$406,984	69	$346,923
Cardiology: Invasive	216	$377,954	266	$347,140
Cardiology: Inv-Intervntnl	276	$414,892	329	$430,504
Cardiology: Noninvasive	176	$350,531	266	$321,872
Critical Care: Intensivist	2	*	13	$200,914
Dentistry	11	$130,727	10	$143,089
Dermatology	59	$225,931	145	$295,000
Dermatology: MOHS Surgery	3	*	14	$461,851
Emergency Medicine	139	$200,440	133	$208,333
Endocrinology/Metabolism	34	$150,034	108	$173,479
Family Practice (w/ OB)	200	$154,690	750	$160,720
Family Practice (w/o OB)	664	$153,011	2,670	$152,916
Family Practice: Sports Med	6	*	19	$171,811
Gastroenterology	135	$320,000	374	$358,574
Gastroenterology: Hepatology	13	$252,600	57	$322,173
Geriatrics	11	$146,016	26	$146,824
Hematology/Oncology	73	$309,962	209	$336,859
Hem/Onc: Oncology (only)	10	$235,687	60	$373,195
Infectious Disease	23	$154,865	79	$201,801
Internal Medicine: General	595	$151,000	2,303	$155,986
Internal Med: Hospitalist	39	$150,000	223	$165,970
Internal Med: Pediatric	1	*	77	$143,147
Nephrology	60	$203,000	116	$230,000
Neurology	100	$178,518	275	$187,508
OBGYN: General	242	$245,157	792	$235,767
OBGYN: Gynecology (only)	42	$191,225	122	$212,255
OBGYN: Gyn Oncology	1	*	13	$265,000
OBGYN: Maternal & Fetal Med	5	*	35	$341,557
OBGYN: Repro Endocrinology	9	*	18	$265,854
Occupational Medicine	19	$168,008	73	$167,275
Ophthalmology	117	$248,764	256	$307,503
Ophthalmology: Pediatric	7	*	13	$320,262
Ophthalmology: Retina	15	$620,000	45	$495,619
Orthopedic (Non-surgical)	6	*	34	$205,387
Orthopedic Surgery: General	170	$379,032	478	$387,639
Ortho Surg: Foot & Ankle	15	$440,696	33	$349,953
Ortho Surg: Hand	43	$398,154	77	$462,523
Ortho Surg: Hip & Joint	40	$445,258	69	$410,305
Ortho Surg: Oncology	*	*	3	*
Ortho Surg: Pediatric	5	*	33	$281,567
Ortho Surg: Spine	34	$470,883	79	$588,748
Ortho Surg: Trauma	8	*	15	$354,814
Ortho Surg: Sports Med	51	$428,080	138	$408,023
Otorhinolaryngology	54	$277,478	256	$282,522
Otorhinolaryngology: Pediatric	4	*	10	$290,835
Pathology: Anatomic & Clinical	67	$463,299	77	$286,068
Pathology: Anatomic	29	$254,225	28	$348,907
Pathology: Clinical	13	$282,780	38	$167,319

Table 12: Physician Compensation by Weeks Worked per Year (continued)

	Less than 46 weeks		46 weeks or more	
	Physicians	Median	Physicians	Median
Pediatrics: General	288	$150,736	1,288	$156,388
Ped: Adolescent Medicine	7	*	38	$154,766
Ped: Allergy/Immunology	4	*	3	*
Ped: Cardiology	11	$293,572	26	$234,444
Ped: Child Development	*	*	9	*
Ped: Critical Care/Intensivist	20	$279,511	36	$252,665
Ped: Emergency Medicine	*	*	8	*
Ped: Endocrinology	3	*	13	$144,839
Ped: Gastroenterology	2	*	13	$185,016
Ped: Genetics	*	*	10	$150,000
Ped: Hematology/Oncology	5	*	32	$185,623
Ped: Hospitalist	2	*	18	$148,375
Ped: Infectious Disease	*	*	5	*
Ped: Neonatal Medicine	20	$395,120	29	$271,047
Ped: Nephrology	*	*	7	*
Ped: Neurology	4	*	15	$174,400
Ped: Pulmonology	7	*	8	*
Ped: Rheumatology	*	*	4	*
Ped: Sports Medicine	*	*	1	*
Physiatry (Phys Med & Rehab)	19	$208,100	98	$203,021
Podiatry: General	28	$145,087	50	$147,101
Podiatry: Surg-Foot & Ankle	10	$150,346	29	$150,303
Podiatry: Surg-Forefoot Only	0	*	12	$168,497
Psychiatry: General	94	$149,514	97	$154,623
Psychiatry: Child & Adolescent	8	*	13	$172,078
Psychiatry: Geriatric	3	*	8	*
Pulmonary Medicine	57	$179,861	152	$224,326
Pulmonary Med: Critical Care	26	$226,257	108	$237,105
Radiation Oncology	52	$457,623	29	$354,066
Radiology: Diagnostic-Inv	228	$436,241	54	$375,000
Radiology: Diagnostic-Noninv	321	$366,190	84	$374,479
Radiology: Nuclear Medicine	21	$374,416	16	$216,915
Rheumatology	38	$177,591	151	$211,882
Sleep Medicine	2	*	12	$169,700
Surgery: General	188	$254,502	485	$257,987
Surg: Cardiovascular	62	$489,281	59	$460,000
Surg: Cardiovascular-Pediatric	1	*	4	*
Surg: Colon and Rectal	12	$334,503	16	$229,985
Surg: Neurological	44	$510,000	113	$473,495
Surg: Oncology	*	*	3	*
Surg: Oral	4	*	13	$246,263
Surg: Pediatric	4	*	9	*
Surg: Plastic & Reconstruction	15	$324,868	44	$290,213
Surg: Plastic & Recon-Hand	3	*	12	$221,000
Surg: Plastic & Recon-Pediatric	1	*	3	*
Surg: Thoracic (primary)	3	*	34	$352,205
Surg: Transplant	*	*	12	$376,730
Surg: Trauma	4	*	16	$213,640
Surg: Trauma-Burn	3	*	9	*
Surg: Vascular (primary)	37	$328,670	60	$274,751
Urgent Care	44	$160,883	237	$154,043
Urology	89	$313,397	250	$312,370
Urology: Pediatric	*	*	13	$149,623

MEDICAL GROUP MANAGEMENT ASSOCIATION™

Table 13: Physician Retirement Benefits

	Physicians	Medical Practices	Mean	Std. Dev.	25th %tile	Median	75th %tile	90th %tile
Allergy/Immunology	124	69	$20,646	$10,609	$11,517	$20,881	$29,000	$35,000
Anesthesiology	1,320	102	$29,484	$9,823	$24,000	$30,000	$40,000	$40,000
Anesth: Pain Management	83	32	$24,624	$11,387	$14,000	$29,000	$32,056	$35,000
Anesth: Pediatric	32	5	$32,428	$5,610	$29,000	$35,000	$35,000	$40,000
Cardiology: Electrophysiology	129	74	$25,641	$8,770	$18,561	$25,500	$29,250	$40,000
Cardiology: Invasive	491	131	$24,630	$9,351	$18,561	$25,000	$30,000	$40,000
Cardiology: Inv-Intervntnl	643	145	$27,178	$8,631	$23,000	$29,000	$30,560	$40,000
Cardiology: Noninvasive	470	145	$23,501	$9,624	$18,000	$24,000	$29,000	$35,000
Critical Care: Intensivist	20	10	$17,527	$9,505	$10,815	$16,705	$28,418	$29,000
Dentistry	40	9	$10,667	$4,313	$6,905	$11,000	$13,560	$15,871
Dermatology	231	119	$21,257	$11,515	$10,759	$20,260	$29,000	$40,000
Dermatology: MOHS Surgery	17	15	$19,620	$9,724	$11,600	$18,604	$25,619	$36,800
Emergency Medicine	366	42	$17,673	$10,316	$8,000	$14,822	$25,701	$30,872
Endocrinology/Metabolism	141	89	$15,422	$8,935	$7,868	$14,725	$22,489	$27,980
Family Practice (w/ OB)	955	166	$14,812	$9,639	$6,218	$12,855	$20,742	$28,947
Family Practice (w/o OB)	3,292	403	$13,427	$8,622	$6,827	$11,218	$18,380	$24,682
Family Practice: Sports Med	24	18	$18,846	$9,365	$9,050	$20,512	$28,618	$30,550
Gastroenterology	537	166	$23,874	$9,558	$18,340	$24,060	$29,000	$35,232
Gastroenterology: Hepatology	60	13	$27,406	$10,304	$23,450	$28,992	$37,500	$40,000
Geriatrics	42	19	$13,770	$9,375	$6,153	$12,025	$16,316	$32,006
Hematology/Oncology	278	101	$21,961	$10,953	$11,466	$20,839	$29,333	$39,663
Hem/Onc: Oncology (only)	81	34	$20,945	$10,499	$12,000	$21,261	$29,000	$30,000
Infectious Disease	98	54	$17,932	$9,740	$9,694	$17,025	$28,000	$29,000
Internal Medicine: General	3,026	358	$14,263	$8,846	$7,043	$12,262	$19,342	$27,732
Internal Med: Hospitalist	278	63	$14,834	$8,830	$8,431	$12,039	$20,608	$27,260
Internal Med: Pediatric	82	26	$13,688	$9,370	$6,893	$10,022	$19,675	$29,000
Nephrology	189	71	$21,338	$11,027	$11,470	$21,000	$29,000	$40,000
Neurology	386	125	$18,664	$9,797	$10,770	$17,722	$24,636	$32,518
OBGYN: General	1,157	242	$19,502	$10,456	$10,678	$19,500	$28,259	$32,555
OBGYN: Gynecology (only)	139	53	$15,306	$7,506	$10,686	$14,464	$19,710	$25,637
OBGYN: Gyn Oncology	13	8	$26,089	$16,854	$7,730	$34,411	$40,000	$47,000
OBGYN: Maternal & Fetal Med	45	12	$26,958	$15,559	$12,000	$29,000	$40,250	$47,000
OBGYN: Repro Endocrinology	25	10	$21,166	$12,629	$6,060	$20,000	$35,000	$35,574
Occupational Medicine	101	42	$16,450	$10,925	$8,500	$12,480	$24,292	$35,000
Ophthalmology	384	123	$21,410	$11,103	$11,899	$21,400	$29,000	$36,858
Ophthalmology: Pediatric	18	13	$24,217	$10,430	$16,043	$26,251	$30,820	$40,000
Ophthalmology: Retina	45	19	$25,558	$9,578	$16,840	$23,000	$33,280	$40,000
Orthopedic (Non-surgical)	40	22	$18,560	$8,430	$11,500	$19,023	$29,000	$29,000
Orthopedic Surgery: General	660	187	$26,115	$10,414	$18,640	$28,924	$33,166	$40,000
Ortho Surg: Foot & Ankle	39	34	$30,241	$7,501	$24,612	$29,000	$38,432	$40,000
Ortho Surg: Hand	103	61	$30,932	$7,842	$29,000	$30,000	$40,000	$40,000
Ortho Surg: Hip & Joint	96	52	$28,519	$8,701	$24,000	$29,000	$35,000	$40,000
Ortho Surg: Oncology	2	2	*	*	*	*	*	*
Ortho Surg: Pediatric	32	23	$30,222	$9,992	$24,773	$29,000	$40,000	$42,580
Ortho Surg: Spine	104	67	$28,723	$8,753	$24,000	$29,000	$34,903	$40,000
Ortho Surg: Trauma	24	13	$29,682	$10,104	$23,127	$30,491	$40,000	$40,000
Ortho Surg: Sports Med	170	84	$27,246	$10,139	$20,763	$29,000	$35,855	$40,000
Otorhinolaryngology	329	121	$21,870	$10,277	$14,000	$21,750	$29,000	$33,000
Otorhinolaryngology: Pediatric	15	2	*	*	*	*	*	*
Pathology: Anatomic & Clinical	187	41	$24,387	$9,940	$18,046	$25,637	$29,000	$40,000
Pathology: Anatomic	47	9	$24,687	$8,613	$22,234	$29,000	$29,000	$38,449
Pathology: Clinical	58	12	$16,795	$10,322	$9,142	$13,951	$27,000	$30,000

Table 13: Physician Retirement Benefits (continued)

	Physicians	Medical Practices	Mean	Std. Dev.	25th %tile	Median	75th %tile	90th %tile
Pediatrics: General	1,564	273	$14,107	$8,751	$6,615	$12,096	$19,820	$27,807
Ped: Adolescent Medicine	44	10	$13,241	$7,304	$6,825	$12,062	$19,273	$25,776
Ped: Allergy/Immunology	7	6	*	*	*	*	*	*
Ped: Cardiology	35	17	$15,685	$10,470	$6,491	$10,703	$25,000	$28,686
Ped: Child Development	10	6	$6,625	$2,457	$3,764	$6,584	$9,201	$9,926
Ped: Critical Care/Intensivist	55	16	$20,455	$10,454	$10,000	$22,843	$29,000	$31,400
Ped: Emergency Medicine	8	2	*	*	*	*	*	*
Ped: Endocrinology	17	12	$10,245	$7,357	$3,611	$7,628	$13,692	$24,983
Ped: Gastroenterology	19	9	$16,120	$8,421	$10,116	$17,000	$22,000	$23,960
Ped: Genetics	8	4	*	*	*	*	*	*
Ped: Hematology/Oncology	33	15	$15,266	$9,413	$5,800	$15,163	$22,000	$27,261
Ped: Hospitalist	19	10	$12,898	$5,949	$10,166	$12,646	$19,308	$20,572
Ped: Infectious Disease	5	3	*	*	*	*	*	*
Ped: Neonatal Medicine	70	13	$24,145	$13,112	$12,198	$21,990	$40,000	$40,275
Ped: Nephrology	8	5	*	*	*	*	*	*
Ped: Neurology	26	17	$15,608	$10,283	$8,263	$13,717	$20,005	$28,463
Ped: Pulmonology	17	9	$17,840	$12,193	$5,790	$22,000	$28,006	$31,733
Ped: Rheumatology	4	3	*	*	*	*	*	*
Ped: Sports Medicine	1	1	*	*	*	*	*	*
Physiatry (Phys Med & Rehab)	122	64	$20,908	$11,574	$11,389	$20,428	$29,000	$40,000
Podiatry: General	94	53	$13,909	$9,004	$6,756	$11,050	$20,714	$26,982
Podiatry: Surg-Foot & Ankle	34	17	$17,858	$10,280	$6,630	$18,529	$29,000	$31,468
Podiatry: Surg-Forefoot Only	11	5	$10,907	$6,079	$5,805	$12,040	$13,074	$23,116
Psychiatry: General	213	54	$14,444	$9,631	$5,875	$13,618	$19,822	$29,145
Psychiatry: Child & Adolescent	18	11	$19,087	$9,679	$13,970	$18,145	$21,190	$36,666
Psychiatry: Geriatric	11	5	$13,638	$8,076	$5,777	$12,500	$23,164	$23,565
Pulmonary Medicine	237	108	$19,424	$9,491	$10,910	$20,000	$27,842	$29,000
Pulmonary Med: Critical Care	140	41	$25,840	$9,264	$20,503	$28,488	$30,843	$36,561
Radiation Oncology	85	30	$26,343	$10,247	$16,793	$27,961	$30,013	$40,000
Radiology: Diagnostic-Inv	306	52	$28,656	$10,362	$26,989	$30,000	$40,000	$40,000
Radiology: Diagnostic-Noninv	442	80	$27,047	$10,643	$20,348	$29,000	$35,000	$40,000
Radiology: Nuclear Medicine	40	22	$21,731	$13,072	$8,590	$20,348	$29,000	$42,322
Rheumatology	201	107	$20,024	$9,774	$12,500	$19,338	$29,000	$31,128
Sleep Medicine	12	5	$17,070	$8,006	$11,000	$15,944	$24,176	$29,700
Surgery: General	712	211	$22,033	$10,552	$12,913	$22,000	$29,000	$39,550
Surg: Cardiovascular	134	37	$22,954	$9,233	$16,329	$27,000	$29,000	$32,500
Surg: Cardiovascular-Pediatric	5	5	*	*	*	*	*	*
Surg: Colon and Rectal	17	11	$21,617	$9,554	$14,302	$24,500	$26,730	$31,716
Surg: Neurological	151	55	$24,608	$10,214	$17,000	$25,582	$30,413	$39,662
Surg: Oncology	10	6	$21,405	$7,638	$18,714	$24,500	$25,112	$27,859
Surg: Oral	23	11	$24,498	$12,592	$12,500	$20,000	$40,000	$40,000
Surg: Pediatric	18	8	$20,088	$13,436	$8,705	$16,064	$35,901	$40,000
Surg: Plastic & Reconstruction	52	37	$17,998	$11,660	$8,563	$15,376	$27,808	$36,391
Surg: Plastic & Recon-Hand	10	4	$27,800	$5,692	$26,750	$29,000	$29,000	$37,100
Surg: Plastic & Recon-Pediatric	2	1	*	*	*	*	*	*
Surg: Thoracic (primary)	24	12	$26,391	$10,175	$18,201	$27,961	$30,563	$40,000
Surg: Transplant	9	5	*	*	*	*	*	*
Surg: Trauma	22	7	$23,390	$12,327	$13,950	$22,937	$33,753	$40,629
Surg: Trauma-Burn	13	6	$20,949	$12,710	$12,500	$18,000	$30,545	$41,281
Surg: Vascular (primary)	91	42	$24,203	$10,630	$16,000	$28,787	$29,500	$40,000
Urgent Care	255	74	$15,667	$8,713	$8,465	$14,811	$21,411	$27,350
Urology	357	121	$25,051	$11,256	$15,600	$25,637	$34,645	$40,000
Urology: Pediatric	3	2	*	*	*	*	*	*

MEDICAL GROUP MANAGEMENT ASSOCIATION™

Table 14: Physician Retirement Benefits by Group Type

	Single-specialty			Multispecialty		
	Physicians	Medical Practices	Median	Physicians	Medical Practices	Median
Allergy/Immunology	30	7	$24,791	94	62	$20,251
Anesthesiology	1,086	62	$30,000	234	40	$19,259
Anesth: Pain Management	63	20	$29,000	20	12	$24,587
Anesth: Pediatric	20	2	*	12	3	$29,000
Cardiology: Electrophysiology	96	54	$26,056	33	20	$19,000
Cardiology: Invasive	247	64	$29,000	244	67	$18,831
Cardiology: Inv-Intervntnl	423	87	$29,000	220	58	$26,488
Cardiology: Noninvasive	287	75	$27,387	183	70	$19,211
Critical Care: Intensivist	5	2	*	15	8	$11,845
Dentistry	10	2	*	30	7	$11,000
Dermatology	23	10	$36,000	208	109	$19,198
Dermatology: MOHS Surgery	4	3	*	13	12	$18,604
Emergency Medicine	120	9	$13,750	246	33	$14,932
Endocrinology/Metabolism	8	5	*	133	84	$14,725
Family Practice (w/ OB)	205	52	$8,000	750	114	$14,035
Family Practice (w/o OB)	546	150	$10,099	2,746	253	$11,463
Family Practice: Sports Med	12	9	$24,087	12	9	$18,725
Gastroenterology	197	27	$28,726	340	139	$21,238
Gastroenterology: Hepatology	47	8	$30,000	13	5	$14,996
Geriatrics	0	*	*	42	19	$12,025
Hematology/Oncology	114	26	$28,000	164	75	$20,000
Hem/Onc: Oncology (only)	37	6	$28,903	44	28	$19,802
Infectious Disease	31	10	$28,000	67	44	$15,152
Internal Medicine: General	247	56	$11,846	2,779	302	$12,353
Internal Med: Hospitalist	6	2	*	272	61	$12,973
Internal Med: Pediatric	4	2	*	78	24	$10,182
Nephrology	64	10	$29,000	125	61	$18,584
Neurology	112	19	$17,257	274	106	$17,809
OBGYN: General	372	74	$21,733	785	168	$19,198
OBGYN: Gynecology (only)	32	17	$11,558	107	36	$14,771
OBGYN: Gyn Oncology	1	1	*	12	7	$34,888
OBGYN: Maternal & Fetal Med	10	4	$12,000	35	8	$30,944
OBGYN: Repro Endocrinology	9	4	*	16	6	$9,561
Occupational Medicine	8	3	*	93	39	$11,167
Ophthalmology	143	26	$23,432	241	97	$21,000
Ophthalmology: Pediatric	13	9	$29,000	5	4	*
Ophthalmology: Retina	36	12	$23,000	9	7	*
Orthopedic (Non-surgical)	16	7	$20,084	24	15	$15,365
Orthopedic Surgery: General	328	87	$29,000	332	100	$23,086
Ortho Surg: Foot & Ankle	33	29	$29,000	6	5	*
Ortho Surg: Hand	86	50	$30,000	17	11	$29,000
Ortho Surg: Hip & Joint	79	44	$29,000	17	8	$29,000
Ortho Surg: Oncology	2	2	*	0	*	*
Ortho Surg: Pediatric	21	17	$29,000	11	6	$41,497
Ortho Surg: Spine	81	51	$29,000	23	16	$29,000
Ortho Surg: Trauma	20	12	$33,300	4	1	*
Ortho Surg: Sports Med	136	66	$29,000	34	18	$16,376
Otorhinolaryngology	84	16	$24,000	245	105	$21,214
Otorhinolaryngology: Pediatric	7	1	*	8	1	*
Pathology: Anatomic & Clinical	100	14	$29,000	87	27	$20,659
Pathology: Anatomic	40	6	$29,000	7	3	*
Pathology: Clinical	18	5	$18,910	40	7	$13,262

Table 14: Physician Retirement Benefits by Group Type (continued)

	Single-specialty			Multispecialty		
	Physicians	Medical Practices	Median	Physicians	Medical Practices	Median
Pediatrics: General	436	70	$11,000	1,128	203	$12,523
Ped: Adolescent Medicine	3	1	*	41	9	$12,560
Ped: Allergy/Immunology	3	2	*	4	4	*
Ped: Cardiology	21	8	$8,000	14	9	$10,759
Ped: Child Development	*	*	*	10	6	$6,584
Ped: Critical Care/Intensivist	30	7	$29,000	25	9	$10,301
Ped: Emergency Medicine	2	1	*	6	1	*
Ped: Endocrinology	2	2	*	15	10	$7,475
Ped: Gastroenterology	8	4	*	11	5	$10,643
Ped: Genetics	*	*	*	8	4	*
Ped: Hematology/Oncology	11	4	$13,500	22	11	$15,235
Ped: Hospitalist	1	1	*	18	9	$12,966
Ped: Infectious Disease	2	1	*	3	2	*
Ped: Neonatal Medicine	28	3	$33,578	42	10	$17,000
Ped: Nephrology	2	1	*	6	4	*
Ped: Neurology	7	5	*	19	12	$11,782
Ped: Pulmonology	8	3	*	9	6	*
Ped: Rheumatology	1	1	*	3	2	*
Ped: Sports Medicine	*	*	*	1	1	*
Physiatry (Phys Med & Rehab)	41	23	$25,500	81	41	$16,293
Podiatry: General	2	2	*	92	51	$11,050
Podiatry: Surg-Foot & Ankle	5	3	*	29	14	$21,486
Podiatry: Surg-Forefoot Only	1	1	*	10	4	$9,752
Psychiatry: General	10	3	$18,226	203	51	$12,460
Psychiatry: Child & Adolescent	1	1	*	17	10	$17,000
Psychiatry: Geriatric	*	*	*	11	5	$12,500
Pulmonary Medicine	32	10	$27,715	205	98	$17,871
Pulmonary Med: Critical Care	48	8	$30,000	92	33	$23,780
Radiation Oncology	48	12	$29,000	37	18	$27,104
Radiology: Diagnostic-Inv	218	30	$30,000	88	22	$17,630
Radiology: Diagnostic-Noninv	229	28	$30,000	213	52	$21,214
Radiology: Nuclear Medicine	20	10	$24,367	20	12	$11,522
Rheumatology	28	7	$29,500	173	100	$18,675
Sleep Medicine	6	2	*	6	3	*
Surgery: General	165	39	$29,000	547	172	$21,214
Surg: Cardiovascular	66	15	$29,000	68	22	$20,000
Surg: Cardiovascular-Pediatric	3	3	*	2	2	*
Surg: Colon and Rectal	7	3	*	10	8	$23,424
Surg: Neurological	73	18	$25,722	78	37	$24,590
Surg: Oncology	1	1	*	9	5	*
Surg: Oral	13	3	$19,600	10	8	$20,000
Surg: Pediatric	7	3	*	11	5	$11,740
Surg: Plastic & Reconstruction	2	2	*	50	35	$13,846
Surg: Plastic & Recon-Hand	8	2	*	2	2	*
Surg: Plastic & Recon-Pediatric	0	*	*	2	1	*
Surg: Thoracic (primary)	2	1	*	22	11	$27,961
Surg: Transplant	4	1	*	5	4	*
Surg: Trauma	5	2	*	17	5	$27,960
Surg: Trauma-Burn	8	3	*	5	3	*
Surg: Vascular (primary)	26	8	$28,894	65	34	$26,480
Urgent Care	1	1	*	254	73	$14,741
Urology	138	28	$30,000	219	93	$21,261
Urology: Pediatric	1	1	*	2	1	*

MEDICAL GROUP MANAGEMENT ASSOCIATION™

THIS PAGE INTENTIONALLY LEFT BLANK

PHYSICIAN PRODUCTIVITY

Table 15: Collections for Professional Charges (TC Excluded)

	Physicians	Medical Practices	Mean	Std. Dev.	25th %tile	Median	75th %tile	90th %tile
Allergy/Immunology	56	38	$595,660	$299,686	$329,880	$537,529	$817,471	$1,032,422
Anesthesiology	297	34	$413,006	$166,646	$313,230	$397,213	$466,085	$576,645
Anesth: Pain Management	24	10	$561,475	$310,747	$389,670	$516,785	$697,535	$882,449
Anesth: Pediatric	13	1	*	*	*	*	*	*
Cardiology: Electrophysiology	22	16	$775,521	$448,264	$487,853	$697,185	$889,695	$1,324,237
Cardiology: Invasive	74	32	$695,487	$344,991	$432,448	$630,770	$793,351	$1,250,895
Cardiology: Inv-Intervntnl	118	38	$760,013	$351,071	$547,434	$673,705	$859,255	$1,368,579
Cardiology: Noninvasive	97	41	$590,353	$333,119	$391,152	$536,916	$674,877	$924,373
Critical Care: Intensivist	13	7	$282,982	$206,810	$171,918	$234,122	$331,667	$684,176
Dentistry	9	3	*	*	*	*	*	*
Dermatology	113	58	$635,421	$340,393	$416,386	$572,675	$748,691	$985,627
Dermatology: MOHS Surgery	10	8	$1,120,925	$415,813	$831,911	$999,778	$1,409,070	$1,856,143
Emergency Medicine	145	14	$322,761	$98,777	$274,637	$315,389	$386,623	$440,749
Endocrinology/Metabolism	72	46	$343,421	$181,321	$236,239	$309,290	$372,589	$537,264
Family Practice (w/ OB)	404	73	$339,729	$112,252	$264,170	$329,277	$404,000	$479,284
Family Practice (w/o OB)	1,204	148	$313,345	$104,437	$241,928	$301,136	$369,827	$448,521
Family Practice: Sports Med	2	2	*	*	*	*	*	*
Gastroenterology	302	88	$722,466	$305,298	$536,286	$658,991	$833,001	$1,011,886
Gastroenterology: Hepatology	21	5	$608,388	$129,039	$514,373	$569,339	$669,780	$834,483
Geriatrics	23	11	$271,183	$108,639	$177,140	$240,164	$330,042	$456,212
Hematology/Oncology	144	50	$505,751	$428,534	$255,345	$372,110	$563,145	$949,304
Hem/Onc: Oncology (only)	47	17	$417,810	$182,107	$289,691	$357,858	$520,924	$688,114
Infectious Disease	67	31	$378,964	$173,551	$233,516	$354,771	$516,954	$617,265
Internal Medicine: General	1,266	153	$308,322	$116,517	$234,603	$296,034	$362,426	$448,582
Internal Med: Hospitalist	82	27	$214,806	$88,126	$141,602	$196,343	$278,956	$348,389
Internal Med: Pediatric	24	9	$315,131	$112,050	$214,716	$288,516	$394,235	$502,218
Nephrology	109	39	$430,572	$166,756	$342,888	$404,239	$474,733	$622,773
Neurology	207	65	$423,498	$237,313	$278,500	$374,813	$483,152	$773,804
OBGYN: General	383	89	$559,506	$269,954	$399,041	$512,459	$642,312	$823,656
OBGYN: Gynecology (only)	41	26	$376,923	$202,921	$235,534	$324,264	$480,246	$625,007
OBGYN: Gyn Oncology	11	7	$567,245	$286,150	$311,712	$498,436	$834,546	$964,528
OBGYN: Maternal & Fetal Med	24	8	$691,364	$349,720	$423,510	$610,827	$846,671	$1,430,670
OBGYN: Repro Endocrinology	12	4	$609,170	$305,588	$376,544	$470,715	$861,877	$1,140,801
Occupational Medicine	23	16	$379,750	$138,270	$259,897	$378,525	$486,775	$581,018
Ophthalmology	120	47	$708,148	$342,617	$490,588	$645,558	$869,100	$1,097,381
Ophthalmology: Pediatric	3	3	*	*	*	*	*	*
Ophthalmology: Retina	6	6	*	*	*	*	*	*
Orthopedic (Non-surgical)	21	10	$669,925	$311,102	$385,708	$628,513	$876,610	$1,085,604
Orthopedic Surgery: General	209	60	$792,078	$306,650	$591,383	$747,395	$941,836	$1,182,617
Ortho Surg: Foot & Ankle	12	9	$732,799	$163,273	$553,443	$746,130	$829,588	$980,845
Ortho Surg: Hand	30	19	$856,662	$268,133	$627,727	$890,790	$1,089,110	$1,239,161
Ortho Surg: Hip & Joint	29	12	$762,775	$213,381	$603,561	$685,015	$919,379	$1,083,092
Ortho Surg: Oncology	0	*	*	*	*	*	*	*
Ortho Surg: Pediatric	6	6	*	*	*	*	*	*
Ortho Surg: Spine	31	19	$1,253,268	$584,705	$819,443	$1,213,597	$1,600,456	$1,709,722
Ortho Surg: Trauma	14	8	$690,479	$374,081	$449,051	$527,830	$893,278	$1,403,090
Ortho Surg: Sports Med	49	25	$838,011	$287,626	$587,476	$883,271	$1,071,551	$1,206,054
Otorhinolaryngology	153	56	$688,149	$338,972	$478,334	$598,569	$810,844	$1,041,050
Otorhinolaryngology: Pediatric	0	*	*	*	*	*	*	*
Pathology: Anatomic & Clinical	40	12	$383,205	$156,535	$260,465	$386,312	$453,195	$538,740
Pathology: Anatomic	10	3	$553,665	$202,280	$453,195	$474,111	$721,293	$918,365
Pathology: Clinical	31	6	$391,138	$85,005	$334,550	$384,484	$462,119	$515,483

Table 15: Collections for Professional Charges (TC Excluded) (continued)

	Physicians	Medical Practices	Mean	Std. Dev.	25th %tile	Median	75th %tile	90th %tile
Pediatrics: General	721	119	$348,285	$122,314	$265,120	$334,297	$415,055	$509,033
Ped: Adolescent Medicine	16	3	$281,377	$79,250	$211,147	$273,139	$340,023	$416,900
Ped: Allergy/Immunology	5	4	*	*	*	*	*	*
Ped: Cardiology	18	8	$345,005	$135,101	$233,440	$362,204	$418,641	$522,318
Ped: Child Development	9	5	*	*	*	*	*	*
Ped: Critical Care/Intensivist	34	9	$361,130	$165,397	$219,224	$306,624	$536,289	$596,582
Ped: Emergency Medicine	6	1	*	*	*	*	*	*
Ped: Endocrinology	9	8	*	*	*	*	*	*
Ped: Gastroenterology	9	5	*	*	*	*	*	*
Ped: Genetics	7	3	*	*	*	*	*	*
Ped: Hematology/Oncology	16	9	$318,800	$226,372	$171,394	$272,468	$387,626	$665,049
Ped: Hospitalist	11	4	$166,923	$66,801	$110,954	$153,331	$182,044	$290,927
Ped: Infectious Disease	0	*	*	*	*	*	*	*
Ped: Neonatal Medicine	45	12	$504,755	$196,895	$342,784	$464,535	$676,554	$750,437
Ped: Nephrology	6	4	*	*	*	*	*	*
Ped: Neurology	21	11	$283,813	$184,899	$154,713	$213,701	$361,868	$671,412
Ped: Pulmonology	8	7	*	*	*	*	*	*
Ped: Rheumatology	3	2	*	*	*	*	*	*
Ped: Sports Medicine	0	*	*	*	*	*	*	*
Physiatry (Phys Med & Rehab)	36	23	$477,754	$214,828	$324,992	$395,799	$614,397	$805,689
Podiatry: General	49	31	$421,448	$159,368	$311,606	$379,629	$493,974	$701,610
Podiatry: Surg-Foot & Ankle	14	8	$449,915	$203,352	$279,112	$416,040	$537,664	$817,048
Podiatry: Surg-Forefoot Only	4	1	*	*	*	*	*	*
Psychiatry: General	96	29	$230,289	$92,236	$169,087	$211,874	$277,895	$347,243
Psychiatry: Child & Adolescent	16	9	$199,065	$58,141	$151,454	$186,008	$254,112	$292,003
Psychiatry: Geriatric	10	6	$409,693	$202,110	$213,752	$399,631	$621,589	$718,768
Pulmonary Medicine	96	49	$443,781	$288,890	$316,641	$399,461	$486,160	$623,743
Pulmonary Med: Critical Care	45	18	$385,879	$157,930	$265,930	$317,801	$471,788	$625,825
Radiation Oncology	57	17	$666,487	$242,112	$499,466	$613,214	$781,891	$978,556
Radiology: Diagnostic-Inv	145	19	$663,596	$203,799	$513,690	$639,193	$799,969	$937,067
Radiology: Diagnostic-Noninv	160	28	$608,674	$207,237	$477,167	$611,721	$759,537	$854,825
Radiology: Nuclear Medicine	13	9	$462,529	$218,958	$316,837	$435,459	$553,011	$875,094
Rheumatology	96	47	$397,536	$211,256	$263,230	$340,650	$452,655	$646,406
Sleep Medicine	2	1	*	*	*	*	*	*
Surgery: General	337	101	$567,084	$232,940	$424,996	$516,040	$670,029	$831,380
Surg: Cardiovascular	85	24	$763,301	$244,345	$593,934	$708,613	$887,868	$1,090,509
Surg: Cardiovascular-Pediatric	4	4	*	*	*	*	*	*
Surg: Colon and Rectal	19	10	$621,163	$263,435	$372,557	$674,598	$794,144	$998,791
Surg: Neurological	92	27	$1,040,884	$564,369	$691,609	$930,451	$1,182,625	$1,610,457
Surg: Oncology	7	3	*	*	*	*	*	*
Surg: Oral	20	7	$806,958	$284,819	$638,838	$800,000	$1,067,285	$1,155,550
Surg: Pediatric	10	5	$374,862	$108,374	$268,290	$393,396	$457,929	$533,428
Surg: Plastic & Reconstruction	47	24	$790,143	$542,058	$465,121	$641,568	$960,623	$1,592,012
Surg: Plastic & Recon-Hand	2	1	*	*	*	*	*	*
Surg: Plastic & Recon-Pediatric	2	1	*	*	*	*	*	*
Surg: Thoracic (primary)	21	4	$752,216	$275,440	$537,400	$800,206	$942,031	$1,127,166
Surg: Transplant	9	5	*	*	*	*	*	*
Surg: Trauma	11	4	$459,277	$297,339	$197,386	$515,148	$620,885	$1,056,138
Surg: Trauma-Burn	8	3	*	*	*	*	*	*
Surg: Vascular (primary)	43	22	$598,636	$245,906	$378,702	$599,344	$758,819	$943,487
Urgent Care	118	34	$378,652	$135,460	$289,754	$370,942	$459,754	$525,310
Urology	132	49	$744,067	$279,417	$570,004	$704,495	$856,121	$1,159,293
Urology: Pediatric	2	1	*	*	*	*	*	*

Table 16: Collections for Professional Charges (TC Excluded) by Hours Worked per Week

	Less than 40 hours		40 hours or more	
	Physicians	Median	Physicians	Median
Allergy/Immunology	7	*	32	$619,083
Anesthesiology	19	$330,899	235	$394,896
Anesth: Pain Management	1	*	18	$461,375
Anesth: Pediatric	0	*	13	*
Cardiology: Electrophysiology	1	*	18	$713,388
Cardiology: Invasive	0	*	65	$626,539
Cardiology: Inv-Intervntnl	0	*	98	$673,705
Cardiology: Noninvasive	4	*	64	$510,725
Critical Care: Intensivist	1	*	9	*
Dentistry	0	*	6	*
Dermatology	11	$604,018	65	$534,245
Dermatology: MOHS Surgery	2	*	6	*
Emergency Medicine	65	$281,512	42	$330,211
Endocrinology/Metabolism	6	*	38	$329,387
Family Practice (w/ OB)	34	$340,106	216	$310,831
Family Practice (w/o OB)	200	$329,467	734	$291,020
Family Practice: Sports Med	0	*	2	*
Gastroenterology	8	*	207	$648,084
Gastroenterology: Hepatology	0	*	21	$569,339
Geriatrics	6	*	12	$281,876
Hematology/Oncology	4	*	106	$383,751
Hem/Onc: Oncology (only)	1	*	28	$336,616
Infectious Disease	5	*	45	$372,847
Internal Medicine: General	130	$282,341	841	$306,000
Internal Med: Hospitalist	5	*	42	$198,515
Internal Med: Pediatric	3	*	20	$326,993
Nephrology	3	*	83	$404,239
Neurology	17	$326,165	149	$373,800
OBGYN: General	34	$596,827	248	$489,641
OBGYN: Gynecology (only)	4	*	27	$408,679
OBGYN: Gyn Oncology	1	*	6	*
OBGYN: Maternal & Fetal Med	2	*	21	$672,223
OBGYN: Repro Endocrinology	0	*	12	$470,715
Occupational Medicine	3	*	13	$386,309
Ophthalmology	16	$734,655	64	$639,549
Ophthalmology: Pediatric	1	*	2	*
Ophthalmology: Retina	0	*	4	*
Orthopedic (Non-surgical)	8	*	12	$682,677
Orthopedic Surgery: General	10	$786,325	105	$729,212
Ortho Surg: Foot & Ankle	2	*	8	*
Ortho Surg: Hand	3	*	23	$906,555
Ortho Surg: Hip & Joint	3	*	21	$644,117
Ortho Surg: Oncology	0	*	0	*
Ortho Surg: Pediatric	1	*	5	*
Ortho Surg: Spine	2	*	22	$1,219,643
Ortho Surg: Trauma	1	*	11	$511,731
Ortho Surg: Sports Med	5	*	41	$883,271
Otorhinolaryngology	18	$521,813	90	$633,012
Otorhinolaryngology: Pediatric	0	*	0	*
Pathology: Anatomic & Clinical	3	*	22	$345,521
Pathology: Anatomic	*	*	10	$474,111
Pathology: Clinical	2	*	29	$386,329

Table 16: Collections for Professional Charges (TC Excluded) by Hours Worked per Week (continued)

	Less than 40 hours		40 hours or more	
	Physicians	Median	Physicians	Median
Pathology: Clinical	2	*	29	$386,329
Pediatrics: General	132	$312,504	416	$344,993
Ped: Adolescent Medicine	0	*	2	*
Ped: Allergy/Immunology	*	*	4	*
Ped: Cardiology	0	*	17	$372,323
Ped: Child Development	0	*	3	*
Ped: Critical Care/Intensivist	4	*	30	$379,985
Ped: Emergency Medicine	0	*	5	*
Ped: Endocrinology	1	*	7	*
Ped: Gastroenterology	1	*	8	*
Ped: Genetics	2	*	5	*
Ped: Hematology/Oncology	1	*	15	$280,966
Ped: Hospitalist	1	*	10	$146,409
Ped: Infectious Disease	0	*	0	*
Ped: Neonatal Medicine	2	*	36	$587,016
Ped: Nephrology	0	*	5	*
Ped: Neurology	1	*	17	$213,701
Ped: Pulmonology	*	*	7	*
Ped: Rheumatology	0	*	3	*
Ped: Sports Medicine	*	*	0	*
Physiatry (Phys Med & Rehab)	0	*	29	$378,844
Podiatry: General	5	*	22	$341,567
Podiatry: Surg-Foot & Ankle	2	*	9	*
Podiatry: Surg-Forefoot Only	0	*	4	*
Psychiatry: General	11	$180,555	52	$190,644
Psychiatry: Child & Adolescent	2	*	11	$185,450
Psychiatry: Geriatric	*	*	10	$399,631
Pulmonary Medicine	5	*	58	$424,788
Pulmonary Med: Critical Care	5	*	23	$421,307
Radiation Oncology	3	*	45	$651,969
Radiology: Diagnostic-Inv	3	*	114	$617,562
Radiology: Diagnostic-Noninv	9	*	132	$614,218
Radiology: Nuclear Medicine	3	*	7	*
Rheumatology	12	$307,929	58	$380,214
Sleep Medicine	0	*	2	*
Surgery: General	12	$541,070	231	$508,961
Surg: Cardiovascular	0	*	57	$716,261
Surg: Cardiovascular-Pediatric	*	*	4	*
Surg: Colon and Rectal	2	*	12	$541,081
Surg: Neurological	1	*	74	$913,781
Surg: Oncology	*	*	1	*
Surg: Oral	4	*	13	$715,124
Surg: Pediatric	0	*	10	$393,396
Surg: Plastic & Reconstruction	1	*	28	$730,897
Surg: Plastic & Recon-Hand	*	*	0	*
Surg: Plastic & Recon-Pediatric	*	*	2	*
Surg: Thoracic (primary)	0	*	20	$809,124
Surg: Transplant	0	*	9	*
Surg: Trauma	0	*	6	*
Surg: Trauma-Burn	0	*	8	*
Surg: Vascular (primary)	1	*	31	$556,029
Urgent Care	25	$406,678	40	$358,759
Urology	10	$711,810	85	$711,811
Urology: Pediatric	*	*	2	*

Table 17: Collections for Professional Charges (TC Excluded) by Weeks Worked per Year

	Less than 46 weeks		46 weeks or more	
	Physicians	Median	Physicians	Median
Allergy/Immunology	2	*	41	$606,763
Anesthesiology	149	$420,606	98	$360,525
Anesth: Pain Management	8	*	12	$548,818
Anesth: Pediatric	7	*	6	*
Cardiology: Electrophysiology	5	*	13	$704,475
Cardiology: Invasive	18	$528,047	49	$673,396
Cardiology: Inv-Intervntnl	30	$631,930	74	$717,795
Cardiology: Noninvasive	17	$539,994	47	$518,942
Critical Care: Intensivist	1	*	4	*
Dentistry	4	*	5	*
Dermatology	17	$572,675	67	$569,610
Dermatology: MOHS Surgery	2	*	5	*
Emergency Medicine	59	$281,512	25	$307,547
Endocrinology/Metabolism	7	*	46	$341,503
Family Practice (w/ OB)	87	$296,502	210	$330,512
Family Practice (w/o OB)	179	$302,000	723	$307,000
Family Practice: Sports Med	0	*	2	*
Gastroenterology	56	$583,417	187	$674,674
Gastroenterology: Hepatology	0	*	21	$569,339
Geriatrics	2	*	7	*
Hematology/Oncology	12	$270,482	98	$459,313
Hem/Onc: Oncology (only)	2	*	30	$344,674
Infectious Disease	6	*	44	$405,173
Internal Medicine: General	181	$270,010	796	$304,185
Internal Med: Hospitalist	3	*	51	$192,296
Internal Med: Pediatric	0	*	22	$288,516
Nephrology	29	$426,097	56	$397,334
Neurology	47	$429,719	113	$348,665
OBGYN: General	70	$503,418	225	$527,986
OBGYN: Gynecology (only)	8	*	28	$308,480
OBGYN: Gyn Oncology	1	*	9	*
OBGYN: Maternal & Fetal Med	4	*	17	$727,989
OBGYN: Repro Endocrinology	1	*	11	$483,094
Occupational Medicine	2	*	13	$353,913
Ophthalmology	18	$604,985	67	$648,966
Ophthalmology: Pediatric	1	*	1	*
Ophthalmology: Retina	1	*	2	*
Orthopedic (Non-surgical)	0	*	17	$794,281
Orthopedic Surgery: General	46	$757,019	91	$714,866
Ortho Surg: Foot & Ankle	6	*	6	*
Ortho Surg: Hand	14	$803,699	14	$932,262
Ortho Surg: Hip & Joint	9	*	19	$675,127
Ortho Surg: Oncology	*	*	0	*
Ortho Surg: Pediatric	1	*	4	*
Ortho Surg: Spine	7	*	19	$1,202,130
Ortho Surg: Trauma	5	*	3	*
Ortho Surg: Sports Med	14	$913,774	30	$876,778
Otorhinolaryngology	29	$598,569	81	$597,303
Otorhinolaryngology: Pediatric	0	*	0	*
Pathology: Anatomic & Clinical	1	*	23	$401,478
Pathology: Anatomic	4	*	6	*
Pathology: Clinical	0	*	13	$378,767

Table 17: Collections for Professional Charges (TC Excluded) by Weeks Worked per Year (continued)

	Less than 46 weeks		46 weeks or more	
	Physicians	Median	Physicians	Median
Pediatrics: General	106	$312,672	481	$343,983
Ped: Adolescent Medicine	0	*	1	*
Ped: Allergy/Immunology	3	*	0	*
Ped: Cardiology	4	*	9	*
Ped: Child Development	*	*	2	*
Ped: Critical Care/Intensivist	17	$306,373	13	$536,779
Ped: Emergency Medicine	*	*	6	*
Ped: Endocrinology	2	*	5	*
Ped: Gastroenterology	2	*	4	*
Ped: Genetics	*	*	7	*
Ped: Hematology/Oncology	3	*	11	$280,966
Ped: Hospitalist	1	*	10	$146,409
Ped: Infectious Disease	*	*	0	*
Ped: Neonatal Medicine	20	$676,554	15	$510,769
Ped: Nephrology	*	*	4	*
Ped: Neurology	3	*	12	$202,062
Ped: Pulmonology	2	*	3	*
Ped: Rheumatology	*	*	3	*
Ped: Sports Medicine	*	*	0	*
Physiatry (Phys Med & Rehab)	4	*	22	$382,165
Podiatry: General	8	*	22	$359,518
Podiatry: Surg-Foot & Ankle	3	*	8	*
Podiatry: Surg-Forefoot Only	1	*	3	*
Psychiatry: General	22	$184,579	38	$249,547
Psychiatry: Child & Adolescent	5	*	8	*
Psychiatry: Geriatric	1	*	8	*
Pulmonary Medicine	10	$355,820	61	$412,671
Pulmonary Med: Critical Care	14	$287,106	22	$437,525
Radiation Oncology	35	$682,907	9	*
Radiology: Diagnostic-Inv	109	$614,371	17	$629,696
Radiology: Diagnostic-Noninv	111	$629,776	16	$574,342
Radiology: Nuclear Medicine	6	*	4	*
Rheumatology	5	*	71	$344,119
Sleep Medicine	2	*	0	*
Surgery: General	55	$525,784	209	$515,861
Surg: Cardiovascular	43	$719,733	25	$746,722
Surg: Cardiovascular-Pediatric	1	*	3	*
Surg: Colon and Rectal	5	*	9	*
Surg: Neurological	23	$1,091,604	61	$879,298
Surg: Oncology	*	*	2	*
Surg: Oral	4	*	10	$991,549
Surg: Pediatric	2	*	6	*
Surg: Plastic & Reconstruction	9	*	22	$648,317
Surg: Plastic & Recon-Hand	0	*	0	*
Surg: Plastic & Recon-Pediatric	0	*	2	*
Surg: Thoracic (primary)	1	*	20	$809,124
Surg: Transplant	*	*	8	*
Surg: Trauma	0	*	9	*
Surg: Trauma-Burn	0	*	8	*
Surg: Vascular (primary)	14	$618,104	19	$559,000
Urgent Care	11	$233,057	82	$366,403
Urology	28	$752,815	76	$703,901
Urology: Pediatric	*	*	2	*

Table 18: Collections for Professional Charges with 1-10% Technical Component

	Physicians	Medical Practices	Mean	Std. Dev.	25th %tile	Median	75th %tile	90th %tile
Allergy/Immunology	19	5	$784,761	$666,020	$303,441	$672,345	$972,843	$1,377,913
Anesthesiology	3	1	*	*	*	*	*	*
Anesth: Pain Management	9	2	*	*	*	*	*	*
Anesth: Pediatric	0	*	*	*	*	*	*	*
Cardiology: Electrophysiology	16	11	$736,601	$174,891	$553,555	$819,490	$870,434	$958,741
Cardiology: Invasive	84	24	$704,641	$339,157	$489,926	$639,137	$870,355	$1,049,528
Cardiology: Inv-Intervntnl	105	24	$940,532	$502,404	$568,729	$834,528	$1,182,538	$1,569,748
Cardiology: Noninvasive	61	27	$597,556	$289,045	$415,462	$528,861	$753,791	$973,018
Critical Care: Intensivist	0	*	*	*	*	*	*	*
Dentistry	0	*	*	*	*	*	*	*
Dermatology	32	19	$667,461	$370,632	$478,012	$611,619	$779,944	$1,102,447
Dermatology: MOHS Surgery	2	2	*	*	*	*	*	*
Emergency Medicine	8	3	*	*	*	*	*	*
Endocrinology/Metabolism	20	14	$377,207	$167,833	$231,215	$318,025	$545,868	$665,275
Family Practice (w/ OB)	184	44	$392,469	$141,453	$291,023	$364,254	$485,245	$599,289
Family Practice (w/o OB)	728	119	$398,510	$182,946	$291,587	$377,862	$470,088	$596,525
Family Practice: Sports Med	8	5	*	*	*	*	*	*
Gastroenterology	54	24	$736,613	$247,305	$619,975	$648,247	$834,172	$1,167,902
Gastroenterology: Hepatology	8	2	*	*	*	*	*	*
Geriatrics	3	2	*	*	*	*	*	*
Hematology/Oncology	21	11	$663,771	$531,474	$328,041	$407,358	$709,461	$1,768,488
Hem/Onc: Oncology (only)	2	2	*	*	*	*	*	*
Infectious Disease	6	4	*	*	*	*	*	*
Internal Medicine: General	498	81	$366,729	$148,338	$273,428	$354,734	$438,561	$531,698
Internal Med: Hospitalist	32	5	$272,409	$82,893	$199,854	$249,440	$358,471	$396,597
Internal Med: Pediatric	20	8	$347,155	$115,254	$246,205	$328,372	$439,700	$528,829
Nephrology	6	4	*	*	*	*	*	*
Neurology	35	16	$420,274	$110,357	$362,896	$401,925	$477,348	$583,145
OBGYN: General	237	39	$641,564	$669,265	$450,817	$558,040	$701,089	$896,000
OBGYN: Gynecology (only)	9	8	*	*	*	*	*	*
OBGYN: Gyn Oncology	0	*	*	*	*	*	*	*
OBGYN: Maternal & Fetal Med	4	2	*	*	*	*	*	*
OBGYN: Repro Endocrinology	1	1	*	*	*	*	*	*
Occupational Medicine	6	3	*	*	*	*	*	*
Ophthalmology	84	23	$813,384	$355,308	$591,198	$748,001	$976,667	$1,257,873
Ophthalmology: Pediatric	6	4	*	*	*	*	*	*
Ophthalmology: Retina	19	4	$1,086,707	$315,445	$860,578	$1,111,125	$1,290,766	$1,500,019
Orthopedic (Non-surgical)	1	1	*	*	*	*	*	*
Orthopedic Surgery: General	167	43	$833,324	$250,152	$658,857	$789,269	$982,799	$1,197,519
Ortho Surg: Foot & Ankle	13	12	$818,834	$272,724	$610,063	$702,243	$1,050,731	$1,286,080
Ortho Surg: Hand	35	18	$875,085	$368,754	$605,059	$797,340	$1,029,820	$1,583,795
Ortho Surg: Hip & Joint	29	18	$915,495	$424,022	$643,025	$782,500	$1,191,038	$1,379,608
Ortho Surg: Oncology	0	*	*	*	*	*	*	*
Ortho Surg: Pediatric	10	7	$773,039	$246,420	$625,793	$732,325	$958,723	$1,228,839
Ortho Surg: Spine	36	24	$1,050,246	$532,398	$741,762	$894,996	$1,349,505	$1,610,450
Ortho Surg: Trauma	6	3	*	*	*	*	*	*
Ortho Surg: Sports Med	62	26	$960,115	$574,567	$591,372	$881,789	$1,077,624	$1,793,285
Otorhinolaryngology	38	15	$600,337	$177,777	$494,908	$573,468	$699,857	$881,359
Otorhinolaryngology: Pediatric	6	2	*	*	*	*	*	*
Pathology: Anatomic & Clinical	4	1	*	*	*	*	*	*
Pathology: Anatomic	3	2	*	*	*	*	*	*
Pathology: Clinical	7	2	*	*	*	*	*	*

Table 18: Collections for Professional Charges with 1-10% Technical Component (continued)

	Physicians	Medical Practices	Mean	Std. Dev.	25th %tile	Median	75th %tile	90th %tile
Pediatrics: General	214	46	$374,662	$121,872	$293,586	$379,486	$447,277	$521,201
Ped: Adolescent Medicine	6	1	*	*	*	*	*	*
Ped: Allergy/Immunology	0	*	*	*	*	*	*	*
Ped: Cardiology	1	1	*	*	*	*	*	*
Ped: Child Development	0	*	*	*	*	*	*	*
Ped: Critical Care/Intensivist	1	1	*	*	*	*	*	*
Ped: Emergency Medicine	0	*	*	*	*	*	*	*
Ped: Endocrinology	0	*	*	*	*	*	*	*
Ped: Gastroenterology	1	1	*	*	*	*	*	*
Ped: Genetics	3	1	*	*	*	*	*	*
Ped: Hematology/Oncology	2	2	*	*	*	*	*	*
Ped: Hospitalist	2	2	*	*	*	*	*	*
Ped: Infectious Disease	2	1	*	*	*	*	*	*
Ped: Neonatal Medicine	1	1	*	*	*	*	*	*
Ped: Nephrology	0	*	*	*	*	*	*	*
Ped: Neurology	1	1	*	*	*	*	*	*
Ped: Pulmonology	5	1	*	*	*	*	*	*
Ped: Rheumatology	0	*	*	*	*	*	*	*
Ped: Sports Medicine	0	*	*	*	*	*	*	*
Physiatry (Phys Med & Rehab)	20	12	$454,471	$251,112	$295,748	$345,008	$531,688	$942,087
Podiatry: General	6	6	*	*	*	*	*	*
Podiatry: Surg-Foot & Ankle	2	2	*	*	*	*	*	*
Podiatry: Surg-Forefoot Only	3	2	*	*	*	*	*	*
Psychiatry: General	6	3	*	*	*	*	*	*
Psychiatry: Child & Adolescent	1	1	*	*	*	*	*	*
Psychiatry: Geriatric	0	*	*	*	*	*	*	*
Pulmonary Medicine	51	18	$444,837	$251,542	$332,793	$389,916	$476,759	$630,790
Pulmonary Med: Critical Care	17	7	$567,167	$291,885	$421,945	$453,722	$555,664	$1,222,934
Radiation Oncology	2	2	*	*	*	*	*	*
Radiology: Diagnostic-Inv	40	9	$768,963	$413,453	$581,494	$678,493	$738,853	$1,375,229
Radiology: Diagnostic-Noninv	9	3	*	*	*	*	*	*
Radiology: Nuclear Medicine	4	3	*	*	*	*	*	*
Rheumatology	28	19	$610,662	$718,818	$309,747	$406,875	$545,686	$1,146,237
Sleep Medicine	0	*	*	*	*	*	*	*
Surgery: General	71	28	$569,505	$225,575	$404,657	$578,098	$712,964	$793,944
Surg: Cardiovascular	7	3	*	*	*	*	*	*
Surg: Cardiovascular-Pediatric	0	*	*	*	*	*	*	*
Surg: Colon and Rectal	0	*	*	*	*	*	*	*
Surg: Neurological	16	10	$762,733	$233,261	$600,096	$768,885	$943,545	$1,042,680
Surg: Oncology	0	*	*	*	*	*	*	*
Surg: Oral	1	1	*	*	*	*	*	*
Surg: Pediatric	0	*	*	*	*	*	*	*
Surg: Plastic & Reconstruction	6	5	*	*	*	*	*	*
Surg: Plastic & Recon-Hand	7	1	*	*	*	*	*	*
Surg: Plastic & Recon-Pediatric	0	*	*	*	*	*	*	*
Surg: Thoracic (primary)	2	1	*	*	*	*	*	*
Surg: Transplant	0	*	*	*	*	*	*	*
Surg: Trauma	0	*	*	*	*	*	*	*
Surg: Trauma-Burn	0	*	*	*	*	*	*	*
Surg: Vascular (primary)	14	7	$573,271	$158,148	$437,266	$544,133	$671,355	$843,470
Urgent Care	62	13	$402,576	$185,106	$284,404	$360,457	$467,843	$608,379
Urology	60	23	$719,735	$270,203	$516,938	$677,573	$875,047	$1,005,032
Urology: Pediatric	1	1	*	*	*	*	*	*

Table 19: Collections for Professional Charges with over 10% Technical Component

	Physicians	Medical Practices	Mean	Std. Dev.	25th %tile	Median	75th %tile	90th %tile
Allergy/Immunology	15	7	$649,674	$405,890	$391,252	$568,025	$892,126	$1,365,975
Anesthesiology	74	3	$388,671	$159,200	$296,550	$353,224	$442,958	$674,583
Anesth: Pain Management	0	*	*	*	*	*	*	*
Anesth: Pediatric	6	2	*	*	*	*	*	*
Cardiology: Electrophysiology	14	13	$890,744	$277,375	$675,664	$904,914	$1,100,260	$1,325,117
Cardiology: Invasive	69	18	$936,689	$371,293	$653,882	$864,261	$1,193,399	$1,434,639
Cardiology: Inv-Intervntnl	118	26	$1,013,405	$504,746	$670,897	$902,286	$1,192,321	$1,738,597
Cardiology: Noninvasive	79	26	$927,451	$513,713	$561,997	$789,854	$1,268,812	$1,625,656
Critical Care: Intensivist	3	2	*	*	*	*	*	*
Dentistry	9	1	*	*	*	*	*	*
Dermatology	4	3	*	*	*	*	*	*
Dermatology: MOHS Surgery	1	1	*	*	*	*	*	*
Emergency Medicine	0	*	*	*	*	*	*	*
Endocrinology/Metabolism	4	2	*	*	*	*	*	*
Family Practice (w/ OB)	122	22	$380,508	$138,626	$287,256	$364,807	$459,131	$560,493
Family Practice (w/o OB)	220	37	$367,618	$141,167	$278,943	$348,472	$417,691	$533,615
Family Practice: Sports Med	3	2	*	*	*	*	*	*
Gastroenterology	22	9	$804,280	$314,515	$672,384	$799,010	$858,295	$1,420,853
Gastroenterology: Hepatology	12	1	*	*	*	*	*	*
Geriatrics	1	1	*	*	*	*	*	*
Hematology/Oncology	10	7	$1,424,513	$1,139,159	$470,659	$1,141,532	$2,184,836	$3,675,338
Hem/Onc: Oncology (only)	1	1	*	*	*	*	*	*
Infectious Disease	5	2	*	*	*	*	*	*
Internal Medicine: General	200	39	$392,441	$126,641	$302,418	$379,489	$459,814	$560,581
Internal Med: Hospitalist	19	5	$229,213	$81,462	$152,458	$210,275	$264,608	$367,829
Internal Med: Pediatric	1	1	*	*	*	*	*	*
Nephrology	8	3	*	*	*	*	*	*
Neurology	36	10	$595,461	$238,821	$397,484	$567,019	$792,156	$978,369
OBGYN: General	64	22	$562,015	$218,383	$440,231	$560,672	$672,418	$842,395
OBGYN: Gynecology (only)	1	1	*	*	*	*	*	*
OBGYN: Gyn Oncology	0	*	*	*	*	*	*	*
OBGYN: Maternal & Fetal Med	1	1	*	*	*	*	*	*
OBGYN: Repro Endocrinology	1	1	*	*	*	*	*	*
Occupational Medicine	0	*	*	*	*	*	*	*
Ophthalmology	10	7	$606,863	$317,814	$328,206	$655,582	$792,052	$1,196,187
Ophthalmology: Pediatric	0	*	*	*	*	*	*	*
Ophthalmology: Retina	15	4	$1,445,227	$330,544	$1,278,432	$1,375,000	$1,550,000	$2,132,320
Orthopedic (Non-surgical)	0	*	*	*	*	*	*	*
Orthopedic Surgery: General	42	16	$739,981	$302,616	$510,449	$653,048	$928,825	$1,280,701
Ortho Surg: Foot & Ankle	5	5	*	*	*	*	*	*
Ortho Surg: Hand	6	6	*	*	*	*	*	*
Ortho Surg: Hip & Joint	4	3	*	*	*	*	*	*
Ortho Surg: Oncology	0	*	*	*	*	*	*	*
Ortho Surg: Pediatric	2	2	*	*	*	*	*	*
Ortho Surg: Spine	2	2	*	*	*	*	*	*
Ortho Surg: Trauma	1	1	*	*	*	*	*	*
Ortho Surg: Sports Med	14	7	$885,597	$218,014	$741,987	$787,895	$1,060,253	$1,272,834
Otorhinolaryngology	12	5	$755,934	$229,553	$545,283	$761,523	$887,512	$1,112,398
Otorhinolaryngology: Pediatric	0	*	*	*	*	*	*	*
Pathology: Anatomic & Clinical	3	1	*	*	*	*	*	*
Pathology: Anatomic	0	*	*	*	*	*	*	*
Pathology: Clinical	0	*	*	*	*	*	*	*

Table 19: Collections for Professional Charges with over 10% Technical Component (continued)

	Physicians	Medical Practices	Mean	Std. Dev.	25th %tile	Median	75th %tile	90th %tile
Pediatrics: General	81	19	$360,494	$121,558	$290,934	$335,467	$409,197	$543,065
Ped: Adolescent Medicine	0	*	*	*	*	*	*	*
Ped: Allergy/Immunology	1	1	*	*	*	*	*	*
Ped: Cardiology	9	3	*	*	*	*	*	*
Ped: Child Development	0	*	*	*	*	*	*	*
Ped: Critical Care/Intensivist	0	*	*	*	*	*	*	*
Ped: Emergency Medicine	0	*	*	*	*	*	*	*
Ped: Endocrinology	0	*	*	*	*	*	*	*
Ped: Gastroenterology	0	*	*	*	*	*	*	*
Ped: Genetics	0	*	*	*	*	*	*	*
Ped: Hematology/Oncology	0	*	*	*	*	*	*	*
Ped: Hospitalist	0	*	*	*	*	*	*	*
Ped: Infectious Disease	0	*	*	*	*	*	*	*
Ped: Neonatal Medicine	0	*	*	*	*	*	*	*
Ped: Nephrology	0	*	*	*	*	*	*	*
Ped: Neurology	1	1	*	*	*	*	*	*
Ped: Pulmonology	0	*	*	*	*	*	*	*
Ped: Rheumatology	0	*	*	*	*	*	*	*
Ped: Sports Medicine	0	*	*	*	*	*	*	*
Physiatry (Phys Med & Rehab)	2	2	*	*	*	*	*	*
Podiatry: General	4	3	*	*	*	*	*	*
Podiatry: Surg-Foot & Ankle	10	2	*	*	*	*	*	*
Podiatry: Surg-Forefoot Only	0	*	*	*	*	*	*	*
Psychiatry: General	5	3	*	*	*	*	*	*
Psychiatry: Child & Adolescent	0	*	*	*	*	*	*	*
Psychiatry: Geriatric	0	*	*	*	*	*	*	*
Pulmonary Medicine	12	8	$476,974	$145,217	$334,419	$456,531	$630,988	$676,924
Pulmonary Med: Critical Care	17	5	$486,835	$190,736	$348,649	$449,738	$721,217	$751,065
Radiation Oncology	4	1	*	*	*	*	*	*
Radiology: Diagnostic-Inv	25	6	$1,880,299	$1,033,470	$805,695	$1,810,806	$2,686,422	$3,429,632
Radiology: Diagnostic-Noninv	34	10	$1,129,160	$463,289	$803,045	$946,394	$1,607,177	$1,892,501
Radiology: Nuclear Medicine	2	2	*	*	*	*	*	*
Rheumatology	13	9	$458,668	$179,385	$322,296	$456,000	$552,346	$772,342
Sleep Medicine	0	*	*	*	*	*	*	*
Surgery: General	37	13	$516,646	$268,612	$387,731	$476,641	$564,203	$674,563
Surg: Cardiovascular	5	1	*	*	*	*	*	*
Surg: Cardiovascular-Pediatric	0	*	*	*	*	*	*	*
Surg: Colon and Rectal	0	*	*	*	*	*	*	*
Surg: Neurological	12	4	$697,123	$230,075	$602,688	$691,059	$766,532	$1,099,876
Surg: Oncology	1	1	*	*	*	*	*	*
Surg: Oral	0	*	*	*	*	*	*	*
Surg: Pediatric	0	*	*	*	*	*	*	*
Surg: Plastic & Reconstruction	1	1	*	*	*	*	*	*
Surg: Plastic & Recon-Hand	1	1	*	*	*	*	*	*
Surg: Plastic & Recon-Pediatric	0	*	*	*	*	*	*	*
Surg: Thoracic (primary)	0	*	*	*	*	*	*	*
Surg: Transplant	0	*	*	*	*	*	*	*
Surg: Trauma	0	*	*	*	*	*	*	*
Surg: Trauma-Burn	0	*	*	*	*	*	*	*
Surg: Vascular (primary)	5	2	*	*	*	*	*	*
Urgent Care	32	6	$549,834	$233,044	$407,372	$468,466	$634,000	$940,900
Urology	19	6	$974,251	$294,817	$678,213	$997,535	$1,281,555	$1,371,379
Urology: Pediatric	0	*	*	*	*	*	*	*

Table 20: Physician Compensation to Collections Ratio (TC Excluded)

	Physicians	Medical Practices	Mean	Std. Dev.	25th %tile	Median	75th %tile	90th %tile
Allergy/Immunology	54	37	.506	.156	.408	.498	.579	.687
Anesthesiology	297	34	.820	.293	.627	.799	.943	1.109
Anesth: Pain Management	23	10	.591	.146	.480	.557	.653	.862
Anesth: Pediatric	13	1	*	*	*	*	*	*
Cardiology: Electrophysiology	22	16	.606	.230	.456	.578	.820	.961
Cardiology: Invasive	74	32	.619	.207	.462	.583	.765	.908
Cardiology: Inv-Intervntnl	116	37	.698	.512	.489	.623	.804	.908
Cardiology: Noninvasive	97	41	.654	.323	.471	.602	.779	.918
Critical Care: Intensivist	13	7	1.009	.580	.608	.849	1.212	2.194
Dentistry	9	3	*	*	*	*	*	*
Dermatology	110	57	.482	.132	.398	.448	.551	.665
Dermatology: MOHS Surgery	9	8	*	*	*	*	*	*
Emergency Medicine	145	14	.800	.272	.651	.746	.903	1.125
Endocrinology/Metabolism	72	46	.599	.193	.467	.588	.687	.797
Family Practice (w/ OB)	404	73	.517	.144	.418	.509	.587	.665
Family Practice (w/o OB)	1,192	147	.541	.156	.429	.523	.623	.722
Family Practice: Sports Med	2	2	*	*	*	*	*	*
Gastroenterology	301	87	.539	.185	.414	.525	.638	.739
Gastroenterology: Hepatology	21	5	.458	.115	.373	.420	.510	.688
Geriatrics	23	11	.631	.236	.392	.689	.836	.928
Hematology/Oncology	143	49	1.141	.654	.702	.929	1.458	2.073
Hem/Onc: Oncology (only)	47	17	.977	.361	.714	.849	1.130	1.602
Infectious Disease	67	31	.651	.267	.466	.587	.775	1.089
Internal Medicine: General	1,259	152	.575	.201	.437	.542	.651	.823
Internal Med: Hospitalist	82	27	.898	.276	.672	.854	1.086	1.271
Internal Med: Pediatric	24	9	.561	.166	.452	.535	.655	.819
Nephrology	108	38	.596	.225	.426	.558	.691	.835
Neurology	205	64	.603	.246	.463	.552	.668	.896
OBGYN: General	380	88	.504	.136	.405	.496	.581	.673
OBGYN: Gynecology (only)	41	26	.615	.324	.447	.525	.676	1.044
OBGYN: Gyn Oncology	11	7	.709	.228	.550	.609	.786	1.222
OBGYN: Maternal & Fetal Med	24	8	.592	.325	.425	.527	.748	1.014
OBGYN: Repro Endocrinology	12	4	.529	.183	.368	.545	.672	.796
Occupational Medicine	23	16	.549	.199	.422	.483	.661	.909
Ophthalmology	118	46	.443	.117	.372	.426	.521	.580
Ophthalmology: Pediatric	3	3	*	*	*	*	*	*
Ophthalmology: Retina	5	5	*	*	*	*	*	*
Orthopedic (Non-surgical)	20	10	.454	.105	.371	.425	.543	.581
Orthopedic Surgery: General	207	59	.520	.130	.430	.497	.586	.724
Ortho Surg: Foot & Ankle	12	9	.608	.259	.459	.548	.732	1.132
Ortho Surg: Hand	30	19	.568	.143	.440	.583	.675	.756
Ortho Surg: Hip & Joint	29	12	.585	.203	.459	.543	.667	.938
Ortho Surg: Oncology	0	*	*	*	*	*	*	*
Ortho Surg: Pediatric	6	6	*	*	*	*	*	*
Ortho Surg: Spine	31	19	.543	.151	.437	.560	.635	.716
Ortho Surg: Trauma	14	8	.580	.222	.381	.559	.684	.982
Ortho Surg: Sports Med	49	25	.485	.115	.390	.491	.580	.611
Otorhinolaryngology	151	55	.484	.124	.394	.449	.564	.652
Otorhinolaryngology: Pediatric	0	*	*	*	*	*	*	*
Pathology: Anatomic & Clinical	40	12	.755	.353	.497	.708	.856	1.185
Pathology: Anatomic	10	3	.620	.401	.320	.558	.771	1.510
Pathology: Clinical	31	6	.428	.117	.340	.400	.479	.641

Table 20: Physician Compensation to Collections Ratio (TC Excluded) (continued)

	Physicians	Medical Practices	Mean	Std. Dev.	25th %tile	Median	75th %tile	90th %tile
Pediatrics: General	717	118	.497	.151	.399	.475	.569	.664
Ped: Adolescent Medicine	16	3	.578	.110	.531	.566	.680	.713
Ped: Allergy/Immunology	5	4	*	*	*	*	*	*
Ped: Cardiology	18	8	.671	.224	.514	.627	.799	1.052
Ped: Child Development	9	5	*	*	*	*	*	*
Ped: Critical Care/Intensivist	34	9	.931	.426	.634	.895	1.157	1.520
Ped: Emergency Medicine	6	1	*	*	*	*	*	*
Ped: Endocrinology	9	8	*	*	*	*	*	*
Ped: Gastroenterology	9	5	*	*	*	*	*	*
Ped: Genetics	7	3	*	*	*	*	*	*
Ped: Hematology/Oncology	16	9	.715	.256	.459	.727	.911	1.101
Ped: Hospitalist	11	4	1.081	.294	.702	1.214	1.269	1.369
Ped: Infectious Disease	0	*	*	*	*	*	*	*
Ped: Neonatal Medicine	45	12	.683	.236	.503	.658	.892	.986
Ped: Nephrology	6	4	*	*	*	*	*	*
Ped: Neurology	21	11	.807	.236	.559	.881	1.009	1.103
Ped: Pulmonology	8	7	*	*	*	*	*	*
Ped: Rheumatology	3	2	*	*	*	*	*	*
Ped: Sports Medicine	0	*	*	*	*	*	*	*
Physiatry (Phys Med & Rehab)	36	23	.572	.176	.447	.513	.674	.825
Podiatry: General	48	30	.423	.069	.383	.422	.461	.508
Podiatry: Surg-Foot & Ankle	14	8	.383	.090	.328	.413	.440	.493
Podiatry: Surg-Forefoot Only	3	1	*	*	*	*	*	*
Psychiatry: General	96	29	.785	.379	.584	.677	.869	1.235
Psychiatry: Child & Adolescent	16	9	.947	.374	.730	.873	1.074	1.449
Psychiatry: Geriatric	10	6	.719	.397	.479	.549	.878	1.659
Pulmonary Medicine	94	48	.571	.174	.464	.555	.625	.825
Pulmonary Med: Critical Care	45	18	.674	.172	.556	.666	.748	.940
Radiation Oncology	57	17	.671	.210	.501	.689	.783	.894
Radiology: Diagnostic-Inv	145	19	.701	.353	.522	.631	.843	1.005
Radiology: Diagnostic-Noninv	160	28	.688	.221	.510	.680	.849	.968
Radiology: Nuclear Medicine	13	9	.786	.499	.414	.605	1.132	1.735
Rheumatology	95	46	.596	.214	.454	.580	.722	.853
Sleep Medicine	2	1	*	*	*	*	*	*
Surgery: General	334	100	.565	.218	.436	.525	.635	.755
Surg: Cardiovascular	85	24	.657	.168	.570	.626	.758	.866
Surg: Cardiovascular-Pediatric	4	4	*	*	*	*	*	*
Surg: Colon and Rectal	19	10	.518	.148	.413	.472	.567	.726
Surg: Neurological	91	27	.542	.146	.467	.544	.635	.700
Surg: Oncology	7	3	*	*	*	*	*	*
Surg: Oral	20	7	.364	.114	.268	.355	.423	.570
Surg: Pediatric	9	4	*	*	*	*	*	*
Surg: Plastic & Reconstruction	47	24	.488	.133	.403	.485	.575	.641
Surg: Plastic & Recon-Hand	2	1	*	*	*	*	*	*
Surg: Plastic & Recon-Pediatric	2	1	*	*	*	*	*	*
Surg: Thoracic (primary)	21	4	.722	.227	.494	.725	.906	1.033
Surg: Transplant	9	5	*	*	*	*	*	*
Surg: Trauma	11	4	.915	.378	.585	.833	1.169	1.683
Surg: Trauma-Burn	8	3	*	*	*	*	*	*
Surg: Vascular (primary)	43	22	.644	.318	.449	.529	.733	1.178
Urgent Care	118	34	.458	.185	.385	.465	.515	.615
Urology	130	48	.476	.178	.358	.461	.575	.676
Urology: Pediatric	2	1	*	*	*	*	*	*

Table 21: Physician Gross Charges (TC Excluded)

	Physicians	Medical Practices	Mean	Std. Dev.	25th %tile	Median	75th %tile	90th %tile
Allergy/Immunology	75	52	$755,485	$387,550	$468,718	$692,340	$910,459	$1,288,175
Anesthesiology	350	42	$832,548	$400,004	$601,119	$769,094	$951,775	$1,133,038
Anesth: Pain Management	30	13	$1,355,567	$579,056	$895,388	$1,301,730	$1,746,365	$1,951,394
Anesth: Pediatric	0	*	*	*	*	*	*	*
Cardiology: Electrophysiology	24	17	$1,746,033	$989,168	$1,064,283	$1,702,206	$2,200,150	$3,270,973
Cardiology: Invasive	106	41	$1,520,015	$736,571	$963,416	$1,438,519	$1,977,603	$2,459,859
Cardiology: Inv-Intervntnl	135	44	$1,766,340	$733,792	$1,318,414	$1,627,381	$2,022,512	$3,077,450
Cardiology: Noninvasive	107	45	$1,301,793	$735,311	$712,437	$1,177,541	$1,616,884	$2,202,524
Critical Care: Intensivist	17	9	$531,227	$300,002	$260,864	$530,557	$635,592	$1,007,931
Dentistry	10	4	$390,095	$235,253	$254,498	$350,597	$435,327	$955,195
Dermatology	143	74	$968,470	$390,432	$697,902	$910,607	$1,235,982	$1,433,257
Dermatology: MOHS Surgery	13	11	$1,852,717	$437,597	$1,427,761	$1,961,733	$2,139,445	$2,511,120
Emergency Medicine	182	18	$638,688	$248,863	$450,732	$612,001	$814,959	$979,533
Endocrinology/Metabolism	93	57	$535,439	$342,352	$368,910	$452,417	$579,287	$881,686
Family Practice (w/ OB)	625	91	$471,771	$148,217	$373,947	$442,429	$549,518	$666,733
Family Practice (w/o OB)	1,745	186	$470,099	$193,994	$342,647	$431,376	$550,066	$717,076
Family Practice: Sports Med	3	3	*	*	*	*	*	*
Gastroenterology	331	102	$1,478,564	$544,511	$1,130,255	$1,433,899	$1,732,198	$2,213,022
Gastroenterology: Hepatology	19	3	$1,201,670	$263,782	$983,657	$1,192,009	$1,409,847	$1,504,202
Geriatrics	20	13	$317,059	$121,133	$243,002	$295,628	$406,360	$520,468
Hematology/Oncology	171	59	$701,389	$430,746	$427,039	$612,245	$849,100	$1,191,675
Hem/Onc: Oncology (only)	47	21	$641,365	$297,624	$452,393	$551,103	$786,568	$1,087,317
Infectious Disease	77	39	$557,042	$276,458	$343,041	$515,902	$743,323	$1,014,818
Internal Medicine: General	1,535	181	$460,411	$192,357	$338,669	$426,044	$539,407	$678,261
Internal Med: Hospitalist	154	37	$374,521	$148,930	$264,142	$345,936	$452,784	$604,887
Internal Med: Pediatric	31	13	$414,232	$181,243	$303,945	$351,818	$505,863	$705,941
Nephrology	134	47	$754,814	$292,372	$535,890	$732,353	$944,198	$1,083,826
Neurology	224	75	$709,576	$398,689	$489,938	$624,120	$820,499	$1,076,906
OBGYN: General	538	115	$923,820	$405,281	$679,740	$874,092	$1,079,366	$1,361,118
OBGYN: Gynecology (only)	90	33	$781,265	$352,902	$489,832	$773,066	$986,809	$1,258,014
OBGYN: Gyn Oncology	12	8	$1,092,466	$598,515	$633,575	$980,179	$1,672,686	$1,973,738
OBGYN: Maternal & Fetal Med	31	10	$1,067,299	$601,300	$645,160	$1,001,744	$1,352,110	$1,861,095
OBGYN: Repro Endocrinology	11	4	$869,943	$184,985	$754,999	$850,336	$952,649	$1,231,033
Occupational Medicine	47	25	$408,614	$139,782	$281,161	$390,492	$525,102	$610,423
Ophthalmology	152	63	$1,302,468	$667,296	$852,996	$1,150,407	$1,633,727	$2,111,403
Ophthalmology: Pediatric	3	3	*	*	*	*	*	*
Ophthalmology: Retina	6	6	*	*	*	*	*	*
Orthopedic (Non-surgical)	11	9	$1,036,759	$413,199	$611,433	$995,923	$1,417,713	$1,582,801
Orthopedic Surgery: General	252	71	$1,521,862	$804,769	$1,072,485	$1,378,255	$1,750,987	$2,294,463
Ortho Surg: Foot & Ankle	13	10	$1,905,254	$931,375	$1,282,172	$1,501,757	$2,340,019	$3,780,114
Ortho Surg: Hand	30	20	$1,854,479	$983,492	$1,276,909	$1,515,303	$2,186,714	$2,929,992
Ortho Surg: Hip & Joint	29	12	$1,645,848	$419,835	$1,247,930	$1,641,946	$2,059,012	$2,156,468
Ortho Surg: Oncology	0	*	*	*	*	*	*	*
Ortho Surg: Pediatric	7	7	*	*	*	*	*	*
Ortho Surg: Spine	34	22	$2,847,291	$1,706,175	$1,442,619	$2,479,173	$3,670,969	$6,174,830
Ortho Surg: Trauma	12	7	$1,348,342	$270,222	$1,159,577	$1,289,043	$1,406,925	$1,921,094
Ortho Surg: Sports Med	55	28	$1,613,278	$769,165	$1,089,216	$1,587,659	$2,022,237	$2,440,954
Otorhinolaryngology	195	76	$1,276,567	$620,772	$841,208	$1,122,047	$1,624,108	$2,037,970
Otorhinolaryngology: Pediatric	1	1	*	*	*	*	*	*
Pathology: Anatomic & Clinical	48	15	$799,155	$427,265	$603,383	$754,221	$991,174	$1,074,398
Pathology: Anatomic	10	3	$1,045,398	$497,351	$754,221	$857,718	$1,381,126	$1,994,277
Pathology: Clinical	16	6	$643,198	$283,955	$409,960	$613,418	$905,889	$998,085

Table 21: Physician Gross Charges (TC Excluded) (continued)

	Physicians	Medical Practices	Mean	Std. Dev.	25th %tile	Median	75th %tile	90th %tile
Pediatrics: General	925	148	$495,593	$178,520	$369,984	$465,456	$585,898	$732,941
Ped: Adolescent Medicine	38	8	$474,974	$129,376	$391,003	$469,359	$556,059	$625,726
Ped: Allergy/Immunology	6	5	*	*	*	*	*	*
Ped: Cardiology	20	10	$748,122	$224,628	$593,113	$720,420	$912,041	$1,028,563
Ped: Child Development	11	5	$318,144	$153,437	$185,767	$307,206	$411,086	$612,149
Ped: Critical Care/Intensivist	29	11	$471,204	$171,979	$329,324	$413,278	$575,459	$765,424
Ped: Emergency Medicine	6	1	*	*	*	*	*	*
Ped: Endocrinology	11	9	$311,007	$188,017	$140,147	$270,989	$522,976	$633,689
Ped: Gastroenterology	10	6	$528,454	$79,943	$438,290	$564,379	$590,366	$609,242
Ped: Genetics	7	3	*	*	*	*	*	*
Ped: Hematology/Oncology	18	11	$637,069	$407,274	$326,252	$513,822	$867,426	$1,252,958
Ped: Hospitalist	13	5	$284,488	$55,052	$242,782	$276,284	$304,178	$393,308
Ped: Infectious Disease	1	1	*	*	*	*	*	*
Ped: Neonatal Medicine	55	15	$881,715	$365,025	$573,204	$865,323	$1,180,344	$1,411,387
Ped: Nephrology	6	4	*	*	*	*	*	*
Ped: Neurology	25	14	$480,344	$300,260	$278,238	$361,038	$622,034	$1,095,804
Ped: Pulmonology	8	7	*	*	*	*	*	*
Ped: Rheumatology	3	2	*	*	*	*	*	*
Ped: Sports Medicine	0	*	*	*	*	*	*	*
Physiatry (Phys Med & Rehab)	51	28	$666,964	$369,586	$412,227	$597,948	$785,164	$1,111,239
Podiatry: General	69	40	$670,728	$262,759	$510,496	$614,746	$737,139	$1,080,044
Podiatry: Surg-Foot & Ankle	17	10	$695,154	$198,308	$569,381	$682,368	$782,058	$1,085,994
Podiatry: Surg-Forefoot Only	5	2	*	*	*	*	*	*
Psychiatry: General	128	39	$359,497	$134,253	$269,633	$366,232	$439,668	$533,266
Psychiatry: Child & Adolescent	21	12	$412,131	$177,072	$292,964	$393,442	$494,268	$705,279
Psychiatry: Geriatric	10	6	$681,612	$310,853	$380,123	$650,160	$1,014,136	$1,177,503
Pulmonary Medicine	115	60	$799,620	$473,850	$595,007	$707,168	$865,272	$1,089,870
Pulmonary Med: Critical Care	60	22	$718,312	$255,915	$492,760	$728,715	$880,582	$1,003,246
Radiation Oncology	61	20	$1,614,727	$648,299	$1,200,000	$1,476,232	$1,887,515	$2,444,247
Radiology: Diagnostic-Inv	175	25	$1,444,019	$464,443	$1,120,530	$1,407,022	$1,744,226	$2,048,597
Radiology: Diagnostic-Noninv	194	34	$1,345,207	$560,114	$1,021,512	$1,245,714	$1,600,279	$2,041,540
Radiology: Nuclear Medicine	16	12	$1,002,853	$579,475	$643,969	$843,392	$1,271,604	$1,902,925
Rheumatology	120	60	$639,077	$346,176	$409,855	$546,275	$770,796	$987,897
Sleep Medicine	3	2	*	*	*	*	*	*
Surgery: General	446	126	$1,138,140	$471,440	$816,346	$1,052,897	$1,351,551	$1,718,915
Surg: Cardiovascular	102	30	$1,906,038	$678,614	$1,380,940	$1,886,190	$2,419,399	$2,840,865
Surg: Cardiovascular-Pediatric	4	4	*	*	*	*	*	*
Surg: Colon and Rectal	19	11	$1,151,040	$498,794	$733,686	$1,052,342	$1,572,265	$1,882,798
Surg: Neurological	97	31	$2,423,761	$1,265,495	$1,543,798	$2,133,091	$3,014,513	$4,410,126
Surg: Oncology	7	3	*	*	*	*	*	*
Surg: Oral	21	8	$1,129,282	$294,797	$886,885	$1,110,567	$1,381,778	$1,635,179
Surg: Pediatric	10	5	$960,301	$221,912	$786,082	$902,677	$1,154,193	$1,305,585
Surg: Plastic & Reconstruction	51	27	$1,463,797	$1,091,733	$769,363	$1,089,633	$1,949,950	$2,786,554
Surg: Plastic & Recon-Hand	3	2	*	*	*	*	*	*
Surg: Plastic & Recon-Pediatric	2	1	*	*	*	*	*	*
Surg: Thoracic (primary)	23	6	$2,645,653	$1,008,972	$2,027,195	$2,485,360	$3,513,582	$4,078,354
Surg: Transplant	10	6	$1,218,106	$723,389	$411,557	$1,309,925	$1,816,359	$2,323,714
Surg: Trauma	11	4	$1,152,644	$552,669	$735,066	$1,021,689	$1,519,484	$2,187,998
Surg: Trauma-Burn	8	3	*	*	*	*	*	*
Surg: Vascular (primary)	50	26	$1,364,787	$733,139	$829,556	$1,241,860	$1,760,380	$2,489,975
Urgent Care	194	47	$492,241	$169,730	$375,057	$489,225	$586,088	$673,530
Urology	167	66	$1,323,482	$499,079	$1,028,802	$1,290,095	$1,547,929	$1,962,198
Urology: Pediatric	2	1	*	*	*	*	*	*

MEDICAL GROUP MANAGEMENT ASSOCIATION™

Table 22: Physician Gross Charges (TC Excluded) by Group Type

	Single-specialty			Multispecialty		
	Physicians	Medical Practices	Median	Physicians	Medical Practices	Median
Allergy/Immunology	8	4	*	67	48	$621,905
Anesthesiology	157	12	$780,719	193	30	$753,665
Anesth: Pain Management	20	5	$1,479,020	10	8	$1,226,667
Anesth: Pediatric	0	*	*	0	*	*
Cardiology: Electrophysiology	11	7	$1,713,010	13	10	$1,148,161
Cardiology: Invasive	31	11	$1,028,511	75	30	$1,502,760
Cardiology: Inv-Intervntnl	64	16	$1,604,131	71	28	$1,653,642
Cardiology: Noninvasive	26	10	$1,045,657	81	35	$1,274,158
Critical Care: Intensivist	0	*	*	17	9	$530,557
Dentistry	2	1	*	8	3	*
Dermatology	8	5	*	135	69	$924,862
Dermatology: MOHS Surgery	3	2	*	10	9	$1,725,871
Emergency Medicine	68	5	$793,065	114	13	$538,102
Endocrinology/Metabolism	1	1	*	92	56	$454,747
Family Practice (w/ OB)	89	24	$378,508	536	67	$452,174
Family Practice (w/o OB)	180	43	$412,776	1,565	143	$434,075
Family Practice: Sports Med	1	1	*	2	2	*
Gastroenterology	122	16	$1,404,389	209	86	$1,444,512
Gastroenterology: Hepatology	19	3	$1,192,009	0	*	*
Geriatrics	0	*	*	20	13	$295,628
Hematology/Oncology	57	9	$685,000	114	50	$568,557
Hem/Onc: Oncology (only)	15	2	*	32	19	$598,797
Infectious Disease	34	9	$627,104	43	30	$404,419
Internal Medicine: General	56	20	$461,764	1,479	161	$425,866
Internal Med: Hospitalist	0	*	*	154	37	$345,936
Internal Med: Pediatric	0	*	*	31	13	$351,818
Nephrology	45	6	$844,672	89	41	$631,881
Neurology	60	9	$648,053	164	66	$598,657
OBGYN: General	110	23	$945,543	428	92	$871,501
OBGYN: Gynecology (only)	9	5	*	81	28	$765,937
OBGYN: Gyn Oncology	0	*	*	12	8	$980,179
OBGYN: Maternal & Fetal Med	5	3	*	26	7	$1,056,561
OBGYN: Repro Endocrinology	0	*	*	11	4	$850,336
Occupational Medicine	0	*	*	47	25	$390,492
Ophthalmology	13	4	$1,300,000	139	59	$1,132,797
Ophthalmology: Pediatric	1	1	*	2	2	*
Ophthalmology: Retina	1	1	*	5	5	*
Orthopedic (Non-surgical)	0	*	*	11	9	$995,923
Orthopedic Surgery: General	47	13	$1,380,350	205	58	$1,371,537
Ortho Surg: Foot & Ankle	9	7	*	4	3	*
Ortho Surg: Hand	18	11	$1,635,231	12	9	$1,374,585
Ortho Surg: Hip & Joint	16	7	$1,820,579	13	5	$1,271,569
Ortho Surg: Oncology	0	*	*	0	*	*
Ortho Surg: Pediatric	3	3	*	4	4	*
Ortho Surg: Spine	18	11	$2,609,076	16	11	$2,186,873
Ortho Surg: Trauma	7	5	*	5	2	*
Ortho Surg: Sports Med	33	13	$1,663,865	22	15	$1,120,796
Otorhinolaryngology	42	6	$1,103,652	153	70	$1,131,272
Otorhinolaryngology: Pediatric	0	*	*	1	1	*
Pathology: Anatomic & Clinical	6	1	*	42	14	$735,707
Pathology: Anatomic	5	1	*	5	2	*
Pathology: Clinical	0	*	*	16	6	$613,418

Table 22: Physician Gross Charges (TC Excluded) by Group Type (continued)

	Single-specialty			Multispecialty		
	Physicians	Medical Practices	Median	Physicians	Medical Practices	Median
Pediatrics: General	228	28	$468,051	697	120	$465,198
Ped: Adolescent Medicine	4	1	*	34	7	$453,453
Ped: Allergy/Immunology	2	1	*	4	4	*
Ped: Cardiology	1	1	*	19	9	$715,123
Ped: Child Development	*	*	*	11	5	$307,206
Ped: Critical Care/Intensivist	15	4	$413,278	14	7	$406,782
Ped: Emergency Medicine	0	*	*	6	1	*
Ped: Endocrinology	1	1	*	10	8	$270,427
Ped: Gastroenterology	1	1	*	9	5	*
Ped: Genetics	*	*	*	7	3	*
Ped: Hematology/Oncology	5	2	*	13	9	$395,747
Ped: Hospitalist	0	*	*	13	5	$276,284
Ped: Infectious Disease	0	*	*	1	1	*
Ped: Neonatal Medicine	17	3	$865,323	38	12	$977,745
Ped: Nephrology	0	*	*	6	4	*
Ped: Neurology	5	3	*	20	11	$357,512
Ped: Pulmonology	1	1	*	7	6	*
Ped: Rheumatology	0	*	*	3	2	*
Ped: Sports Medicine	*	*	*	0	*	*
Physiatry (Phys Med & Rehab)	4	3	*	47	25	$589,360
Podiatry: General	0	*	*	69	40	$614,746
Podiatry: Surg-Foot & Ankle	2	1	*	15	9	$614,675
Podiatry: Surg-Forefoot Only	0	*	*	5	2	*
Psychiatry: General	3	1	*	125	38	$364,914
Psychiatry: Child & Adolescent	6	2	*	15	10	$425,847
Psychiatry: Geriatric	*	*	*	10	6	$650,160
Pulmonary Medicine	1	1	*	114	59	$706,953
Pulmonary Med: Critical Care	17	3	$737,919	43	19	$719,510
Radiation Oncology	35	8	$1,475,324	26	12	$1,599,418
Radiology: Diagnostic-Inv	106	10	$1,321,230	69	15	$1,680,404
Radiology: Diagnostic-Noninv	97	10	$1,324,922	97	24	$1,187,151
Radiology: Nuclear Medicine	4	3	*	12	9	$873,977
Rheumatology	15	3	$808,002	105	57	$540,258
Sleep Medicine	2	1	*	1	1	*
Surgery: General	78	16	$1,161,840	368	110	$1,022,114
Surg: Cardiovascular	65	14	$2,055,099	37	16	$1,518,199
Surg: Cardiovascular-Pediatric	3	3	*	1	1	*
Surg: Colon and Rectal	8	4	*	11	7	$1,339,761
Surg: Neurological	49	9	$2,837,582	48	22	$1,661,478
Surg: Oncology	0	*	*	7	3	*
Surg: Oral	13	3	$1,110,567	8	5	*
Surg: Pediatric	3	2	*	7	3	*
Surg: Plastic & Reconstruction	7	2	*	44	25	$992,296
Surg: Plastic & Recon-Hand	0	*	*	3	2	*
Surg: Plastic & Recon-Pediatric	2	1	*	0	*	*
Surg: Thoracic (primary)	18	2	*	5	4	*
Surg: Transplant	4	1	*	6	5	*
Surg: Trauma	3	1	*	8	3	*
Surg: Trauma-Burn	7	2	*	1	1	*
Surg: Vascular (primary)	7	3	*	43	23	$1,350,966
Urgent Care	22	2	*	172	45	$494,033
Urology	37	9	$1,544,169	130	57	$1,166,227
Urology: Pediatric	0	*	*	2	1	*

Table 23A: Physician Gross Charges (TC Excluded) by Size of Multispecialty Practice (50 or Less FTE Physicians)

	10 FTE or less		11 to 25 FTE		26 to 50 FTE	
	Physicians	Median	Physicians	Median	Physicians	Median
Allergy/Immunology	0	*	0	*	11	$550,772
Anesthesiology	*	*	0	*	20	$556,215
Anesth: Pain Management	0	*	0	*	3	*
Anesth: Pediatric	*	*	0	*	0	*
Cardiology: Electrophysiology	0	*	1	*	0	*
Cardiology: Invasive	*	*	2	*	12	$1,415,050
Cardiology: Inv-Intervntnl	0	*	7	*	13	$1,458,300
Cardiology: Noninvasive	0	*	0	*	17	$810,122
Critical Care: Intensivist	1	*	1	*	2	*
Dentistry	0	*	1	*	0	*
Dermatology	*	*	1	*	21	$750,720
Dermatology: MOHS Surgery	*	*	1	*	2	*
Emergency Medicine	0	*	1	*	0	*
Endocrinology/Metabolism	2	*	6	*	11	$417,968
Family Practice (w/ OB)	22	$404,261	63	$504,391	27	$425,816
Family Practice (w/o OB)	66	$299,541	113	$400,170	224	$419,552
Family Practice: Sports Med	0	*	0	*	0	*
Gastroenterology	0	*	18	$1,371,147	37	$1,208,035
Gastroenterology: Hepatology	0	*	0	*	0	*
Geriatrics	*	*	2	*	2	*
Hematology/Oncology	4	*	6	*	18	$519,198
Hem/Onc: Oncology (only)	*	*	2	*	3	*
Infectious Disease	1	*	8	*	2	*
Internal Medicine: General	50	$351,899	175	$418,634	178	$445,110
Internal Med: Hospitalist	0	*	2	*	16	$382,339
Internal Med: Pediatric	4	*	5	*	0	*
Nephrology	5	*	4	*	6	*
Neurology	1	*	6	*	15	$729,811
OBGYN: General	9	*	19	$768,165	69	$810,957
OBGYN: Gynecology (only)	1	*	0	*	5	*
OBGYN: Gyn Oncology	0	*	0	*	3	*
OBGYN: Maternal & Fetal Med	0	*	*	*	2	*
OBGYN: Repro Endocrinology	0	*	*	*	7	*
Occupational Medicine	2	*	5	*	2	*
Ophthalmology	0	*	5	*	11	$1,094,816
Ophthalmology: Pediatric	*	*	0	*	*	*
Ophthalmology: Retina	*	*	0	*	*	*
Orthopedic (Non-surgical)	0	*	1	*	2	*
Orthopedic Surgery: General	0	*	12	$1,128,650	23	$1,043,501
Ortho Surg: Foot & Ankle	*	*	1	*	0	*
Ortho Surg: Hand	0	*	2	*	0	*
Ortho Surg: Hip & Joint	0	*	5	*	0	*
Ortho Surg: Oncology	*	*	0	*	*	*
Ortho Surg: Pediatric	*	*	1	*	0	*
Ortho Surg: Spine	2	*	2	*	0	*
Ortho Surg: Sports Med	0	*	1	*	2	*
Otorhinolaryngology	0	*	6	*	21	$1,021,853
Pathology: Anatomic & Clinical	4	*	4	*	2	*
Pathology: Anatomic	*	*	*	*	2	*
Pathology: Clinical	*	*	*	*	7	*

Table 23A: Physician Gross Charges (TC Excluded) by Size of Multispecialty Practice (50 or Less FTE Physicians) (continued)

	10 FTE or less		11 to 25 FTE		26 to 50 FTE	
	Physicians	Median	Physicians	Median	Physicians	Median
Pediatrics: General	23	$559,876	66	$415,061	87	$445,733
Ped: Adolescent Medicine	1	*	2	*	5	*
Ped: Allergy/Immunology	*	*	*	*	0	*
Ped: Cardiology	1	*	0	*	4	*
Ped: Child Development	*	*	1	*	2	*
Ped: Critical Care/Intensivist	*	*	0	*	4	*
Ped: Emergency Medicine	*	*	*	*	6	*
Ped: Endocrinology	*	*	1	*	2	*
Ped: Gastroenterology	*	*	*	*	0	*
Ped: Genetics	*	*	0	*	2	*
Ped: Hematology/Oncology	*	*	0	*	3	*
Ped: Hospitalist	*	*	0	*	0	*
Ped: Infectious Disease	*	*	0	*	*	*
Ped: Neonatal Medicine	*	*	0	*	1	*
Ped: Nephrology	*	*	0	*	*	*
Ped: Neurology	*	*	2	*	2	*
Ped: Pulmonology	*	*	1	*	1	*
Ped: Rheumatology	*	*	*	*	1	*
Physiatry (Phys Med & Rehab)	0	*	1	*	2	*
Podiatry: General	0	*	2	*	5	*
Podiatry: Surg-Foot & Ankle	*	*	0	*	1	*
Podiatry: Surg-Forefoot Only	*	*	*	*	0	*
Psychiatry: General	3	*	0	*	8	*
Psychiatry: Child & Adolescent	*	*	2	*	1	*
Psychiatry: Geriatric	*	*	4	*	4	*
Pulmonary Medicine	1	*	8	*	14	$684,995
Pulmonary Med: Critical Care	2	*	14	$737,650	9	*
Radiation Oncology	*	*	*	*	0	*
Radiology: Diagnostic-Inv	*	*	5	*	4	*
Radiology: Diagnostic-Noninv	*	*	12	$966,749	5	*
Radiology: Nuclear Medicine	0	*	3	*	1	*
Rheumatology	1	*	5	*	15	$759,065
Sleep Medicine	0	*	*	*	*	*
Surgery: General	10	$624,012	27	$1,020,487	54	$990,448
Surg: Cardiovascular	*	*	*	*	2	*
Surg: Cardiovascular-Pediatric	*	*	*	*	1	*
Surg: Colon and Rectal	2	*	*	*	3	*
Surg: Neurological	4	*	8	*	2	*
Surg: Oncology	1	*	*	*	1	*
Surg: Oral	*	*	*	*	1	*
Surg: Pediatric	0	*	0	*	*	*
Surg: Plastic & Reconstruction	*	*	0	*	5	*
Surg: Plastic & Recon-Hand	*	*	0	*	*	*
Surg: Thoracic (primary)	1	*	1	*	*	*
Surg: Transplant	1	*	*	*	0	*
Surg: Trauma	0	*	*	*	*	*
Surg: Vascular (primary)	3	*	5	*	2	*
Urgent Care	0	*	2	*	27	$405,120
Urology	*	*	3	*	12	$1,210,576

　　　MEDICAL GROUP MANAGEMENT ASSOCIATION™

Table 23B: Physician Gross Charges (TC Excluded) by Size of Multispecialty Practice (51 or More FTE Physicians)

	51 to 75 FTE		76 to 150 FTE		151 FTE or more	
	Physicians	Median	Physicians	Median	Physicians	Median
Allergy/Immunology	14	$755,157	21	$592,554	21	$692,340
Anesthesiology	5	*	51	$680,315	117	$837,071
Anesth: Pain Management	1	*	1	*	5	*
Anesth: Pediatric	0	*	*	*	*	*
Cardiology: Electrophysiology	1	*	2	*	9	*
Cardiology: Invasive	11	$1,578,597	26	$2,022,512	24	$1,355,043
Cardiology: Inv-Intervntnl	5	*	21	$1,871,618	25	$1,529,263
Cardiology: Noninvasive	4	*	25	$1,328,789	35	$1,337,692
Critical Care: Intensivist	1	*	0	*	12	$525,684
Dentistry	*	*	*	*	7	*
Dermatology	30	$1,024,278	37	$935,335	46	$903,484
Dermatology: MOHS Surgery	0	*	5	*	2	*
Emergency Medicine	0	*	14	*	99	$537,495
Endocrinology/Metabolism	14	$442,653	30	$477,877	29	$452,417
Family Practice (w/ OB)	85	$467,226	147	$414,476	192	$493,252
Family Practice (w/o OB)	170	$424,366	425	$434,714	565	$479,793
Family Practice: Sports Med	0	*	0	*	2	*
Gastroenterology	23	$1,547,569	71	$1,462,562	60	$1,519,474
Gastroenterology: Hepatology	0	*	*	*	0	*
Geriatrics	0	*	8	*	8	*
Hematology/Oncology	17	$500,278	32	$653,567	37	$536,824
Hem/Onc: Oncology (only)	4	*	15	$896,211	8	*
Infectious Disease	5	*	14	$475,134	13	$406,240
Internal Medicine: General	199	$439,954	492	$422,140	383	$422,245
Internal Med: Hospitalist	8	*	52	$363,311	76	$331,641
Internal Med: Pediatric	5	*	14	$351,326	3	*
Nephrology	13	$771,227	36	$662,115	25	$536,349
Neurology	32	$580,353	54	$615,682	56	$586,318
OBGYN: General	65	$778,985	136	$876,917	130	$901,002
OBGYN: Gynecology (only)	9	*	17	$642,766	49	$914,941
OBGYN: Gyn Oncology	*	*	2	*	7	*
OBGYN: Maternal & Fetal Med	0	*	9	*	15	$1,232,585
OBGYN: Repro Endocrinology	*	*	1	*	3	*
Occupational Medicine	7	*	14	$422,465	17	$390,492
Ophthalmology	26	$1,271,166	50	$1,135,495	47	$1,131,192
Ophthalmology: Pediatric	0	*	*	*	2	*
Ophthalmology: Retina	0	*	1	*	4	*
Orthopedic (Non-surgical)	4	*	3	*	1	*
Orthopedic Surgery: General	20	$1,226,108	58	$1,477,963	92	$1,499,092
Ortho Surg: Foot & Ankle	*	*	*	*	3	*
Ortho Surg: Hand	1	*	1	*	8	*
Ortho Surg: Hip & Joint	0	*	1	*	7	*
Ortho Surg: Pediatric	*	*	0	*	3	*
Ortho Surg: Spine	2	*	2	*	8	*
Ortho Surg: Trauma	*	*	*	*	5	*
Ortho Surg: Sports Med	5	*	7	*	7	*
Otorhinolaryngology	20	$1,125,267	44	$1,012,826	62	$1,395,643
Otorhinolaryngology: Pediatric	1	*	0	*	*	*
Pathology: Anatomic & Clinical	4	*	7	*	21	$723,410
Pathology: Anatomic	*	*	0	*	3	*
Pathology: Clinical	0	*	9	*	0	*

Table 23B: Physician Gross Charges (TC Excluded) by Size of Multispecialty Practice (51 or More FTE Physicians) (continued)

	51 to 75 FTE		76 to 150 FTE		151 FTE or more	
	Physicians	Median	Physicians	Median	Physicians	Median
Pediatrics: General	99	$484,806	223	$482,913	199	$444,693
Ped: Adolescent Medicine	*	*	11	*	15	*
Ped: Allergy/Immunology	*	*	*	*	4	*
Ped: Cardiology	5	*	1	*	8	*
Ped: Child Development	2	*	0	*	6	*
Ped: Critical Care/Intensivist	*	*	1	*	9	*
Ped: Endocrinology	2	*	*	*	5	*
Ped: Gastroenterology	3	*	1	*	5	*
Ped: Genetics	3	*	*	*	2	*
Ped: Hematology/Oncology	4	*	1	*	5	*
Ped: Hospitalist	8	*	1	*	4	*
Ped: Infectious Disease	1	*	*	*	0	*
Ped: Neonatal Medicine	3	*	5	*	29	$1,130,050
Ped: Nephrology	3	*	*	*	3	*
Ped: Neurology	3	*	3	*	10	$476,691
Ped: Pulmonology	*	*	*	*	5	*
Ped: Rheumatology	2	*	*	*	*	*
Ped: Sports Medicine	*	*	0	*	*	*
Physiatry (Phys Med & Rehab)	5	*	19	$517,044	20	$633,926
Podiatry: General	6	*	27	$565,552	29	$651,753
Podiatry: Surg-Foot & Ankle	4	*	3	*	7	*
Podiatry: Surg-Forefoot Only	*	*	4	*	1	*
Psychiatry: General	11	$302,857	44	$370,074	59	$389,604
Psychiatry: Child & Adolescent	3	*	2	*	7	*
Psychiatry: Geriatric	*	*	1	*	1	*
Pulmonary Medicine	19	$699,010	40	$768,861	32	$688,137
Pulmonary Med: Critical Care	6	*	7	*	5	*
Radiation Oncology	0	*	8	*	18	$1,599,418
Radiology: Diagnostic-Inv	0	*	28	$1,792,190	32	$1,279,515
Radiology: Diagnostic-Noninv	5	*	19	$1,446,446	56	$1,239,502
Radiology: Nuclear Medicine	2	*	5	*	1	*
Rheumatology	18	$422,959	35	$495,599	31	$546,107
Sleep Medicine	1	*	0	*	*	*
Surgery: General	48	$1,138,155	116	$1,009,310	113	$1,056,891
Surg: Cardiovascular	1	*	7	*	27	$1,551,620
Surg: Colon and Rectal	0	*	3	*	3	*
Surg: Neurological	5	*	10	$1,773,156	19	$1,740,380
Surg: Oncology	*	*	5	*	*	*
Surg: Oral	*	*	2	*	5	*
Surg: Pediatric	4	*	0	*	3	*
Surg: Plastic & Reconstruction	2	*	11	$1,075,195	26	$1,222,103
Surg: Plastic & Recon-Hand	*	*	2	*	1	*
Surg: Plastic & Recon-Pediatric	*	*	0	*	*	*
Surg: Thoracic (primary)	0	*	1	*	2	*
Surg: Transplant	*	*	*	*	5	*
Surg: Trauma	*	*	0	*	8	*
Surg: Trauma-Burn	*	*	0	*	1	*
Surg: Vascular (primary)	4	*	10	$1,355,686	19	$1,492,783
Urgent Care	10	$470,182	68	$515,632	65	$453,612
Urology	24	$1,069,757	46	$1,103,720	45	$1,290,095
Urology: Pediatric	2	*	*	*	*	*

MEDICAL GROUP MANAGEMENT ASSOCIATION™

Table 24: Physician Gross Charges (TC Excluded) by Hospital Ownership

	Hospital Owned			Non-hospital Owned		
	Physicians	Medical Practices	Median	Physicians	Medical Practices	Median
Allergy/Immunology	16	12	$543,362	59	40	$715,877
Anesthesiology	71	10	$838,927	279	32	$746,370
Anesth: Pain Management	6	4	*	24	9	$1,408,148
Anesth: Pediatric	*	*	*	0	*	*
Cardiology: Electrophysiology	5	3	*	19	14	$1,274,113
Cardiology: Invasive	20	6	$1,740,047	86	35	$1,341,102
Cardiology: Inv-Intervntnl	22	7	$2,049,268	113	37	$1,563,842
Cardiology: Noninvasive	33	10	$1,340,226	74	35	$1,069,024
Critical Care: Intensivist	11	5	$520,812	6	4	*
Dentistry	0	*	*	9	3	*
Dermatology	33	15	$808,238	110	59	$975,326
Dermatology: MOHS Surgery	7	6	*	6	5	*
Emergency Medicine	72	7	$541,370	110	11	$649,258
Endocrinology/Metabolism	37	19	$403,158	56	38	$470,054
Family Practice (w/ OB)	191	31	$421,600	433	59	$461,636
Family Practice (w/o OB)	862	72	$431,368	870	112	$430,860
Family Practice: Sports Med	2	2	*	1	1	*
Gastroenterology	56	18	$1,432,640	275	84	$1,433,899
Gastroenterology: Hepatology	*	*	*	19	3	$1,192,009
Geriatrics	11	6	$293,568	9	7	*
Hematology/Oncology	36	13	$448,119	135	46	$641,888
Hem/Onc: Oncology (only)	7	4	*	40	17	$570,582
Infectious Disease	22	15	$363,503	55	24	$555,625
Internal Medicine: General	522	59	$419,669	1,008	121	$431,216
Internal Med: Hospitalist	97	16	$320,494	57	21	$425,585
Internal Med: Pediatric	12	6	$304,160	19	7	$423,540
Nephrology	32	11	$553,685	102	36	$809,862
Neurology	50	19	$524,043	174	56	$656,551
OBGYN: General	150	29	$770,765	388	86	$901,621
OBGYN: Gynecology (only)	55	10	$893,547	35	23	$538,169
OBGYN: Gyn Oncology	5	3	*	7	5	*
OBGYN: Maternal & Fetal Med	17	5	$1,134,534	14	5	$836,976
OBGYN: Repro Endocrinology	9	2	*	2	2	*
Occupational Medicine	15	5	$428,781	32	20	$346,552
Ophthalmology	33	13	$1,043,483	119	50	$1,167,851
Ophthalmology: Pediatric	1	1	*	2	2	*
Ophthalmology: Retina	2	2	*	4	4	*
Orthopedic (Non-surgical)	4	4	*	7	5	*
Orthopedic Surgery: General	40	11	$1,614,823	212	60	$1,356,728
Ortho Surg: Foot & Ankle	*	*	*	13	10	$1,501,757
Ortho Surg: Hand	3	3	*	27	17	$1,555,276
Ortho Surg: Hip & Joint	3	1	*	26	11	$1,670,417
Ortho Surg: Oncology	*	*	*	0	*	*
Ortho Surg: Pediatric	1	1	*	6	6	*
Ortho Surg: Spine	4	3	*	30	19	$2,479,173
Ortho Surg: Trauma	4	1	*	6	5	*
Ortho Surg: Sports Med	7	5	*	44	22	$1,556,970
Otorhinolaryngology	48	19	$1,090,021	147	57	$1,122,047
Otorhinolaryngology: Pediatric	*	*	*	1	1	*
Pathology: Anatomic & Clinical	21	5	$607,832	27	10	$754,221
Pathology: Anatomic	0	*	*	10	3	$857,718
Pathology: Clinical	3	2	*	13	4	$486,449

Table 24: Physician Gross Charges (TC Excluded) by Hospital Ownership (continued)

	Hospital Owned			Non-hospital Owned		
	Physicians	Medical Practices	Median	Physicians	Medical Practices	Median
Pediatrics: General	316	43	$436,659	603	104	$483,612
Ped: Adolescent Medicine	7	3	*	31	5	$481,963
Ped: Allergy/Immunology	1	1	*	5	4	*
Ped: Cardiology	6	3	*	14	7	$720,420
Ped: Child Development	4	3	*	7	2	*
Ped: Critical Care/Intensivist	7	3	*	22	8	$447,915
Ped: Emergency Medicine	6	1	*	*	*	*
Ped: Endocrinology	6	5	*	5	4	*
Ped: Gastroenterology	5	3	*	5	3	*
Ped: Genetics	2	1	*	5	2	*
Ped: Hematology/Oncology	7	4	*	11	7	$434,692
Ped: Hospitalist	3	2	*	10	3	$280,950
Ped: Infectious Disease	0	*	*	1	1	*
Ped: Neonatal Medicine	30	8	$1,020,646	25	7	$865,323
Ped: Nephrology	2	2	*	4	2	*
Ped: Neurology	13	8	$346,131	12	6	$417,603
Ped: Pulmonology	4	3	*	4	4	*
Ped: Rheumatology	*	*	*	3	2	*
Ped: Sports Medicine	*	*	*	0	*	*
Physiatry (Phys Med & Rehab)	18	7	$568,150	33	21	$605,999
Podiatry: General	21	9	$604,947	48	31	$641,107
Podiatry: Surg-Foot & Ankle	5	3	*	12	7	$651,852
Podiatry: Surg-Forefoot Only	0	*	*	5	2	*
Psychiatry: General	51	17	$323,702	77	22	$379,009
Psychiatry: Child & Adolescent	11	6	$382,936	10	6	$413,801
Psychiatry: Geriatric	2	2	*	8	4	*
Pulmonary Medicine	28	14	$662,606	87	46	$754,335
Pulmonary Med: Critical Care	13	7	$561,748	47	15	$755,790
Radiation Oncology	11	5	$977,326	50	15	$1,522,916
Radiology: Diagnostic-Inv	10	5	$1,719,447	165	20	$1,393,890
Radiology: Diagnostic-Noninv	39	8	$1,024,247	155	26	$1,295,101
Radiology: Nuclear Medicine	6	3	*	10	9	$881,699
Rheumatology	40	17	$486,825	80	43	$592,599
Sleep Medicine	0	*	*	3	2	*
Surgery: General	101	27	$983,045	345	99	$1,071,125
Surg: Cardiovascular	15	6	$1,422,122	87	24	$1,917,281
Surg: Cardiovascular-Pediatric	1	1	*	3	3	*
Surg: Colon and Rectal	0	*	*	19	11	$1,052,342
Surg: Neurological	17	9	$1,803,178	80	22	$2,199,086
Surg: Oncology	*	*	*	7	3	*
Surg: Oral	2	1	*	19	7	$1,110,567
Surg: Pediatric	5	3	*	5	2	*
Surg: Plastic & Reconstruction	12	6	$1,125,216	39	21	$1,089,633
Surg: Plastic & Recon-Hand	1	1	*	2	1	*
Surg: Plastic & Recon-Pediatric	*	*	*	2	1	*
Surg: Thoracic (primary)	3	3	*	20	3	$3,049,699
Surg: Transplant	4	3	*	6	3	*
Surg: Trauma	9	3	*	2	1	*
Surg: Trauma-Burn	1	1	*	7	2	*
Surg: Vascular (primary)	12	7	$1,562,059	38	19	$1,038,398
Urgent Care	67	16	$462,127	127	31	$496,567
Urology	28	11	$1,238,788	139	55	$1,291,034
Urology: Pediatric	0	*	*	2	1	*

Table 25A: Physician Gross Charges (TC Excluded) by Geographic Section for All Practices

	Eastern		Midwest		Southern		Western	
	Physicians	Median	Physicians	Median	Physicians	Median	Physicians	Median
Allergy/Immunology	8	*	29	$618,005	17	$715,877	21	$633,505
Anesthesiology	34	$743,526	158	$810,532	74	$804,216	84	$624,941
Anesth: Pain Management	2	*	8	*	20	$1,529,506	0	*
Anesth: Pediatric	*	*	0	*	0	*	0	*
Cardiology: Electrophysiology	5	*	8	*	6	*	5	*
Cardiology: Invasive	13	$1,500,680	41	$1,279,480	38	$1,589,394	14	$1,426,153
Cardiology: Inv-Intervntnl	21	$1,649,403	49	$1,558,809	51	$1,733,228	14	$1,504,000
Cardiology: Noninvasive	28	$1,103,519	31	$1,338,606	30	$1,243,833	18	$882,303
Critical Care: Intensivist	7	*	7	*	0	*	3	*
Dentistry	5	*	*	*	5	*	0	*
Dermatology	20	$1,069,499	66	$957,562	21	$927,932	36	$733,665
Dermatology: MOHS Surgery	1	*	4	*	5	*	3	*
Emergency Medicine	51	$412,737	58	$588,767	25	*	48	$683,902
Endocrinology/Metabolism	17	$452,417	35	$444,604	24	$468,196	17	$403,158
Family Practice (w/ OB)	49	$393,399	423	$438,782	41	$490,467	112	$446,608
Family Practice (w/o OB)	349	$371,300	859	$447,475	214	$434,376	323	$465,809
Family Practice: Sports Med	0	*	1	*	0	*	2	*
Gastroenterology	48	$1,474,525	132	$1,480,029	91	$1,433,899	60	$1,229,912
Gastroenterology: Hepatology	0	*	0	*	19	$1,192,009	0	*
Geriatrics	3	*	13	$334,685	0	*	4	*
Hematology/Oncology	20	$347,182	74	$633,345	50	$718,491	27	$588,203
Hem/Onc: Oncology (only)	15	$784,721	20	$550,198	5	*	7	*
Infectious Disease	21	$488,272	25	$494,991	16	$748,657	15	$511,981
Internal Medicine: General	322	$420,931	645	$410,707	236	$426,254	332	$459,286
Internal Med: Hospitalist	20	$425,582	87	$346,201	20	$355,811	27	$264,822
Internal Med: Pediatric	5	*	10	$460,359	10	*	6	*
Nephrology	44	$788,774	39	$664,312	37	$787,137	14	$614,056
Neurology	38	$572,156	126	$649,697	28	$671,812	32	$546,578
OBGYN: General	107	$874,616	205	$910,045	98	$972,349	128	$747,962
OBGYN: Gynecology (only)	10	$598,723	57	$926,883	15	$538,169	8	*
OBGYN: Gyn Oncology	3	*	5	*	3	*	1	*
OBGYN: Maternal & Fetal Med	5	*	22	$767,289	2	*	2	*
OBGYN: Repro Endocrinology	3	*	8	*	0	*	0	*
Occupational Medicine	2	*	30	$367,878	3	*	12	$461,083
Ophthalmology	28	$1,222,620	75	$1,194,522	24	$1,264,700	25	$976,107
Ophthalmology: Pediatric	1	*	1	*	0	*	1	*
Ophthalmology: Retina	1	*	3	*	1	*	1	*
Orthopedic (Non-surgical)	0	*	6	*	1	*	4	*
Orthopedic Surgery: General	26	$1,508,895	136	$1,403,171	45	$1,365,610	45	$1,202,314
Ortho Surg: Foot & Ankle	3	*	6	*	2	*	2	*
Ortho Surg: Hand	5	*	15	$1,471,605	3	*	7	*
Ortho Surg: Hip & Joint	10	$2,042,885	15	$1,402,660	0	*	4	*
Ortho Surg: Oncology	0	*	*	*	0	*	*	*
Ortho Surg: Pediatric	1	*	6	*	0	*	0	*
Ortho Surg: Spine	7	*	21	$2,005,745	1	*	5	*
Ortho Surg: Trauma	7	*	3	*	2	*	0	*
Ortho Surg: Sports Med	10	$2,090,864	25	$1,638,852	10	$1,523,107	10	$1,311,967
Otorhinolaryngology	30	$973,681	97	$1,265,686	32	$1,457,037	36	$954,693
Otorhinolaryngology: Pediatric	0	*	1	*	0	*	*	*
Pathology: Anatomic & Clinical	16	$845,604	14	$611,238	14	$754,221	4	*
Pathology: Anatomic	0	*	3	*	5	*	2	*
Pathology: Clinical	5	*	6	*	5	*	0	*

Table 25A: Physician Gross Charges (TC Excluded) by Geographic Section for All Practices (continued)

	Eastern		Midwest		Southern		Western	
	Physicians	Median	Physicians	Median	Physicians	Median	Physicians	Median
Pediatrics: General	179	$488,636	427	$450,044	126	$473,561	193	$488,723
Ped: Adolescent Medicine	2	*	25	*	11	$495,810	0	*
Ped: Allergy/Immunology	1	*	3	*	0	*	2	*
Ped: Cardiology	4	*	7	*	1	*	8	*
Ped: Child Development	1	*	7	*	1	*	2	*
Ped: Critical Care/Intensivist	2	*	19	$442,888	8	*	0	*
Ped: Emergency Medicine	0	*	6	*	*	*	*	*
Ped: Endocrinology	1	*	6	*	1	*	3	*
Ped: Gastroenterology	3	*	3	*	1	*	3	*
Ped: Genetics	0	*	2	*	0	*	5	*
Ped: Hematology/Oncology	2	*	6	*	4	*	6	*
Ped: Hospitalist	0	*	3	*	1	*	9	*
Ped: Infectious Disease	*	*	0	*	0	*	1	*
Ped: Neonatal Medicine	9	*	28	$1,020,646	17	$865,323	1	*
Ped: Nephrology	1	*	2	*	*	*	3	*
Ped: Neurology	3	*	17	$366,624	2	*	3	*
Ped: Pulmonology	3	*	3	*	1	*	1	*
Ped: Rheumatology	1	*	*	*	*	*	2	*
Ped: Sports Medicine	0	*	*	*	*	*	*	*
Physiatry (Phys Med & Rehab)	5	*	36	$556,877	2	*	8	*
Podiatry: General	3	*	40	$609,900	11	$606,377	15	$634,612
Podiatry: Surg-Foot & Ankle	4	*	9	*	0	*	4	*
Podiatry: Surg-Forefoot Only	4	*	1	*	0	*	0	*
Psychiatry: General	21	$265,871	77	$379,009	11	$365,609	19	$340,885
Psychiatry: Child & Adolescent	1	*	12	$454,378	8	*	0	*
Psychiatry: Geriatric	4	*	2	*	4	*	0	*
Pulmonary Medicine	20	$762,376	42	$684,909	35	$793,075	18	$548,774
Pulmonary Med: Critical Care	15	$718,787	19	$691,278	20	$848,224	6	*
Radiation Oncology	3	*	26	$1,406,838	23	$1,504,918	9	*
Radiology: Diagnostic-Inv	22	$1,252,182	83	$1,414,600	40	$1,664,435	30	*
Radiology: Diagnostic-Noninv	49	$1,032,511	71	$1,333,473	70	$1,315,406	4	*
Radiology: Nuclear Medicine	5	*	6	*	4	*	1	*
Rheumatology	19	$528,562	52	$497,513	30	$648,888	19	$646,800
Sleep Medicine	0	*	2	*	0	*	1	*
Surgery: General	74	$1,005,644	191	$1,092,642	102	$1,194,874	79	$877,599
Surg: Cardiovascular	12	$2,147,190	29	$1,551,620	41	$2,030,341	20	$1,807,023
Surg: Cardiovascular-Pediatric	*	*	1	*	2	*	1	*
Surg: Colon and Rectal	9	*	7	*	1	*	2	*
Surg: Neurological	31	$2,333,447	45	$1,967,585	13	$2,301,246	8	*
Surg: Oncology	2	*	5	*	*	*	0	*
Surg: Oral	8	*	6	*	3	*	4	*
Surg: Pediatric	3	*	2	*	0	*	5	*
Surg: Plastic & Reconstruction	9	*	17	$1,432,520	10	$1,629,408	15	$848,914
Surg: Plastic & Recon-Hand	0	*	3	*	0	*	*	*
Surg: Plastic & Recon-Pediatric	0	*	*	*	2	*	*	*
Surg: Thoracic (primary)	3	*	20	$3,049,699	0	*	0	*
Surg: Transplant	4	*	1	*	4	*	1	*
Surg: Trauma	3	*	5	*	3	*	*	*
Surg: Trauma-Burn	1	*	0	*	6	*	1	*
Surg: Vascular (primary)	17	$1,067,051	20	$1,299,213	3	*	10	$860,079
Urgent Care	2	*	78	$419,902	40	$513,115	74	$542,914
Urology	32	$1,583,905	72	$1,265,441	36	$1,381,966	27	$1,076,205
Urology: Pediatric	*	*	0	*	0	*	2	*

Table 25B: Physician Gross Charges (TC Excluded) by Geographic Section for Single-specialty Practices

	Eastern		Midwest		Southern		Western	
	Physicians	Median	Physicians	Median	Physicians	Median	Physicians	Median
Allergy/Immunology	1	*	*	*	2	*	5	*
Anesthesiology	0	*	60	$754,091	47	$899,734	50	$619,573
Anesth: Pain Management	0	*	3	*	17	$1,701,980	0	*
Anesth: Pediatric	*	*	*	*	0	*	0	*
Cardiology: Electrophysiology	2	*	4	*	5	*	0	*
Cardiology: Invasive	2	*	9	*	15	$985,505	5	*
Cardiology: Inv-Intervntnl	11	$1,610,242	22	$1,491,894	25	$1,733,228	6	
Cardiology: Noninvasive	9	*	1	*	15	$1,309,271	1	*
Critical Care: Intensivist	0	*	*	*	0	*	*	*
Dentistry	2	*	*	*	*	*	0	*
Dermatology	3	*	0	*	2	*	3	*
Dermatology: MOHS Surgery	0	*	1	*	2	*	*	*
Emergency Medicine	0	*	*	*	25	*	43	$686,489
Endocrinology/Metabolism	0	*	1	*	0	*	*	*
Family Practice (w/ OB)	11	$380,446	32	$427,740	10	*	36	$348,560
Family Practice (w/o OB)	71	$376,000	44	$365,440	16	$523,323	49	$500,680
Family Practice: Sports Med	0	*	0	*	0	*	1	*
Gastroenterology	10	*	46	$1,402,313	41	$1,549,000	25	$1,207,827
Gastroenterology: Hepatology	0	*	0	*	19	$1,192,009	0	*
Geriatrics	*	*	*	*	*	*	0	*
Hematology/Oncology	0	*	22	$584,000	25	$788,444	10	*
Hem/Onc: Oncology (only)	9	*	0	*	*	*	6	*
Infectious Disease	11	*	5	*	9	*	9	*
Internal Medicine: General	15	$377,293	17	$346,315	7	*	17	$470,534
Internal Med: Hospitalist	*	*	*	*	0	*	0	*
Internal Med: Pediatric	*	*	0	*	*	*	*	*
Nephrology	28	$844,524	1	*	11	*	5	*
Neurology	4	*	45	$665,029	3	*	8	*
OBGYN: General	21	$994,113	10	$894,866	40	$1,080,278	39	$695,000
OBGYN: Gynecology (only)	2	*	0	*	6	*	1	*
OBGYN: Gyn Oncology	0	*	*	*	*	*	*	*
OBGYN: Maternal & Fetal Med	0	*	3	*	2	*	0	*
OBGYN: Repro Endocrinology	*	*	0	*	0	*	0	*
Occupational Medicine	0	*	0	*	0	*	*	*
Ophthalmology	9	*	0	*	3	*	1	*
Ophthalmology: Pediatric	0	*	0	*	0	*	1	*
Ophthalmology: Retina	0	*	0	*	1	*	0	*
Orthopedic (Non-surgical)	0	*	0	*	0	*	0	*
Orthopedic Surgery: General	5	*	16	$1,360,619	8	*	18	$1,213,943
Ortho Surg: Foot & Ankle	3	*	2	*	2	*	2	*
Ortho Surg: Hand	4	*	6	*	3	*	5	*
Ortho Surg: Hip & Joint	10	$2,042,885	5	*	0	*	1	*
Ortho Surg: Oncology	0	*	*	*	0	*	*	*
Ortho Surg: Pediatric	0	*	3	*	0	*	0	*
Ortho Surg: Spine	4	*	11	$1,965,365	1	*	2	*
Ortho Surg: Trauma	3	*	2	*	2	*	0	*
Ortho Surg: Sports Med	8	*	11	$1,814,598	10	$1,523,107	4	*
Otorhinolaryngology	11	*	16	*	8	*	7	*
Otorhinolaryngology: Pediatric	*	*	0	*	0	*	*	*
Pathology: Anatomic & Clinical	0	*	0	*	6	*	0	*
Pathology: Anatomic	*	*	*	*	5	*	0	*
Pathology: Clinical	*	*	0	*	0	*	0	*

Table 25B: Physician Gross Charges (TC Excluded) by Geographic Section for Single-specialty Practices (continued)

	Eastern		Midwest		Southern		Western	
	Physicians	**Median**	**Physicians**	**Median**	**Physicians**	**Median**	**Physicians**	**Median**
Pediatrics: General	46	$550,390	117	$424,771	29	$561,000	36	$491,461
Ped: Adolescent Medicine	*	*	*	*	4	*	0	*
Ped: Allergy/Immunology	*	*	*	*	*	*	2	*
Ped: Cardiology	0	*	1	*	0	*	0	*
Ped: Critical Care/Intensivist	*	*	8	*	7	*	0	*
Ped: Emergency Medicine	0	*	*	*	*	*	*	*
Ped: Endocrinology	*	*	*	*	0	*	1	*
Ped: Gastroenterology	*	*	0	*	1	*	0	*
Ped: Hematology/Oncology	*	*	0	*	3	*	2	*
Ped: Hospitalist	*	*	*	*	*	*	0	*
Ped: Infectious Disease	*	*	*	*	*	*	0	*
Ped: Neonatal Medicine	*	*	*	*	16	*	1	*
Ped: Nephrology	*	*	*	*	*	*	0	*
Ped: Neurology	0	*	4	*	1	*	0	*
Ped: Pulmonology	*	*	0	*	*	*	1	*
Ped: Rheumatology	*	*	*	*	*	*	0	*
Physiatry (Phys Med & Rehab)	2	*	2	*	0	*	0	*
Podiatry: General	*	*	0	*	0	*	*	*
Podiatry: Surg-Foot & Ankle	0	*	2	*	*	*	0	*
Podiatry: Surg-Forefoot Only	*	*	*	*	*	*	0	*
Psychiatry: General	0	*	3	*	*	*	*	*
Psychiatry: Child & Adolescent	0	*	*	*	6	*	*	*
Pulmonary Medicine	0	*	0	*	1	*	0	*
Pulmonary Med: Critical Care	1	*	0	*	10	*	6	*
Radiation Oncology	0	*	8	*	21	$1,504,918	6	*
Radiology: Diagnostic-Inv	6	*	46	$1,119,333	30	$1,588,963	24	
Radiology: Diagnostic-Noninv	23	*	22	$1,573,929	51	$1,386,535	1	*
Radiology: Nuclear Medicine	0	*	2	*	2	*	0	*
Rheumatology	0	*	2	*	9	*	4	*
Sleep Medicine	0	*	2	*	0	*	*	*
Surgery: General	17	*	6	*	42	$1,549,359	13	$815,502
Surg: Cardiovascular	6	*	8	*	36	$2,046,111	15	$1,917,281
Surg: Cardiovascular-Pediatric	*	*	*	*	2	*	1	*
Surg: Colon and Rectal	6	*	0	*	*	*	2	*
Surg: Neurological	16	*	25	$2,974,921	8	*	0	*
Surg: Oncology	*	*	0	*	*	*	*	*
Surg: Oral	6	*	*	*	3	*	4	*
Surg: Pediatric	*	*	2	*	0	*	1	*
Surg: Plastic & Reconstruction	*	*	*	*	6	*	1	*
Surg: Plastic & Recon-Hand	0	*	*	*	0	*	*	*
Surg: Plastic & Recon-Pediatric	*	*	*	*	2	*	*	*
Surg: Thoracic (primary)	2	*	16	*	0	*	*	*
Surg: Transplant	*	*	*	*	4	*	*	*
Surg: Trauma	*	*	0	*	3	*	*	*
Surg: Trauma-Burn	*	*	0	*	6	*	1	*
Surg: Vascular (primary)	3	*	0	*	0	*	4	*
Urgent Care	0	*	3	*	19	*	0	*
Urology	13	*	9	*	12	$1,533,503	3	*
Urology: Pediatric	*	*	*	*	0	*	0	*

Table 25C: Physician Gross Charges (TC Excluded) by Geographic Section for Multispecialty Practices

	Eastern		Midwest		Southern		Western	
	Physicians	Median	Physicians	Median	Physicians	Median	Physicians	Median
Allergy/Immunology	7	*	29	$618,005	15	$674,718	16	$598,925
Anesthesiology	34	$743,526	98	$815,429	27	$554,172	34	$629,812
Anesth: Pain Management	2	*	5	*	3	*	0	*
Anesth: Pediatric	*	*	0	*	0	*	*	*
Cardiology: Electrophysiology	3	*	4	*	1	*	5	*
Cardiology: Invasive	11	$1,500,680	32	$1,463,875	23	$1,724,347	9	*
Cardiology: Inv-Intervntnl	10	$1,683,180	27	$1,635,220	26	$1,709,152	8	*
Cardiology: Noninvasive	19	$1,575,903	30	$1,374,710	15	$1,177,541	17	$853,229
Critical Care: Intensivist	7	*	7	*	*	*	3	*
Dentistry	3	*	*	*	5	*	0	*
Dermatology	17	$1,098,721	66	$957,562	19	$927,119	33	$686,268
Dermatology: MOHS Surgery	1	*	3	*	3	*	3	*
Emergency Medicine	51	$412,737	58	$588,767	0	*	5	*
Endocrinology/Metabolism	17	$452,417	34	$445,604	24	$468,196	17	$403,158
Family Practice (w/ OB)	38	$437,657	391	$439,068	31	$483,134	76	$517,595
Family Practice (w/o OB)	278	$369,598	815	$455,616	198	$432,167	274	$461,262
Family Practice: Sports Med	0	*	1	*	0	*	1	*
Gastroenterology	38	$1,547,860	86	$1,527,835	50	$1,349,499	35	$1,244,685
Gastroenterology: Hepatology	0	*	*	*	0	*	0	*
Geriatrics	3	*	13	$334,685	0	*	4	*
Hematology/Oncology	20	$347,182	52	$636,530	25	$592,267	17	$567,193
Hem/Onc: Oncology (only)	6	*	20	$550,198	5	*	1	*
Infectious Disease	10	$294,244	20	$499,960	7	*	6	*
Internal Medicine: General	307	$421,205	628	$412,459	229	$423,924	315	$457,556
Internal Med: Hospitalist	20	$425,582	87	$346,201	20	$355,811	27	$264,822
Internal Med: Pediatric	5	*	10	$460,359	10	*	6	*
Nephrology	16	$640,682	38	$664,698	26	$622,957	9	*
Neurology	34	$566,567	81	$645,335	25	$730,469	24	$527,694
OBGYN: General	86	$872,083	195	$913,662	58	$922,722	89	$765,636
OBGYN: Gynecology (only)	8	*	57	$926,883	9	*	7	*
OBGYN: Gyn Oncology	3	*	5	*	3	*	1	*
OBGYN: Maternal & Fetal Med	5	*	19	$790,092	0	*	2	*
OBGYN: Repro Endocrinology	3	*	8	*	*	*	0	*
Occupational Medicine	2	*	30	$367,878	3	*	12	$461,083
Ophthalmology	19	$1,179,895	75	$1,194,522	21	$1,168,959	24	$963,098
Ophthalmology: Pediatric	1	*	1	*	0	*	0	*
Ophthalmology: Retina	1	*	3	*	0	*	1	*
Orthopedic (Non-surgical)	0	*	6	*	1	*	4	*
Orthopedic Surgery: General	21	$1,571,880	120	$1,434,522	37	$1,164,216	27	$1,174,034
Ortho Surg: Foot & Ankle	0	*	4	*	0	*	*	*
Ortho Surg: Hand	1	*	9	*	0	*	2	*
Ortho Surg: Hip & Joint	*	*	10	$1,275,672	0	*	3	*
Ortho Surg: Oncology	*	*	*	*	0	*	*	*
Ortho Surg: Pediatric	1	*	3	*	0	*	0	*
Ortho Surg: Spine	3	*	10	$2,186,873	0	*	3	*
Ortho Surg: Trauma	4	*	1	*	*	*	0	*
Ortho Surg: Sports Med	2	*	14	$1,398,115	0	*	6	*
Otorhinolaryngology	19	$1,080,180	81	$1,240,721	24	$1,415,672	29	$930,098
Otorhinolaryngology: Pediatric	0	*	1	*	*	*	*	*
Pathology: Anatomic & Clinical	16	$845,604	14	$611,238	8	*	4	*
Pathology: Anatomic	0	*	3	*	0	*	2	*
Pathology: Clinical	5	*	6	*	5	*	0	*

Table 25C: Physician Gross Charges (TC Excluded) by Geographic Section for Multispecialty Practices (continued)

	Eastern		Midwest		Southern		Western	
	Physicians	Median	Physicians	Median	Physicians	Median	Physicians	Median
Pediatrics: General	133	$455,643	310	$458,114	97	$450,271	157	$487,616
Ped: Adolescent Medicine	2	*	25	*	7	*	*	*
Ped: Allergy/Immunology	1	*	3	*	0	*	*	*
Ped: Cardiology	4	*	6	*	1	*	8	*
Ped: Child Development	1	*	7	*	1	*	2	*
Ped: Critical Care/Intensivist	2	*	11	$370,676	1	*	0	*
Ped: Emergency Medicine	*	*	6	*	*	*	*	*
Ped: Endocrinology	1	*	6	*	1	*	2	*
Ped: Gastroenterology	3	*	3	*	*	*	3	*
Ped: Genetics	0	*	2	*	0	*	5	*
Ped: Hematology/Oncology	2	*	6	*	1	*	4	*
Ped: Hospitalist	0	*	3	*	1	*	9	*
Ped: Infectious Disease	*	*	0	*	0	*	1	*
Ped: Neonatal Medicine	9	*	28	$1,020,646	1	*	0	*
Ped: Nephrology	1	*	2	*	*	*	3	*
Ped: Neurology	3	*	13	$361,038	1	*	3	*
Ped: Pulmonology	3	*	3	*	1	*	0	*
Ped: Rheumatology	1	*	*	*	*	*	2	*
Ped: Sports Medicine	0	*	*	*	*	*	*	*
Physiatry (Phys Med & Rehab)	3	*	34	$543,082	2	*	8	*
Podiatry: General	3	*	40	$609,900	11	$606,377	15	$634,612
Podiatry: Surg-Foot & Ankle	4	*	7	*	0	*	4	*
Podiatry: Surg-Forefoot Only	4	*	1	*	0	*	0	*
Psychiatry: General	21	$265,871	74	$376,774	11	$365,609	19	$340,885
Psychiatry: Child & Adolescent	1	*	12	$454,378	2	*	0	*
Psychiatry: Geriatric	4	*	2	*	4	*	0	*
Pulmonary Medicine	20	$762,376	42	$684,909	34	$793,615	18	$548,774
Pulmonary Med: Critical Care	14	$719,149	19	$691,278	10	$774,642	0	*
Radiation Oncology	3	*	18	$1,798,720	2	*	3	*
Radiology: Diagnostic-Inv	16	$1,252,182	37	$1,744,226	10	$1,906,584	6	*
Radiology: Diagnostic-Noninv	26	*	49	$1,271,510	19	$1,166,925	3	*
Radiology: Nuclear Medicine	5	*	4	*	2	*	1	*
Rheumatology	19	$528,562	50	$501,768	21	$543,919	15	$588,958
Sleep Medicine	0	*	0	*	0	*	1	*
Surgery: General	57	$986,398	185	$1,064,802	60	$1,116,497	66	$881,329
Surg: Cardiovascular	6	*	21	$1,411,571	5	*	5	*
Surg: Cardiovascular-Pediatric	*	*	1	*	*	*	*	*
Surg: Colon and Rectal	3	*	7	*	1	*	0	*
Surg: Neurological	15	$1,722,275	20	$1,447,503	5	*	8	*
Surg: Oncology	2	*	5	*	*	*	0	*
Surg: Oral	2	*	6	*	0	*	0	*
Surg: Pediatric	3	*	*	*	0	*	4	*
Surg: Plastic & Reconstruction	9	*	17	$1,432,520	4	*	14	$823,775
Surg: Plastic & Recon-Hand	0	*	3	*	*	*	*	*
Surg: Plastic & Recon-Pediatric	0	*	*	*	*	*	*	*
Surg: Thoracic (primary)	1	*	4	*	*	*	0	*
Surg: Transplant	4	*	1	*	0	*	1	*
Surg: Trauma	3	*	5	*	0	*	*	*
Surg: Trauma-Burn	1	*	0	*	*	*	*	*
Surg: Vascular (primary)	14	$1,460,948	20	$1,299,213	3	*	6	*
Urgent Care	2	*	75	$419,983	21	$515,418	74	$542,914
Urology	19	$1,206,902	63	$1,185,825	24	$1,223,435	24	$1,055,236
Urology: Pediatric	*	*	0	*	*	*	2	*

　　MEDICAL GROUP MANAGEMENT ASSOCIATION™

Table 26: Physician Gross Charges (TC Excluded) by Percent of Capitation Revenue

	No capitation		10% or less		11% to 50%		51% or more	
	Physicians	Median	Physicians	Median	Physicians	Median	Physicians	Median
Allergy/Immunology	36	$630,709	20	$781,469	13	$621,905	6	*
Anesthesiology	249	$750,956	46	$616,946	48	$903,386	7	*
Anesth: Pain Management	25	$1,375,000	2	*	3	*	0	*
Anesth: Pediatric	0	*	*	*	0	*	*	*
Cardiology: Electrophysiology	14	$1,765,196	5	*	4	*	1	*
Cardiology: Invasive	54	$1,421,660	45	$1,329,419	3	*	4	*
Cardiology: Inv-Intervntnl	78	$1,582,773	46	$1,621,115	7	*	3	*
Cardiology: Noninvasive	48	$1,031,622	28	$1,153,382	25	$1,611,661	6	*
Critical Care: Intensivist	1	*	5	*	8	*	3	*
Dentistry	2	*	3	*	4	*	0	*
Dermatology	69	$831,042	41	$977,590	27	$988,506	6	*
Dermatology: MOHS Surgery	6	*	6	*	1	*	0	*
Emergency Medicine	83	$758,371	41	$577,378	58	$479,234	0	*
Endocrinology/Metabolism	43	$488,298	29	$461,942	17	$397,300	3	*
Family Practice (w/ OB)	268	$446,748	184	$449,088	168	$433,144	4	*
Family Practice (w/o OB)	905	$463,456	411	$404,089	358	$409,132	56	$427,893
Family Practice: Sports Med	1	*	1	*	0	*	*	*
Gastroenterology	221	$1,390,000	57	$1,544,577	44	$1,534,150	8	*
Gastroenterology: Hepatology	16	*	0	*	3	*	0	*
Geriatrics	2	*	8	*	10	$308,418	0	*
Hematology/Oncology	86	$687,165	45	$575,282	28	$364,185	3	*
Hem/Onc: Oncology (only)	35	$572,232	3	*	8	*	1	*
Infectious Disease	42	$529,724	19	$463,032	14	$499,960	2	*
Internal Medicine: General	659	$425,321	432	$431,365	355	$421,734	69	$438,402
Internal Med: Hospitalist	95	$351,638	45	$320,494	10	$402,933	4	*
Internal Med: Pediatric	14	$397,791	13	$346,911	4	*	0	*
Nephrology	83	$761,577	22	$607,664	27	$769,890	1	*
Neurology	115	$646,591	61	$551,773	38	$652,817	10	$482,767
OBGYN: General	268	$871,501	115	$847,564	132	$876,917	23	$888,339
OBGYN: Gynecology (only)	60	$883,010	17	$705,699	8	*	5	*
OBGYN: Gyn Oncology	5	*	3	*	4	*	*	*
OBGYN: Maternal & Fetal Med	20	$704,183	4	*	7	*	*	*
OBGYN: Repro Endocrinology	1	*	8	*	2	*	0	*
Occupational Medicine	21	$390,492	13	$458,907	10	$350,374	3	*
Ophthalmology	76	$1,038,558	31	$1,360,440	32	$1,456,133	13	$900,234
Ophthalmology: Pediatric	1	*	0	*	2	*	0	*
Ophthalmology: Retina	2	*	0	*	4	*	0	*
Orthopedic (Non-surgical)	5	*	3	*	1	*	2	*
Orthopedic Surgery: General	140	$1,360,775	47	$1,144,542	60	$1,567,955	5	*
Ortho Surg: Foot & Ankle	10	$1,479,078	1	*	2	*	*	*
Ortho Surg: Hand	23	$1,555,276	2	*	4	*	1	*
Ortho Surg: Hip & Joint	24	$1,543,571	2	*	2	*	1	*
Ortho Surg: Oncology	0	*	*	*	*	*	*	*
Ortho Surg: Pediatric	4	*	1	*	2	*	0	*
Ortho Surg: Spine	25	$2,116,900	1	*	6	*	2	*
Ortho Surg: Trauma	7	*	*	*	5	*	*	*
Ortho Surg: Sports Med	38	$1,665,606	8	*	5	*	3	*
Otorhinolaryngology	95	$1,103,531	43	$989,343	53	$1,547,970	4	*
Otorhinolaryngology: Pediatric	1	*	*	*	*	*	*	*
Pathology: Anatomic & Clinical	22	$754,221	14	$723,923	9	*	3	*
Pathology: Anatomic	7	*	0	*	3	*	*	*
Pathology: Clinical	6	*	8	*	2	*	*	*

Table 26: Physician Gross Charges (TC Excluded) by Percent of Capitation Revenue (continued)

	No capitation		10% or less		11% to 50%		51% or more	
	Physicians	Median	Physicians	Median	Physicians	Median	Physicians	Median
Pediatrics: General	473	$460,177	208	$446,188	207	$491,745	27	$465,456
Ped: Adolescent Medicine	17	$430,918	1	*	16	$493,922	*	*
Ped: Allergy/Immunology	0	*	1	*	5	*	*	*
Ped: Cardiology	6	*	7	*	7	*	0	*
Ped: Child Development	0	*	5	*	6	*	*	*
Ped: Critical Care/Intensivist	20	$412,628	2	*	7	*	*	*
Ped: Emergency Medicine	6	*	*	*	*	*	*	*
Ped: Endocrinology	4	*	3	*	4	*	*	*
Ped: Gastroenterology	2	*	4	*	4	*	*	*
Ped: Genetics	2	*	5	*	*	*	*	*
Ped: Hematology/Oncology	6	*	7	*	5	*	0	*
Ped: Hospitalist	3	*	9	*	1	*	0	*
Ped: Infectious Disease	*	*	1	*	*	*	*	*
Ped: Neonatal Medicine	16	$1,020,646	28	$865,323	11	$788,037	0	*
Ped: Nephrology	0	*	4	*	2	*	*	*
Ped: Neurology	12	$360,501	7	*	6	*	*	*
Ped: Pulmonology	1	*	1	*	6	*	*	*
Ped: Rheumatology	*	*	2	*	1	*	*	*
Ped: Sports Medicine	0	*	*	*	*	*	*	*
Physiatry (Phys Med & Rehab)	30	$597,680	10	$505,865	9	*	2	*
Podiatry: General	35	$608,727	13	$647,602	15	$684,071	6	*
Podiatry: Surg-Foot & Ankle	6	*	6	*	2	*	3	*
Podiatry: Surg-Forefoot Only	4	*	1	*	*	*	0	*
Psychiatry: General	42	$364,407	34	$332,870	48	$378,609	4	*
Psychiatry: Child & Adolescent	12	$332,287	4	*	4	*	1	*
Psychiatry: Geriatric	5	*	3	*	1	*	*	*
Pulmonary Medicine	52	$706,221	36	$778,004	24	$672,613	3	*
Pulmonary Med: Critical Care	43	$737,919	9	*	8	*	0	*
Radiation Oncology	41	$1,458,566	3	*	16	$2,012,125	1	*
Radiology: Diagnostic-Inv	92	$1,482,251	23	$1,278,906	54	$1,439,997	6	*
Radiology: Diagnostic-Noninv	137	$1,246,644	17	$1,024,247	40	$1,356,218	0	*
Radiology: Nuclear Medicine	8	*	2	*	4	*	1	*
Rheumatology	56	$609,451	46	$536,241	14	$502,074	3	*
Sleep Medicine	2	*	0	*	1	*	*	*
Surgery: General	272	$1,093,703	93	$975,940	71	$1,017,357	10	$854,743
Surg: Cardiovascular	74	$1,968,745	10	$1,522,658	16	$2,029,165	2	*
Surg: Cardiovascular-Pediatric	3	*	1	*	0	*	*	*
Surg: Colon and Rectal	10	$812,487	2	*	6	*	0	*
Surg: Neurological	75	$2,297,215	11	$1,355,646	11	$2,133,091	0	*
Surg: Oncology	1	*	*	*	6	*	*	*
Surg: Oral	16	$1,018,979	1	*	4	*	0	*
Surg: Pediatric	2	*	5	*	3	*	*	*
Surg: Plastic & Reconstruction	11	$843,820	21	$1,089,633	18	$1,543,593	1	*
Surg: Plastic & Recon-Hand	1	*	*	*	2	*	*	*
Surg: Plastic & Recon-Pediatric	0	*	2	*	*	*	*	*
Surg: Thoracic (primary)	21	$2,931,889	2	*	0	*	0	*
Surg: Transplant	6	*	1	*	3	*	*	*
Surg: Trauma	3	*	3	*	5	*	*	*
Surg: Trauma-Burn	6	*	1	*	1	*	*	*
Surg: Vascular (primary)	25	$852,329	7	*	18	$1,419,949	0	*
Urgent Care	99	$510,812	52	$419,732	25	$497,202	16	$522,535
Urology	96	$1,296,017	39	$1,176,142	28	$1,362,293	4	*
Urology: Pediatric	0	*	2	*	0	*	*	*

Table 27A: Physician Gross Charges (TC Excluded) by Method of Compensation (1-2 Years in Specialty)

	Productivity Based		Guaranteed or Base' Salary		Straight Salary	
	Physicians	Median	Physicians	Median	Physicians	Median
Allergy/Immunology	*	*	3	*	0	*
Anesthesiology	0	*	15	$699,247	5	*
Anesth: Pain Management	*	*	1	*	3	*
Anesth: Pediatric	*	*	0	*	*	*
Cardiology: Electrophysiology	*	*	2	*	0	*
Cardiology: Invasive	*	*	0	*	0	*
Cardiology: Inv-Intervntnl	*	*	3	*	2	*
Cardiology: Noninvasive	*	*	2	*	0	*
Critical Care: Intensivist	*	*	*	*	0	*
Dermatology	1	*	5	*	1	*
Dermatology: MOHS Surgery	*	*	*	*	0	*
Emergency Medicine	2	*	8	*	2	*
Endocrinology/Metabolism	*	*	1	*	0	*
Family Practice (w/ OB)	1	*	34	$409,318	22	$466,389
Family Practice (w/o OB)	1	*	50	$350,699	12	$354,076
Family Practice: Sports Med	*	*	0	*	0	*
Gastroenterology	*	*	7	*	6	*
Gastroenterology: Hepatology	*	*	1	*	*	*
Geriatrics	0	*	0	*	*	*
Hematology/Oncology	0	*	5	*	1	*
Infectious Disease	*	*	3	*	2	*
Internal Medicine: General	1	*	55	$371,313	19	$394,999
Internal Med: Hospitalist	0	*	13	$319,850	6	*
Internal Med: Pediatric	*	*	6	*	0	*
Nephrology	0	*	6	*	1	*
Neurology	*	*	5	*	5	*
OBGYN: General	2	*	18	$785,949	6	*
OBGYN: Gynecology (only)	*	*	1	*	0	*
OBGYN: Gyn Oncology	*	*	*	*	0	*
OBGYN: Maternal & Fetal Med	0	*	1	*	0	*
OBGYN: Repro Endocrinology	*	*	*	*	0	*
Occupational Medicine	*	*	2	*	0	*
Ophthalmology	*	*	4	*	1	*
Ophthalmology: Retina	*	*	*	*	0	*
Orthopedic (Non-surgical)	*	*	*	*	0	*
Orthopedic Surgery: General	1	*	6	*	2	*
Ortho Surg: Foot & Ankle	*	*	0	*	2	*
Ortho Surg: Hand	0	*	1	*	0	*
Ortho Surg: Hip & Joint	*	*	1	*	0	*
Ortho Surg: Oncology	*	*	*	*	0	*
Ortho Surg: Pediatric	*	*	*	*	0	*
Ortho Surg: Spine	0	*	1	*	1	*
Ortho Surg: Trauma	*	*	*	*	0	*
Ortho Surg: Sports Med	1	*	1	*	2	*
Otorhinolaryngology	1	*	4	*	2	*
Pathology: Anatomic & Clinical	*	*	1	*	2	*
Pathology: Clinical	*	*	1	*	1	*

Table 27A: Physician Gross Charges (TC Excluded) by Method of Compensation (1-2 Years in Specialty) (continued)

	Productivity Based		Guaranteed or Base Salary		Straight Salary	
	Physicians	Median	Physicians	Median	Physicians	Median
Pediatrics: General	2	*	27	$378,635	17	$412,522
Ped: Adolescent Medicine	*	*	1	*	1	*
Ped: Cardiology	*	*	0	*	*	*
Ped: Critical Care/Intensivist	1	*	1	*	0	*
Ped: Endocrinology	*	*	2	*	0	*
Ped: Gastroenterology	*	*	0	*	0	*
Ped: Genetics	*	*	*	*	0	*
Ped: Hematology/Oncology	*	*	*	*	0	*
Ped: Hospitalist	*	*	1	*	*	*
Ped: Neonatal Medicine	*	*	*	*	1	*
Ped: Neurology	*	*	1	*	*	*
Ped: Pulmonology	*	*	0	*	*	*
Physiatry (Phys Med & Rehab)	*	*	1	*	0	*
Podiatry: General	1	*	1	*	0	*
Podiatry: Surg-Foot & Ankle	*	*	*	*	0	*
Psychiatry: General	*	*	5	*	1	*
Psychiatry: Child & Adolescent	*	*	1	*	0	*
Pulmonary Medicine	*	*	2	*	0	*
Pulmonary Med: Critical Care	0	*	3	*	0	*
Radiation Oncology	*	*	1	*	2	*
Radiology: Diagnostic-Inv	*	*	1	*	6	*
Radiology: Diagnostic-Noninv	*	*	4	*	4	*
Radiology: Nuclear Medicine	*	*	0	*	0	*
Rheumatology	*	*	3	*	0	*
Sleep Medicine	*	*	*	*	1	*
Surgery: General	1	*	13	$871,000	7	*
Surg: Cardiovascular	*	*	1	*	3	*
Surg: Cardiovascular-Pediatric	*	*	*	*	1	*
Surg: Colon and Rectal	*	*	*	*	1	*
Surg: Neurological	*	*	3	*	4	*
Surg: Pediatric	*	*	2	*	*	*
Surg: Plastic & Reconstruction	*	*	4	*	0	*
Surg: Thoracic (primary)	*	*	*	*	0	*
Surg: Transplant	*	*	1	*	1	*
Surg: Trauma	*	*	1	*	*	*
Surg: Trauma-Burn	*	*	*	*	0	*
Surg: Vascular (primary)	*	*	1	*	1	*
Urgent Care	*	*	5	*	1	*
Urology	*	*	4	*	0	*

Table 27B: Physician Gross Charges (TC Excluded) by Method of Compensation (More than 2 Years in Specialty)

	Productivity Based		Guaranteed or Base Salary		Straight Salary	
	Physicians	Median	Physicians	Median	Physicians	Median
Allergy/Immunology	33	$777,739	21	$576,249	0	*
Anesthesiology	91	$766,953	43	$823,949	7	*
Anesth: Pain Management	5	*	2	*	3	*
Anesth: Pediatric	*	*	0	*	*	*
Cardiology: Electrophysiology	9	*	5	*	0	*
Cardiology: Invasive	43	$1,485,284	21	$1,502,760	3	*
Cardiology: Inv-Intervntnl	41	$1,589,545	29	$1,649,403	3	*
Cardiology: Noninvasive	31	$1,039,346	25	$1,106,128	0	*
Critical Care: Intensivist	2	*	7	*	2	*
Dentistry	5	*	3	*	0	*
Dermatology	63	$810,340	28	$1,060,713	2	*
Dermatology: MOHS Surgery	4	*	5	*	0	*
Emergency Medicine	25	$638,159	57	$522,274	0	*
Endocrinology/Metabolism	36	$506,965	19	$374,225	4	*
Family Practice (w/ OB)	227	$461,652	140	$427,997	13	$604,093
Family Practice (w/o OB)	725	$470,650	288	$407,241	48	$359,130
Family Practice: Sports Med	1	*	1	*	0	*
Gastroenterology	129	$1,611,431	45	$1,244,685	17	$1,433,899
Gastroenterology: Hepatology	5	*	13	*	*	*
Geriatrics	8	*	3	*	0	*
Hematology/Oncology	63	$663,827	43	$523,495	0	*
Hem/Onc: Oncology (only)	15	$458,902	2	*	9	*
Infectious Disease	38	$595,310	10	$403,678	4	*
Internal Medicine: General	598	$469,928	329	$413,184	68	$417,704
Internal Med: Hospitalist	55	$360,214	26	$310,744	0	*
Internal Med: Pediatric	4	*	2	*	2	*
Nephrology	29	$722,686	31	$767,800	4	*
Neurology	88	$652,817	31	$557,286	7	*
OBGYN: General	174	$850,035	120	$891,914	15	$683,407
OBGYN: Gynecology (only)	63	$861,134	12	$605,495	2	*
OBGYN: Gyn Oncology	2	*	5	*	*	*
OBGYN: Maternal & Fetal Med	10	*	8	*	2	*
OBGYN: Repro Endocrinology	0	*	2	*	0	*
Occupational Medicine	19	$405,893	9	*	0	*
Ophthalmology	51	$1,234,000	40	$1,160,991	1	*
Ophthalmology: Pediatric	1	*	0	*	*	*
Ophthalmology: Retina	2	*	1	*	0	*
Orthopedic (Non-surgical)	3	*	5	*	0	*
Orthopedic Surgery: General	116	$1,403,783	46	$1,388,077	2	*
Ortho Surg: Foot & Ankle	7	*	1	*	0	*
Ortho Surg: Hand	16	$1,465,412	4	*	0	*
Ortho Surg: Hip & Joint	9	*	6	*	0	*
Ortho Surg: Oncology	0	*	0	*	*	*
Ortho Surg: Pediatric	3	*	0	*	0	*
Ortho Surg: Spine	20	$2,990,963	5	*	0	*
Ortho Surg: Trauma	2	*	0	*	0	*
Ortho Surg: Sports Med	20	$1,640,849	13	$1,144,561	0	*
Otorhinolaryngology	92	$1,147,884	38	$1,022,918	1	*
Otorhinolaryngology: Pediatric	*	*	0	*	0	*
Pathology: Anatomic & Clinical	7	*	16	$663,694	4	*
Pathology: Anatomic	5	*	*	*	0	*
Pathology: Clinical	6	*	1	*	0	*

Table 27B: Physician Gross Charges (TC Excluded) by Method of Compensation (More than 2 Years in Specialty) (continued)

	Productivity Based		Guaranteed or Base Salary		Straight Salary	
	Physicians	Median	Physicians	Median	Physicians	Median
Pediatrics: General	380	$480,926	179	$446,265	48	$532,356
Ped: Adolescent Medicine	0	*	23	*	5	*
Ped: Allergy/Immunology	1	*	1	*	0	*
Ped: Cardiology	7	*	*	*	6	*
Ped: Child Development	0	*	0	*	2	*
Ped: Critical Care/Intensivist	6	*	3	*	0	*
Ped: Emergency Medicine	*	*	6	*	0	*
Ped: Endocrinology	1	*	1	*	2	*
Ped: Gastroenterology	2	*	*	*	3	*
Ped: Genetics	2	*	2	*	3	*
Ped: Hematology/Oncology	3	*	3	*	7	*
Ped: Hospitalist	1	*	0	*	8	*
Ped: Infectious Disease	*	*	0	*	1	*
Ped: Neonatal Medicine	22	$865,323	14	$1,056,841	0	*
Ped: Nephrology	*	*	2	*	2	*
Ped: Neurology	5	*	6	*	4	*
Ped: Pulmonology	2	*	2	*	0	*
Ped: Rheumatology	1	*	*	*	2	*
Physiatry (Phys Med & Rehab)	24	$574,437	14	$601,974	1	*
Podiatry: General	31	$589,481	18	$649,678	0	*
Podiatry: Surg-Foot & Ankle	2	*	8	*	0	*
Podiatry: Surg-Forefoot Only	0	*	*	*	0	*
Psychiatry: General	40	$387,244	26	$303,712	1	*
Psychiatry: Child & Adolescent	6	*	2	*	*	*
Psychiatry: Geriatric	6	*	1	*	*	*
Pulmonary Medicine	53	$694,908	28	$736,981	4	*
Pulmonary Med: Critical Care	23	$641,209	10	*	1	*
Radiation Oncology	10	$1,739,885	5	*	10	*
Radiology: Diagnostic-Inv	15	$1,744,226	22	$1,625,421	54	$1,018,683
Radiology: Diagnostic-Noninv	38	$1,356,218	45	$1,324,922	10	*
Radiology: Nuclear Medicine	3	*	2	*	2	*
Rheumatology	47	$633,666	20	$527,957	4	*
Sleep Medicine	1	*	*	*	*	*
Surgery: General	169	$1,128,040	89	$857,682	9	*
Surg: Cardiovascular	17	$1,458,458	28	$1,924,976	0	*
Surg: Cardiovascular-Pediatric	1	*	1	*	0	*
Surg: Colon and Rectal	8	*	2	*	5	*
Surg: Neurological	19	$2,133,091	9	*	5	*
Surg: Oncology	1	*	1	*	*	*
Surg: Oral	4	*	2	*	6	*
Surg: Pediatric	0	*	1	*	4	*
Surg: Plastic & Reconstruction	21	$1,781,066	15	$783,386	1	*
Surg: Plastic & Recon-Hand	0	*	0	*	0	*
Surg: Plastic & Recon-Pediatric	2	*	*	*	*	*
Surg: Thoracic (primary)	1	*	0	*	1	*
Surg: Transplant	5	*	2	*	*	*
Surg: Trauma	*	*	7	*	3	*
Surg: Trauma-Burn	6	*	1	*	*	*
Surg: Vascular (primary)	14	$1,426,189	11	$1,140,443	4	*
Urgent Care	59	$503,322	53	$429,417	18	*
Urology	71	$1,264,619	37	$1,138,063	7	*
Urology: Pediatric	*	*	0	*	2	*

Table 28: Physician Gross Charges (TC Excluded) by Years in Specialty

	1 to 2 years		3 to 7 years		8 to 17 years		18 years or more	
	Physicians	Median	Physicians	Median	Physicians	Median	Physicians	Median
Allergy/Immunology	3	*	9	*	29	$819,879	26	$705,973
Anesthesiology	21	$685,046	60	$724,767	124	$761,458	85	$783,134
Anesth: Pain Management	5	*	9	*	8	*	4	*
Anesth: Pediatric	0	*	0	*	0	*	0	*
Cardiology: Electrophysiology	2	*	8	*	12	$1,482,758	2	*
Cardiology: Invasive	0	*	22	$1,358,787	40	$1,540,059	33	$1,389,640
Cardiology: Inv-Intervntnl	5	*	22	$1,535,812	53	$1,716,956	42	$1,593,782
Cardiology: Noninvasive	2	*	19	$1,309,181	31	$1,292,349	44	$975,285
Critical Care: Intensivist	0	*	2	*	11	$533,710	4	*
Dentistry	0	*	0	*	6	*	4	*
Dermatology	8	*	20	$927,526	46	$923,171	49	$872,700
Dermatology: MOHS Surgery	0	*	4	*	6	*	2	*
Emergency Medicine	13	$619,601	51	$693,837	69	$562,346	39	$547,915
Endocrinology/Metabolism	1	*	12	$419,956	34	$464,891	32	$472,809
Family Practice (w/ OB)	58	$412,793	153	$411,478	191	$474,500	142	$443,347
Family Practice (w/o OB)	67	$347,761	330	$409,804	496	$423,235	581	$461,072
Family Practice: Sports Med	0	*	0	*	2	*	1	*
Gastroenterology	18	$1,203,231	52	$1,438,957	112	$1,442,256	115	$1,389,574
Gastroenterology: Hepatology	1	*	3	*	5	*	10	$1,156,673
Geriatrics	0	*	3	*	7	*	4	*
Hematology/Oncology	6	*	25	$599,040	53	$567,193	71	$612,245
Hem/Onc: Oncology (only)	0	*	4	*	14	$532,025	15	$603,008
Infectious Disease	6	*	15	$450,686	22	$542,892	21	$511,981
Internal Medicine: General	84	$381,625	321	$426,026	448	$460,336	450	$434,522
Internal Med: Hospitalist	24	$314,182	46	$362,013	35	$304,212	19	$425,585
Internal Med: Pediatric	6	*	10	$311,383	10	$367,786	1	*
Nephrology	8	*	23	$712,096	34	$770,559	42	$780,971
Neurology	10	$595,574	34	$527,823	80	$673,014	68	$600,633
OBGYN: General	27	$762,113	126	$846,853	170	$911,394	127	$843,689
OBGYN: Gynecology (only)	1	*	5	*	25	$950,939	56	$727,413
OBGYN: Gyn Oncology	1	*	1	*	4	*	2	*
OBGYN: Maternal & Fetal Med	1	*	7	*	11	$1,199,490	6	*
OBGYN: Repro Endocrinology	0	*	0	*	3	*	1	*
Occupational Medicine	2	*	9	*	13	$452,964	13	$369,880
Ophthalmology	5	*	24	$1,080,900	58	$1,255,823	41	$1,179,895
Ophthalmology: Pediatric	*	*	0	*	2	*	1	*
Ophthalmology: Retina	0	*	3	*	2	*	0	*
Orthopedic (Non-surgical)	0	*	3	*	2	*	5	*
Orthopedic Surgery: General	10	$1,450,892	28	$1,513,632	74	$1,424,816	96	$1,304,656
Ortho Surg: Foot & Ankle	2	*	4	*	5	*	2	*
Ortho Surg: Hand	1	*	4	*	13	$1,376,398	11	$1,934,838
Ortho Surg: Hip & Joint	1	*	2	*	15	$1,701,373	11	$1,445,196
Ortho Surg: Oncology	0	*	*	*	0	*	0	*
Ortho Surg: Pediatric	0	*	2	*	2	*	3	*
Ortho Surg: Spine	2	*	5	*	18	$2,989,471	9	*
Ortho Surg: Trauma	0	*	6	*	4	*	2	*
Ortho Surg: Sports Med	4	*	11	$1,663,865	30	$1,703,631	9	*
Otorhinolaryngology	8	*	38	$1,018,322	50	$1,391,574	72	$961,154
Otorhinolaryngology: Pediatric	0	*	0	*	0	*	0	*
Pathology: Anatomic & Clinical	3	*	5	*	19	$754,221	19	$723,841
Pathology: Anatomic	*	*	1	*	0	*	9	*
Pathology: Clinical	2	*	4	*	5	*	5	*

Table 28: Physician Gross Charges (TC Excluded) by Years in Specialty (continued)

	1 to 2 years		3 to 7 years		8 to 17 years		18 years or more	
	Physicians	Median	Physicians	Median	Physicians	Median	Physicians	Median
Pediatrics: General	51	$402,162	204	$428,735	279	$488,723	276	$481,236
Ped: Adolescent Medicine	2	*	6	*	11	$411,052	14	$490,308
Ped: Allergy/Immunology	*	*	1	*	1	*	4	*
Ped: Cardiology	0	*	7	*	5	*	6	*
Ped: Child Development	0	*	3	*	0	*	1	*
Ped: Critical Care/Intensivist	2	*	7	*	16	$447,915	3	*
Ped: Emergency Medicine	*	*	0	*	4	*	2	*
Ped: Endocrinology	2	*	2	*	1	*	4	*
Ped: Gastroenterology	0	*	4	*	1	*	4	*
Ped: Genetics	0	*	3	*	1	*	3	*
Ped: Hematology/Oncology	0	*	6	*	5	*	6	*
Ped: Hospitalist	1	*	5	*	3	*	1	*
Ped: Infectious Disease	0	*	0	*	1	*	0	*
Ped: Neonatal Medicine	1	*	9	*	21	$865,323	13	$1,132,991
Ped: Nephrology	*	*	1	*	3	*	1	*
Ped: Neurology	1	*	8	*	9	*	5	*
Ped: Pulmonology	0	*	3	*	5	*	0	*
Ped: Rheumatology	*	*	2	*	1	*	*	*
Ped: Sports Medicine	*	*	*	*	0	*	*	*
Physiatry (Phys Med & Rehab)	1	*	19	$521,407	22	$637,397	6	*
Podiatry: General	3	*	12	$607,552	24	$561,280	15	$676,329
Podiatry: Surg-Foot & Ankle	0	*	2	*	8	*	4	*
Podiatry: Surg-Forefoot Only	0	*	0	*	2	*	3	*
Psychiatry: General	7	*	17	$274,971	37	$379,009	39	$374,539
Psychiatry: Child & Adolescent	1	*	3	*	6	*	4	*
Psychiatry: Geriatric	*	*	0	*	5	*	5	*
Pulmonary Medicine	2	*	14	$848,839	48	$706,953	35	$681,365
Pulmonary Med: Critical Care	4	*	13	$773,435	21	$719,510	14	$711,581
Radiation Oncology	3	*	12	$1,508,119	23	$1,480,629	14	$1,617,859
Radiology: Diagnostic-Inv	8	*	32	$1,200,982	59	$1,374,120	56	$1,447,263
Radiology: Diagnostic-Noninv	9	*	35	$1,123,000	70	$1,255,607	73	$1,261,504
Radiology: Nuclear Medicine	0	*	3	*	4	*	8	*
Rheumatology	5	*	16	$444,097	34	$546,275	44	$579,027
Sleep Medicine	1	*	0	*	1	*	1	*
Surgery: General	21	$871,000	70	$1,103,487	134	$1,114,466	154	$1,072,171
Surg: Cardiovascular	4	*	20	$2,141,074	42	$2,068,213	23	$1,831,683
Surg: Cardiovascular-Pediatric	1	*	1	*	2	*	*	*
Surg: Colon and Rectal	1	*	3	*	7	*	5	*
Surg: Neurological	8	*	21	$2,333,447	31	$2,297,215	32	$2,155,661
Surg: Oncology	*	*	0	*	2	*	*	*
Surg: Oral	1	*	3	*	8	*	8	*
Surg: Pediatric	2	*	3	*	2	*	3	*
Surg: Plastic & Reconstruction	4	*	8	*	13	$1,437,636	20	$813,603
Surg: Plastic & Recon-Hand	*	*	0	*	0	*	0	*
Surg: Plastic & Recon-Pediatric	*	*	1	*	1	*	*	*
Surg: Thoracic (primary)	1	*	6	*	10	$3,200,487	5	*
Surg: Transplant	2	*	1	*	5	*	2	*
Surg: Trauma	1	*	2	*	5	*	3	*
Surg: Trauma-Burn	0	*	1	*	2	*	5	*
Surg: Vascular (primary)	3	*	8	*	20	$1,636,984	12	$1,088,385
Urgent Care	6	*	42	$464,799	65	$469,961	50	$511,882
Urology	4	*	36	$1,346,486	47	$1,362,773	59	$1,138,063
Urology: Pediatric	*	*	1	*	1	*	*	*

MEDICAL GROUP MANAGEMENT ASSOCIATION™

Table 29: Physician Gross Charges (TC Excluded) by Gender

	Male			Female		
	Physicians	Medical Practices	Median	Physicians	Medical Practices	Median
Allergy/Immunology	57	42	$722,210	12	10	$410,442
Anesthesiology	286	38	$785,103	47	20	$669,111
Anesth: Pain Management	22	9	$1,479,020	6	3	*
Anesth: Pediatric	0	*	*	0	*	*
Cardiology: Electrophysiology	20	15	$1,765,196	3	3	*
Cardiology: Invasive	93	38	$1,470,000	8	8	*
Cardiology: Inv-Intervntnl	127	42	$1,627,381	2	2	*
Cardiology: Noninvasive	92	41	$1,193,292	12	8	$1,031,592
Critical Care: Intensivist	13	8	$530,557	2	2	*
Dentistry	7	3	*	3	3	*
Dermatology	99	58	$982,220	34	26	$778,601
Dermatology: MOHS Surgery	10	8	$2,003,177	3	3	*
Emergency Medicine	152	17	$612,001	19	9	$619,601
Endocrinology/Metabolism	67	46	$467,238	18	16	$387,598
Family Practice (w/ OB)	424	73	$463,791	162	59	$395,706
Family Practice (w/o OB)	1,211	173	$424,221	296	115	$363,898
Family Practice: Sports Med	2	2	*	1	1	*
Gastroenterology	298	96	$1,422,635	22	19	$1,145,000
Gastroenterology: Hepatology	17	3	$1,290,018	2	1	*
Geriatrics	14	10	$310,477	5	4	*
Hematology/Oncology	142	55	$595,654	22	16	$675,198
Hem/Onc: Oncology (only)	38	19	$560,017	7	6	*
Infectious Disease	58	32	$529,170	15	8	$488,272
Internal Medicine: General	1,113	170	$433,551	319	112	$377,829
Internal Med: Hospitalist	88	32	$343,669	30	21	$290,762
Internal Med: Pediatric	19	12	$373,087	12	5	$298,913
Nephrology	107	43	$764,745	20	14	$616,087
Neurology	167	68	$640,675	47	29	$524,337
OBGYN: General	331	105	$906,301	190	79	$782,364
OBGYN: Gynecology (only)	38	28	$556,630	10	8	$702,753
OBGYN: Gyn Oncology	10	6	$1,196,143	2	2	*
OBGYN: Maternal & Fetal Med	21	7	$790,092	8	4	*
OBGYN: Repro Endocrinology	5	4	*	6	2	*
Occupational Medicine	28	18	$355,499	10	7	$442,021
Ophthalmology	125	57	$1,159,324	16	16	$1,091,903
Ophthalmology: Pediatric	3	3	*	0	*	*
Ophthalmology: Retina	5	5	*	0	*	*
Orthopedic (Non-surgical)	10	8	$1,149,127	1	1	*
Orthopedic Surgery: General	221	67	$1,357,526	5	4	*
Ortho Surg: Foot & Ankle	12	9	$1,546,196	1	1	*
Ortho Surg: Hand	28	18	$1,581,840	1	1	*
Ortho Surg: Hip & Joint	29	12	$1,641,946	*	*	*
Ortho Surg: Oncology	0	*	*	*	*	*
Ortho Surg: Pediatric	7	7	*	0	*	*
Ortho Surg: Spine	34	22	$2,479,173	*	*	*
Ortho Surg: Trauma	8	6	*	4	2	*
Ortho Surg: Sports Med	50	26	$1,651,359	3	3	*
Otorhinolaryngology	168	71	$1,118,447	12	9	$991,839
Otorhinolaryngology: Pediatric	1	1	*	0	*	*
Pathology: Anatomic & Clinical	32	13	$740,487	13	8	$754,221
Pathology: Anatomic	8	3	*	2	1	*
Pathology: Clinical	12	6	$613,418	4	3	*

Table 29: Physician Gross Charges (TC Excluded) by Gender (continued)

	Male			Female		
	Physicians	Medical Practices	Median	Physicians	Medical Practices	Median
Pediatrics: General	531	129	$490,345	352	122	$419,031
Ped: Adolescent Medicine	17	6	$449,764	7	4	*
Ped: Allergy/Immunology	5	4	*	0	*	*
Ped: Cardiology	18	10	$789,960	2	1	*
Ped: Child Development	7	4	*	4	3	*
Ped: Critical Care/Intensivist	23	11	$442,888	6	5	*
Ped: Emergency Medicine	4	1	*	2	1	*
Ped: Endocrinology	8	8	*	3	3	*
Ped: Gastroenterology	10	6	$564,379	0	*	*
Ped: Genetics	2	1	*	5	2	*
Ped: Hematology/Oncology	13	10	$434,692	5	3	*
Ped: Hospitalist	8	4	*	5	3	*
Ped: Infectious Disease	0	*	*	1	1	*
Ped: Neonatal Medicine	38	12	$865,323	15	9	$865,323
Ped: Nephrology	4	2	*	1	1	*
Ped: Neurology	19	12	$366,624	3	3	*
Ped: Pulmonology	6	5	*	1	1	*
Ped: Rheumatology	3	2	*	0	*	*
Ped: Sports Medicine	*	*	*	0	*	*
Physiatry (Phys Med & Rehab)	28	19	$637,397	19	13	$457,490
Podiatry: General	52	35	$624,679	8	8	*
Podiatry: Surg-Foot & Ankle	16	10	$689,214	1	1	*
Podiatry: Surg-Forefoot Only	4	2	*	1	1	*
Psychiatry: General	94	35	$371,218	26	14	$322,854
Psychiatry: Child & Adolescent	17	9	$393,442	3	3	*
Psychiatry: Geriatric	10	6	$650,160	0	*	*
Pulmonary Medicine	95	54	$728,427	10	9	$573,803
Pulmonary Med: Critical Care	53	21	$739,499	7	6	*
Radiation Oncology	47	17	$1,460,194	8	7	*
Radiology: Diagnostic-Inv	148	23	$1,381,393	12	4	$1,193,785
Radiology: Diagnostic-Noninv	147	30	$1,305,889	38	17	$980,581
Radiology: Nuclear Medicine	12	10	$874,485	4	4	*
Rheumatology	94	50	$557,625	20	16	$501,095
Sleep Medicine	2	2	*	1	1	*
Surgery: General	392	119	$1,057,317	31	28	$950,752
Surg: Cardiovascular	95	27	$1,875,513	2	2	*
Surg: Cardiovascular-Pediatric	4	4	*	*	*	*
Surg: Colon and Rectal	17	9	$1,318,069	2	2	*
Surg: Neurological	91	30	$2,167,565	5	4	*
Surg: Oncology	5	3	*	2	1	*
Surg: Oral	18	7	$1,073,842	1	1	*
Surg: Pediatric	9	4	*	1	1	*
Surg: Plastic & Reconstruction	44	25	$1,132,435	5	5	*
Surg: Plastic & Recon-Hand	1	1	*	0	*	*
Surg: Plastic & Recon-Pediatric	2	1	*	*	*	*
Surg: Thoracic (primary)	22	6	$2,651,390	1	1	*
Surg: Transplant	10	6	$1,309,925	*	*	*
Surg: Trauma	8	3	*	1	1	*
Surg: Trauma-Burn	8	3	*	0	*	*
Surg: Vascular (primary)	44	24	$1,219,399	4	3	*
Urgent Care	141	43	$503,738	45	26	$424,959
Urology	150	62	$1,290,756	5	5	*
Urology: Pediatric	2	1	*	0	*	*

MEDICAL GROUP MANAGEMENT ASSOCIATION™

Table 30: Physician Professional Gross Charges (TC Excluded) by Hours Worked per Week

	Less than 40 hours			40 hours or more		
	Physicians	Medical Practices	Median	Physicians	Medical Practices	Median
Allergy/Immunology	10	9	$513,593	39	28	$785,198
Anesthesiology	28	9	$667,040	223	23	$798,611
Anesth: Pain Management	1	1	*	22	9	$1,301,730
Anesth: Pediatric	0	*	*	0	*	*
Cardiology: Electrophysiology	2	2	*	17	11	$1,832,291
Cardiology: Invasive	4	1	*	77	32	$1,470,000
Cardiology: Inv-Intervntnl	0	*	*	96	31	$1,644,431
Cardiology: Noninvasive	8	4	*	61	28	$1,309,181
Critical Care: Intensivist	3	1	*	9	4	*
Dentistry	0	*	*	7	3	*
Dermatology	22	14	$804,295	71	37	$927,119
Dermatology: MOHS Surgery	4	3	*	6	5	*
Emergency Medicine	67	9	$604,000	43	6	$681,315
Endocrinology/Metabolism	14	8	$435,198	41	28	$533,962
Family Practice (w/ OB)	84	23	$393,254	280	56	$472,925
Family Practice (w/o OB)	488	62	$502,491	838	120	$415,033
Family Practice: Sports Med	0	*	*	3	3	*
Gastroenterology	16	11	$1,468,068	210	64	$1,424,638
Gastroenterology: Hepatology	0	*	*	19	3	$1,192,009
Geriatrics	9	5	*	4	4	*
Hematology/Oncology	9	5	*	116	37	$643,201
Hem/Onc: Oncology (only)	1	1	*	31	15	$513,100
Infectious Disease	9	6	*	47	22	$530,159
Internal Medicine: General	277	56	$445,202	836	119	$436,326
Internal Med: Hospitalist	47	6	$346,899	48	16	$355,811
Internal Med: Pediatric	4	3	*	23	9	$351,818
Nephrology	4	4	*	90	30	$816,256
Neurology	27	10	$526,118	143	43	$660,298
OBGYN: General	69	19	$822,661	312	70	$876,083
OBGYN: Gynecology (only)	48	7	$914,418	34	21	$710,540
OBGYN: Gyn Oncology	1	1	*	7	5	*
OBGYN: Maternal & Fetal Med	2	2	*	23	8	$1,134,534
OBGYN: Repro Endocrinology	0	*	*	10	3	$853,628
Occupational Medicine	11	4	$452,964	14	11	$380,923
Ophthalmology	28	14	$993,923	66	27	$1,307,590
Ophthalmology: Pediatric	1	1	*	2	2	*
Ophthalmology: Retina	0	*	*	4	4	*
Orthopedic (Non-surgical)	3	3	*	8	6	*
Orthopedic Surgery: General	23	7	$1,262,744	106	35	$1,399,368
Ortho Surg: Foot & Ankle	2	2	*	9	8	*
Ortho Surg: Hand	3	2	*	23	16	$1,798,643
Ortho Surg: Hip & Joint	3	3	*	22	9	$1,670,417
Ortho Surg: Oncology	0	*	*	0	*	*
Ortho Surg: Pediatric	1	1	*	5	5	*
Ortho Surg: Spine	3	3	*	23	13	$2,988,111
Ortho Surg: Trauma	1	1	*	11	6	$1,298,558
Ortho Surg: Sports Med	7	4	*	44	24	$1,653,356
Otorhinolaryngology	25	11	$885,987	103	38	$1,265,686
Otorhinolaryngology: Pediatric	0	*	*	0	*	*
Pathology: Anatomic & Clinical	6	2	*	21	7	$754,221
Pathology: Anatomic	*	*	*	10	3	$857,718
Pathology: Clinical	0	*	*	14	5	$525,374

Table 30: Physician Professional Gross Charges (TC Excluded) by Hours Worked per Week (continued)

	Less than 40 hours			40 hours or more		
	Physicians	Medical Practices	Median	Physicians	Medical Practices	Median
Pediatrics: General	209	53	$430,199	483	97	$491,745
Ped: Adolescent Medicine	0	*	*	12	6	$511,336
Ped: Allergy/Immunology	*	*	*	4	3	*
Ped: Cardiology	0	*	*	18	8	$789,960
Ped: Child Development	0	*	*	6	4	*
Ped: Critical Care/Intensivist	4	2	*	22	8	$412,953
Ped: Emergency Medicine	0	*	*	5	1	*
Ped: Endocrinology	1	1	*	8	7	*
Ped: Gastroenterology	1	1	*	8	5	*
Ped: Genetics	2	1	*	5	2	*
Ped: Hematology/Oncology	1	1	*	15	8	$537,193
Ped: Hospitalist	1	1	*	9	2	*
Ped: Infectious Disease	0	*	*	1	1	*
Ped: Neonatal Medicine	2	1	*	37	9	$865,323
Ped: Nephrology	0	*	*	5	3	*
Ped: Neurology	1	1	*	17	10	$359,963
Ped: Pulmonology	*	*	*	7	6	*
Ped: Rheumatology	0	*	*	3	2	*
Ped: Sports Medicine	*	*	*	0	*	*
Physiatry (Phys Med & Rehab)	0	*	*	28	18	$636,031
Podiatry: General	11	5	$693,191	28	18	$571,212
Podiatry: Surg-Foot & Ankle	5	2	*	7	5	*
Podiatry: Surg-Forefoot Only	0	*	*	4	1	*
Psychiatry: General	18	8	$248,104	67	23	$382,909
Psychiatry: Child & Adolescent	2	1	*	13	9	$363,256
Psychiatry: Geriatric	*	*	*	10	6	$650,160
Pulmonary Medicine	7	4	*	66	36	$728,707
Pulmonary Med: Critical Care	5	2	*	35	14	$751,316
Radiation Oncology	4	4	*	45	13	$1,504,918
Radiology: Diagnostic-Inv	9	3	*	119	14	$1,393,890
Radiology: Diagnostic-Noninv	11	5	$1,206,090	143	24	$1,321,448
Radiology: Nuclear Medicine	3	3	*	7	5	*
Rheumatology	20	11	$468,587	62	32	$584,982
Sleep Medicine	1	1	*	2	1	*
Surgery: General	31	13	$1,102,715	267	79	$1,099,484
Surg: Cardiovascular	0	*	*	70	20	$1,862,905
Surg: Cardiovascular-Pediatric	*	*	*	4	4	*
Surg: Colon and Rectal	2	2	*	13	9	$1,318,069
Surg: Neurological	1	1	*	74	22	$2,257,429
Surg: Oncology	*	*	*	1	1	*
Surg: Oral	4	1	*	13	4	$1,160,250
Surg: Pediatric	0	*	*	10	5	$902,677
Surg: Plastic & Reconstruction	1	1	*	29	14	$1,738,656
Surg: Plastic & Recon-Hand	*	*	*	0	*	*
Surg: Plastic & Recon-Pediatric	*	*	*	2	1	*
Surg: Thoracic (primary)	0	*	*	20	5	$3,049,699
Surg: Transplant	0	*	*	9	5	*
Surg: Trauma	0	*	*	6	2	*
Surg: Trauma-Burn	0	*	*	8	3	*
Surg: Vascular (primary)	1	1	*	35	16	$1,251,312
Urgent Care	42	12	$483,315	62	23	$500,538
Urology	18	9	$1,186,529	96	36	$1,395,319
Urology: Pediatric	*	*	*	2	1	*

Table 31: Physician Gross Charges (TC Excluded) by Weeks Worked per Year

	Less than 46 weeks		46 weeks or more	
	Physicians	Median	Physicians	Median
Allergy/Immunology	7	*	49	$705,281
Anesthesiology	137	$831,421	121	$657,001
Anesth: Pain Management	13	$1,542,269	11	$1,375,000
Anesth: Pediatric	0	*	0	*
Cardiology: Electrophysiology	5	*	15	$1,255,936
Cardiology: Invasive	31	$1,109,000	58	$1,487,516
Cardiology: Inv-Intervntnl	44	$1,631,300	71	$1,589,545
Cardiology: Noninvasive	18	$1,219,076	48	$1,056,922
Critical Care: Intensivist	1	*	6	*
Dentistry	4	*	6	*
Dermatology	21	$1,013,202	86	$901,173
Dermatology: MOHS Surgery	2	*	8	*
Emergency Medicine	64	$551,973	26	$623,029
Endocrinology/Metabolism	10	$391,410	58	$471,307
Family Practice (w/ OB)	116	$423,192	311	$446,069
Family Practice (w/o OB)	267	$409,914	1,092	$455,556
Family Practice: Sports Med	0	*	3	*
Gastroenterology	73	$1,353,715	189	$1,526,699
Gastroenterology: Hepatology	0	*	19	$1,192,009
Geriatrics	2	*	12	$270,971
Hematology/Oncology	18	$545,344	107	$612,245
Hem/Onc: Oncology (only)	4	*	27	$483,462
Infectious Disease	8	*	51	$555,625
Internal Medicine: General	226	$413,606	999	$435,486
Internal Med: Hospitalist	6	*	99	$346,899
Internal Med: Pediatric	1	*	25	$350,834
Nephrology	33	$813,514	60	$808,743
Neurology	47	$732,640	132	$567,966
OBGYN: General	88	$877,903	318	$875,703
OBGYN: Gynecology (only)	10	$561,860	75	$833,339
OBGYN: Gyn Oncology	1	*	10	$1,160,765
OBGYN: Maternal & Fetal Med	4	*	19	$1,001,744
OBGYN: Repro Endocrinology	1	*	9	*
Occupational Medicine	4	*	24	$398,930
Ophthalmology	23	$1,167,851	81	$1,127,459
Ophthalmology: Pediatric	1	*	1	*
Ophthalmology: Retina	1	*	2	*
Orthopedic (Non-surgical)	0	*	9	*
Orthopedic Surgery: General	52	$1,350,504	109	$1,364,025
Ortho Surg: Foot & Ankle	6	*	7	*
Ortho Surg: Hand	14	$1,424,002	14	$1,800,421
Ortho Surg: Hip & Joint	9	*	20	$1,440,273
Ortho Surg: Oncology	*	*	0	*
Ortho Surg: Pediatric	1	*	4	*
Ortho Surg: Spine	8	*	22	$2,497,904
Ortho Surg: Trauma	5	*	3	*
Ortho Surg: Sports Med	16	$1,613,256	34	$1,653,356
Otorhinolaryngology	33	$1,287,906	105	$1,122,047
Otorhinolaryngology: Pediatric	0	*	0	*
Pathology: Anatomic & Clinical	1	*	28	$754,221
Pathology: Anatomic	4	*	6	*
Pathology: Clinical	0	*	14	$525,374

Table 31: Physician Gross Charges (TC Excluded) by Weeks Worked per Year (continued)

	Less than 46 weeks		46 weeks or more	
	Physicians	Median	Physicians	Median
Pediatrics: General	146	$460,596	599	$479,697
Ped: Adolescent Medicine	1	*	22	$453,453
Ped: Allergy/Immunology	3	*	0	*
Ped: Cardiology	4	*	11	$706,252
Ped: Child Development	*	*	5	*
Ped: Critical Care/Intensivist	17	$452,942	6	*
Ped: Emergency Medicine	*	*	6	*
Ped: Endocrinology	2	*	6	*
Ped: Gastroenterology	2	*	4	*
Ped: Genetics	*	*	7	*
Ped: Hematology/Oncology	3	*	12	$604,680
Ped: Hospitalist	2	*	9	*
Ped: Infectious Disease	*	*	1	*
Ped: Neonatal Medicine	20	$865,323	16	$977,745
Ped: Nephrology	*	*	4	*
Ped: Neurology	3	*	12	$340,178
Ped: Pulmonology	2	*	3	*
Ped: Rheumatology	*	*	3	*
Ped: Sports Medicine	*	*	0	*
Physiatry (Phys Med & Rehab)	5	*	27	$589,360
Podiatry: General	10	$604,066	32	$606,837
Podiatry: Surg-Foot & Ankle	4	*	9	*
Podiatry: Surg-Forefoot Only	1	*	3	*
Psychiatry: General	26	$364,060	54	$374,539
Psychiatry: Child & Adolescent	5	*	10	$378,349
Psychiatry: Geriatric	1	*	8	*
Pulmonary Medicine	17	$674,910	69	$728,427
Pulmonary Med: Critical Care	15	$441,556	33	$797,967
Radiation Oncology	35	$1,560,322	10	$1,320,381
Radiology: Diagnostic-Inv	114	$1,377,605	23	$1,680,404
Radiology: Diagnostic-Noninv	125	$1,304,419	14	$1,129,284
Radiology: Nuclear Medicine	6	*	4	*
Rheumatology	9	*	81	$567,209
Sleep Medicine	2	*	1	*
Surgery: General	68	$1,008,189	268	$1,077,390
Surg: Cardiovascular	44	$2,146,480	37	$1,680,139
Surg: Cardiovascular-Pediatric	1	*	3	*
Surg: Colon and Rectal	5	*	11	$1,031,114
Surg: Neurological	23	$2,230,606	61	$2,284,252
Surg: Oncology	*	*	2	*
Surg: Oral	4	*	10	$1,268,467
Surg: Pediatric	2	*	6	*
Surg: Plastic & Reconstruction	10	$1,570,880	24	$1,129,364
Surg: Plastic & Recon-Hand	0	*	0	*
Surg: Plastic & Recon-Pediatric	0	*	2	*
Surg: Thoracic (primary)	1	*	20	$3,049,699
Surg: Transplant	*	*	8	*
Surg: Trauma	0	*	9	*
Surg: Trauma-Burn	0	*	8	*
Surg: Vascular (primary)	15	$1,347,114	25	$1,067,051
Urgent Care	20	$476,950	126	$518,312
Urology	34	$1,455,175	95	$1,238,000
Urology: Pediatric	*	*	2	*

MEDICAL GROUP MANAGEMENT ASSOCIATION™

Table 32: Physician Gross Charges with 1-10% Technical Component

	Physicians	Medical Practices	Mean	Std. Dev.	25th %tile	Median	75th %tile	90th %tile
Allergy/Immunology	28	6	$1,065,593	$712,826	$558,475	$919,150	$1,225,329	$1,781,720
Anesthesiology	3	1	*	*	*	*	*	*
Anesth: Pain Management	2	1	*	*	*	*	*	*
Anesth: Pediatric	0	*	*	*	*	*	*	*
Cardiology: Electrophysiology	18	11	$1,854,685	$630,208	$1,365,854	$1,807,159	$2,281,460	$2,918,472
Cardiology: Invasive	83	24	$1,343,579	$553,303	$948,673	$1,218,404	$1,570,324	$2,043,724
Cardiology: Inv-Intervntnl	96	23	$1,888,328	$705,444	$1,353,391	$1,859,889	$2,408,696	$2,885,638
Cardiology: Noninvasive	65	27	$1,200,566	$680,216	$789,673	$1,070,241	$1,487,636	$2,171,743
Critical Care: Intensivist	0	*	*	*	*	*	*	*
Dentistry	0	*	*	*	*	*	*	*
Dermatology	30	16	$908,352	$252,821	$747,387	$892,028	$1,047,359	$1,337,190
Dermatology: MOHS Surgery	2	2	*	*	*	*	*	*
Emergency Medicine	8	3	*	*	*	*	*	*
Endocrinology/Metabolism	26	17	$581,906	$250,970	$399,641	$513,622	$753,251	$1,020,670
Family Practice (w/ OB)	189	48	$564,496	$178,370	$428,422	$526,605	$663,863	$832,385
Family Practice (w/o OB)	838	129	$560,748	$229,941	$396,366	$519,864	$681,843	$861,482
Family Practice: Sports Med	8	5	*	*	*	*	*	*
Gastroenterology	60	28	$1,264,641	$386,372	$1,018,490	$1,215,000	$1,491,264	$1,918,839
Gastroenterology: Hepatology	8	2	*	*	*	*	*	*
Geriatrics	6	3	*	*	*	*	*	*
Hematology/Oncology	20	9	$799,404	$254,441	$645,937	$768,380	$898,652	$1,174,028
Hem/Onc: Oncology (only)	2	2	*	*	*	*	*	*
Infectious Disease	7	5	*	*	*	*	*	*
Internal Medicine: General	602	93	$569,731	$245,980	$407,022	$544,125	$670,817	$872,707
Internal Med: Hospitalist	36	5	$501,698	$179,845	$383,523	$467,934	$657,031	$747,181
Internal Med: Pediatric	20	8	$528,139	$218,182	$381,229	$454,903	$654,468	$899,315
Nephrology	7	5	*	*	*	*	*	*
Neurology	41	19	$778,893	$353,238	$619,730	$704,065	$833,831	$1,079,632
OBGYN: General	274	47	$935,614	$320,064	$712,407	$885,105	$1,115,458	$1,394,912
OBGYN: Gynecology (only)	9	8	*	*	*	*	*	*
OBGYN: Gyn Oncology	0	*	*	*	*	*	*	*
OBGYN: Maternal & Fetal Med	4	2	*	*	*	*	*	*
OBGYN: Repro Endocrinology	1	1	*	*	*	*	*	*
Occupational Medicine	7	4	*	*	*	*	*	*
Ophthalmology	93	27	$1,295,256	$641,177	$827,167	$1,157,163	$1,693,822	$2,233,167
Ophthalmology: Pediatric	8	5	*	*	*	*	*	*
Ophthalmology: Retina	25	6	$2,042,657	$677,970	$1,462,169	$2,100,000	$2,717,182	$2,869,198
Orthopedic (Non-surgical)	8	2	*	*	*	*	*	*
Orthopedic Surgery: General	168	46	$1,670,850	$657,348	$1,202,110	$1,543,019	$2,041,369	$2,739,432
Ortho Surg: Foot & Ankle	14	13	$1,741,504	$702,885	$1,243,362	$1,560,763	$2,341,820	$2,823,374
Ortho Surg: Hand	36	19	$1,800,118	$805,295	$1,234,814	$1,576,865	$2,338,726	$3,150,224
Ortho Surg: Hip & Joint	26	19	$2,079,828	$778,025	$1,436,340	$2,037,519	$2,601,560	$3,268,987
Ortho Surg: Oncology	0	*	*	*	*	*	*	*
Ortho Surg: Pediatric	10	7	$1,931,716	$779,527	$1,231,717	$1,903,593	$2,532,200	$3,237,684
Ortho Surg: Spine	35	23	$2,559,424	$1,352,058	$1,892,451	$2,372,494	$3,216,711	$3,700,867
Ortho Surg: Trauma	8	4	*	*	*	*	*	*
Ortho Surg: Sports Med	66	27	$2,072,752	$1,195,547	$1,328,263	$1,903,869	$2,661,886	$3,598,010
Otorhinolaryngology	41	16	$1,180,705	$470,223	$860,214	$1,122,275	$1,414,804	$1,863,220
Otorhinolaryngology: Pediatric	6	2	*	*	*	*	*	*
Pathology: Anatomic & Clinical	4	1	*	*	*	*	*	*
Pathology: Anatomic	3	2	*	*	*	*	*	*
Pathology: Clinical	7	2	*	*	*	*	*	*

Table 32: Physician Gross Charges with 1-10% Technical Component (continued)

	Physicians	Medical Practices	Mean	Std. Dev.	25th %tile	Median	75th %tile	90th %tile
Pediatrics: General	271	55	$535,863	$166,340	$408,430	$526,538	$628,953	$771,065
Ped: Adolescent Medicine	6	1	*	*	*	*	*	*
Ped: Allergy/Immunology	0	*	*	*	*	*	*	*
Ped: Cardiology	1	1	*	*	*	*	*	*
Ped: Child Development	0	*	*	*	*	*	*	*
Ped: Critical Care/Intensivist	1	1	*	*	*	*	*	*
Ped: Emergency Medicine	0	*	*	*	*	*	*	*
Ped: Endocrinology	0	*	*	*	*	*	*	*
Ped: Gastroenterology	1	1	*	*	*	*	*	*
Ped: Genetics	3	1	*	*	*	*	*	*
Ped: Hematology/Oncology	3	2	*	*	*	*	*	*
Ped: Hospitalist	3	2	*	*	*	*	*	*
Ped: Infectious Disease	2	1	*	*	*	*	*	*
Ped: Neonatal Medicine	1	1	*	*	*	*	*	*
Ped: Nephrology	0	*	*	*	*	*	*	*
Ped: Neurology	1	1	*	*	*	*	*	*
Ped: Pulmonology	5	1	*	*	*	*	*	*
Ped: Rheumatology	0	*	*	*	*	*	*	*
Ped: Sports Medicine	0	*	*	*	*	*	*	*
Physiatry (Phys Med & Rehab)	23	14	$953,625	$637,018	$522,536	$714,164	$1,143,000	$2,166,827
Podiatry: General	8	6	*	*	*	*	*	*
Podiatry: Surg-Foot & Ankle	9	4	*	*	*	*	*	*
Podiatry: Surg-Forefoot Only	3	2	*	*	*	*	*	*
Psychiatry: General	8	3	*	*	*	*	*	*
Psychiatry: Child & Adolescent	1	1	*	*	*	*	*	*
Psychiatry: Geriatric	0	*	*	*	*	*	*	*
Pulmonary Medicine	60	24	$746,790	$532,638	$549,139	$628,578	$759,984	$1,144,092
Pulmonary Med: Critical Care	17	7	$879,966	$311,751	$695,913	$794,085	$1,016,714	$1,588,228
Radiation Oncology	1	1	*	*	*	*	*	*
Radiology: Diagnostic-Inv	31	7	$1,892,694	$972,411	$1,445,301	$1,709,785	$2,140,000	$3,619,033
Radiology: Diagnostic-Noninv	9	3	*	*	*	*	*	*
Radiology: Nuclear Medicine	3	2	*	*	*	*	*	*
Rheumatology	26	19	$911,188	$950,025	$578,208	$682,539	$775,663	$1,634,993
Sleep Medicine	0	*	*	*	*	*	*	*
Surgery: General	75	30	$1,146,248	$509,700	$745,852	$1,114,213	$1,391,515	$1,875,327
Surg: Cardiovascular	9	4	*	*	*	*	*	*
Surg: Cardiovascular-Pediatric	0	*	*	*	*	*	*	*
Surg: Colon and Rectal	0	*	*	*	*	*	*	*
Surg: Neurological	21	9	$1,973,674	$891,246	$1,376,832	$1,816,483	$2,423,129	$3,075,675
Surg: Oncology	0	*	*	*	*	*	*	*
Surg: Oral	1	1	*	*	*	*	*	*
Surg: Pediatric	2	1	*	*	*	*	*	*
Surg: Plastic & Reconstruction	7	6	*	*	*	*	*	*
Surg: Plastic & Recon-Hand	7	1	*	*	*	*	*	*
Surg: Plastic & Recon-Pediatric	0	*	*	*	*	*	*	*
Surg: Thoracic (primary)	2	1	*	*	*	*	*	*
Surg: Transplant	0	*	*	*	*	*	*	*
Surg: Trauma	0	*	*	*	*	*	*	*
Surg: Trauma-Burn	0	*	*	*	*	*	*	*
Surg: Vascular (primary)	18	8	$1,476,071	$522,060	$1,130,793	$1,627,494	$1,812,587	$2,154,235
Urgent Care	72	17	$561,173	$249,561	$373,620	$524,222	$694,332	$914,400
Urology	54	23	$1,237,370	$513,179	$855,611	$1,146,321	$1,454,805	$2,196,406
Urology: Pediatric	1	1	*	*	*	*	*	*

MEDICAL GROUP MANAGEMENT ASSOCIATION™

Table 33: Physician Gross Charges with 1-10% Technical Component by Group Type

	Single-specialty			Multispecialty		
	Physicians	Medical Practices	Median	Physicians	Medical Practices	Median
Allergy/Immunology	19	2	*	9	4	*
Anesthesiology	0	*	*	3	1	*
Anesth: Pain Management	2	1	*	0	*	*
Anesth: Pediatric	0	*	*	0	*	*
Cardiology: Electrophysiology	14	8	$1,807,159	4	3	*
Cardiology: Invasive	49	13	$1,277,793	34	11	$1,199,970
Cardiology: Inv-Intervntnl	65	17	$1,868,737	31	6	$1,851,040
Cardiology: Noninvasive	48	19	$1,047,076	17	8	$1,243,260
Critical Care: Intensivist	0	*	*	0	*	*
Dentistry	0	*	*	0	*	*
Dermatology	9	3	*	21	13	$926,936
Dermatology: MOHS Surgery	1	1	*	1	1	*
Emergency Medicine	0	*	*	8	3	*
Endocrinology/Metabolism	5	4	*	21	13	$514,418
Family Practice (w/ OB)	64	18	$492,719	125	30	$547,550
Family Practice (w/o OB)	242	59	$552,205	596	70	$514,013
Family Practice: Sports Med	6	3	*	2	2	*
Gastroenterology	20	6	$1,215,000	40	22	$1,283,638
Gastroenterology: Hepatology	5	1	*	3	1	*
Geriatrics	0	*	*	6	3	*
Hematology/Oncology	5	2	*	15	7	$822,642
Hem/Onc: Oncology (only)	1	1	*	1	1	*
Infectious Disease	1	1	*	6	4	*
Internal Medicine: General	138	25	$502,948	464	68	$556,512
Internal Med: Hospitalist	0	*	*	36	5	$467,934
Internal Med: Pediatric	3	1	*	17	7	$453,485
Nephrology	1	1	*	6	4	*
Neurology	24	7	$720,514	17	12	$692,810
OBGYN: General	115	17	$967,204	159	30	$839,748
OBGYN: Gynecology (only)	6	5	*	3	3	*
OBGYN: Gyn Oncology	0	*	*	0	*	*
OBGYN: Maternal & Fetal Med	3	1	*	1	1	*
OBGYN: Repro Endocrinology	1	1	*	0	*	*
Occupational Medicine	4	1	*	3	3	*
Ophthalmology	60	10	$1,150,973	33	17	$1,207,129
Ophthalmology: Pediatric	8	5	*	0	*	*
Ophthalmology: Retina	25	6	$2,100,000	0	*	*
Orthopedic (Non-surgical)	7	1	*	1	1	*
Orthopedic Surgery: General	126	29	$1,543,019	42	17	$1,553,739
Ortho Surg: Foot & Ankle	11	11	$1,526,795	3	2	*
Ortho Surg: Hand	27	15	$1,563,148	9	4	*
Ortho Surg: Hip & Joint	20	16	$1,957,341	6	3	*
Ortho Surg: Oncology	0	*	*	0	*	*
Ortho Surg: Pediatric	8	5	*	2	2	*
Ortho Surg: Spine	28	18	$2,454,988	7	5	*
Ortho Surg: Trauma	8	4	*	0	*	*
Ortho Surg: Sports Med	52	22	$2,108,129	14	5	$726,045
Otorhinolaryngology	12	4	$1,069,063	29	12	$1,155,641
Otorhinolaryngology: Pediatric	1	1	*	5	1	*
Pathology: Anatomic & Clinical	4	1	*	0	*	*
Pathology: Anatomic	1	1	*	2	1	*
Pathology: Clinical	7	2	*	0	*	*

Table 33: Physician Gross Charges with 1-10% Technical Component by Group Type (continued)

	Single-specialty			Multispecialty		
	Physicians	Medical Practices	Median	Physicians	Medical Practices	Median
Pediatrics: General	98	22	$507,799	173	33	$558,995
Ped: Adolescent Medicine	0	*	*	6	1	*
Ped: Allergy/Immunology	0	*	*	0	*	*
Ped: Cardiology	1	1	*	0	*	*
Ped: Child Development	*	*	*	0	*	*
Ped: Critical Care/Intensivist	0	*	*	1	1	*
Ped: Emergency Medicine	0	*	*	0	*	*
Ped: Endocrinology	0	*	*	0	*	*
Ped: Gastroenterology	1	1	*	0	*	*
Ped: Genetics	*	*	*	3	1	*
Ped: Hematology/Oncology	2	1	*	1	1	*
Ped: Hospitalist	0	*	*	3	2	*
Ped: Infectious Disease	0	*	*	2	1	*
Ped: Neonatal Medicine	0	*	*	1	1	*
Ped: Nephrology	0	*	*	0	*	*
Ped: Neurology	1	1	*	0	*	*
Ped: Pulmonology	5	1	*	0	*	*
Ped: Rheumatology	0	*	*	0	*	*
Ped: Sports Medicine	*	*	*	0	*	*
Physiatry (Phys Med & Rehab)	16	9	$726,559	7	5	*
Podiatry: General	0	*	*	8	6	*
Podiatry: Surg-Foot & Ankle	2	1	*	7	3	*
Podiatry: Surg-Forefoot Only	1	1	*	2	1	*
Psychiatry: General	0	*	*	8	3	*
Psychiatry: Child & Adolescent	0	*	*	1	1	*
Psychiatry: Geriatric	*	*	*	0	*	*
Pulmonary Medicine	22	7	$604,425	38	17	$665,881
Pulmonary Med: Critical Care	7	2	*	10	5	$817,081
Radiation Oncology	0	*	*	1	1	*
Radiology: Diagnostic-Inv	29	6	$1,662,025	2	1	*
Radiology: Diagnostic-Noninv	9	3	*	0	*	*
Radiology: Nuclear Medicine	1	1	*	2	1	*
Rheumatology	2	2	*	24	17	$682,539
Sleep Medicine	0	*	*	0	*	*
Surgery: General	15	7	$1,114,213	60	23	$1,120,025
Surg: Cardiovascular	2	1	*	7	3	*
Surg: Cardiovascular-Pediatric	0	*	*	0	*	*
Surg: Colon and Rectal	0	*	*	0	*	*
Surg: Neurological	6	3	*	15	6	$1,840,320
Surg: Oncology	0	*	*	0	*	*
Surg: Oral	0	*	*	1	1	*
Surg: Pediatric	0	*	*	2	1	*
Surg: Plastic & Reconstruction	4	3	*	3	3	*
Surg: Plastic & Recon-Hand	7	1	*	0	*	*
Surg: Plastic & Recon-Pediatric	0	*	*	0	*	*
Surg: Thoracic (primary)	0	*	*	2	1	*
Surg: Transplant	0	*	*	0	*	*
Surg: Trauma	0	*	*	0	*	*
Surg: Trauma-Burn	0	*	*	0	*	*
Surg: Vascular (primary)	8	2	*	10	6	$1,663,686
Urgent Care	2	1	*	70	16	$519,983
Urology	28	7	$1,108,722	26	16	$1,403,418
Urology: Pediatric	1	1	*	0	*	*

Table 34: Physician Gross Charges with over 10% Technical Component

	Physicians	Medical Practices	Mean	Std. Dev.	25th %tile	Median	75th %tile	90th %tile
Allergy/Immunology	8	5	*	*	*	*	*	*
Anesthesiology	78	2	*	*	*	*	*	*
Anesth: Pain Management	5	1	*	*	*	*	*	*
Anesth: Pediatric	6	2	*	*	*	*	*	*
Cardiology: Electrophysiology	16	13	$2,180,754	$790,851	$1,659,997	$2,525,060	$2,868,498	$3,031,658
Cardiology: Invasive	79	22	$2,007,726	$970,032	$1,156,727	$1,798,001	$2,772,554	$3,322,251
Cardiology: Inv-Intervntnl	139	31	$2,429,989	$1,088,044	$1,666,453	$2,263,467	$2,972,000	$4,013,276
Cardiology: Noninvasive	83	30	$1,825,490	$1,005,527	$1,008,200	$1,659,395	$2,688,594	$3,214,592
Critical Care: Intensivist	1	1	*	*	*	*	*	*
Dentistry	9	1	*	*	*	*	*	*
Dermatology	4	3	*	*	*	*	*	*
Dermatology: MOHS Surgery	0	*	*	*	*	*	*	*
Emergency Medicine	0	*	*	*	*	*	*	*
Endocrinology/Metabolism	5	3	*	*	*	*	*	*
Family Practice (w/ OB)	136	25	$561,257	$229,048	$387,507	$502,053	$688,794	$921,428
Family Practice (w/o OB)	214	33	$581,380	$260,619	$390,853	$522,737	$722,068	$933,192
Family Practice: Sports Med	3	2	*	*	*	*	*	*
Gastroenterology	29	10	$1,441,005	$376,389	$1,199,095	$1,425,149	$1,700,918	$1,900,655
Gastroenterology: Hepatology	14	2	*	*	*	*	*	*
Geriatrics	1	1	*	*	*	*	*	*
Hematology/Oncology	7	5	*	*	*	*	*	*
Hem/Onc: Oncology (only)	1	1	*	*	*	*	*	*
Infectious Disease	3	1	*	*	*	*	*	*
Internal Medicine: General	275	39	$676,001	$273,977	$481,990	$653,273	$803,425	$997,224
Internal Med: Hospitalist	20	5	$354,263	$162,409	$265,053	$326,990	$375,484	$660,161
Internal Med: Pediatric	1	1	*	*	*	*	*	*
Nephrology	7	2	*	*	*	*	*	*
Neurology	34	10	$999,461	$449,200	$616,624	$991,981	$1,330,357	$1,594,037
OBGYN: General	59	23	$885,737	$321,756	$674,372	$872,011	$1,052,113	$1,257,361
OBGYN: Gynecology (only)	5	3	*	*	*	*	*	*
OBGYN: Gyn Oncology	0	*	*	*	*	*	*	*
OBGYN: Maternal & Fetal Med	1	1	*	*	*	*	*	*
OBGYN: Repro Endocrinology	3	2	*	*	*	*	*	*
Occupational Medicine	0	*	*	*	*	*	*	*
Ophthalmology	10	6	$1,093,742	$827,064	$479,484	$990,365	$1,428,842	$2,963,683
Ophthalmology: Pediatric	0	*	*	*	*	*	*	*
Ophthalmology: Retina	8	3	*	*	*	*	*	*
Orthopedic (Non-surgical)	5	2	*	*	*	*	*	*
Orthopedic Surgery: General	41	15	$1,588,038	$830,559	$1,061,804	$1,341,824	$1,740,625	$3,057,340
Ortho Surg: Foot & Ankle	4	4	*	*	*	*	*	*
Ortho Surg: Hand	6	6	*	*	*	*	*	*
Ortho Surg: Hip & Joint	4	3	*	*	*	*	*	*
Ortho Surg: Oncology	0	*	*	*	*	*	*	*
Ortho Surg: Pediatric	2	2	*	*	*	*	*	*
Ortho Surg: Spine	3	3	*	*	*	*	*	*
Ortho Surg: Trauma	1	1	*	*	*	*	*	*
Ortho Surg: Sports Med	15	7	$2,196,271	$726,888	$1,637,320	$1,818,000	$2,686,644	$3,459,527
Otorhinolaryngology	10	4	$1,458,052	$731,477	$862,361	$1,521,174	$2,010,054	$2,461,946
Otorhinolaryngology: Pediatric	0	*	*	*	*	*	*	*
Pathology: Anatomic & Clinical	0	*	*	*	*	*	*	*
Pathology: Anatomic	0	*	*	*	*	*	*	*
Pathology: Clinical	0	*	*	*	*	*	*	*

Table 34: Physician Gross Charges with over 10% Technical Component (continued)

	Physicians	Medical Practices	Mean	Std. Dev.	25th %tile	Median	75th %tile	90th %tile
Pediatrics: General	88	20	$564,670	$230,630	$436,252	$511,373	$651,567	$909,585
Ped: Adolescent Medicine	0	*	*	*	*	*	*	*
Ped: Allergy/Immunology	1	1	*	*	*	*	*	*
Ped: Cardiology	9	3	*	*	*	*	*	*
Ped: Child Development	0	*	*	*	*	*	*	*
Ped: Critical Care/Intensivist	0	*	*	*	*	*	*	*
Ped: Emergency Medicine	0	*	*	*	*	*	*	*
Ped: Endocrinology	0	*	*	*	*	*	*	*
Ped: Gastroenterology	0	*	*	*	*	*	*	*
Ped: Genetics	0	*	*	*	*	*	*	*
Ped: Hematology/Oncology	0	*	*	*	*	*	*	*
Ped: Hospitalist	0	*	*	*	*	*	*	*
Ped: Infectious Disease	0	*	*	*	*	*	*	*
Ped: Neonatal Medicine	0	*	*	*	*	*	*	*
Ped: Nephrology	0	*	*	*	*	*	*	*
Ped: Neurology	1	1	*	*	*	*	*	*
Ped: Pulmonology	0	*	*	*	*	*	*	*
Ped: Rheumatology	0	*	*	*	*	*	*	*
Ped: Sports Medicine	0	*	*	*	*	*	*	*
Physiatry (Phys Med & Rehab)	6	4	*	*	*	*	*	*
Podiatry: General	2	2	*	*	*	*	*	*
Podiatry: Surg-Foot & Ankle	8	1	*	*	*	*	*	*
Podiatry: Surg-Forefoot Only	0	*	*	*	*	*	*	*
Psychiatry: General	4	3	*	*	*	*	*	*
Psychiatry: Child & Adolescent	0	*	*	*	*	*	*	*
Psychiatry: Geriatric	0	*	*	*	*	*	*	*
Pulmonary Medicine	9	8	*	*	*	*	*	*
Pulmonary Med: Critical Care	17	5	$795,396	$265,997	$641,263	$779,767	$1,083,845	$1,163,634
Radiation Oncology	4	1	*	*	*	*	*	*
Radiology: Diagnostic-Inv	30	6	$2,071,828	$1,637,982	$918,923	$1,349,942	$2,853,046	$4,707,265
Radiology: Diagnostic-Noninv	57	13	$2,709,492	$1,134,923	$1,544,317	$2,833,677	$3,314,785	$4,265,679
Radiology: Nuclear Medicine	2	2	*	*	*	*	*	*
Rheumatology	13	9	$734,878	$304,366	$491,670	$747,624	$896,609	$1,250,928
Sleep Medicine	0	*	*	*	*	*	*	*
Surgery: General	33	15	$926,938	$481,677	$709,628	$883,873	$1,012,764	$1,272,398
Surg: Cardiovascular	5	1	*	*	*	*	*	*
Surg: Cardiovascular-Pediatric	0	*	*	*	*	*	*	*
Surg: Colon and Rectal	0	*	*	*	*	*	*	*
Surg: Neurological	14	5	$1,979,882	$985,376	$1,289,252	$1,659,292	$2,375,870	$3,820,825
Surg: Oncology	1	1	*	*	*	*	*	*
Surg: Oral	0	*	*	*	*	*	*	*
Surg: Pediatric	0	*	*	*	*	*	*	*
Surg: Plastic & Reconstruction	0	*	*	*	*	*	*	*
Surg: Plastic & Recon-Hand	1	1	*	*	*	*	*	*
Surg: Plastic & Recon-Pediatric	0	*	*	*	*	*	*	*
Surg: Thoracic (primary)	0	*	*	*	*	*	*	*
Surg: Transplant	0	*	*	*	*	*	*	*
Surg: Trauma	0	*	*	*	*	*	*	*
Surg: Trauma-Burn	0	*	*	*	*	*	*	*
Surg: Vascular (primary)	5	2	*	*	*	*	*	*
Urgent Care	19	4	$952,888	$368,904	$740,000	$912,000	$1,225,000	$1,395,000
Urology	15	4	$1,569,654	$522,511	$1,237,014	$1,543,636	$2,011,071	$2,413,254
Urology: Pediatric	0	*	*	*	*	*	*	*

Table 35: Physician Gross Charges with over 10% Technical Component by Group Type

	Single-specialty			Multispecialty		
	Physicians	Medical Practices	Median	Physicians	Medical Practices	Median
Allergy/Immunology	2	1	*	6	4	*
Anesthesiology	63	1	*	15	1	*
Anesth: Pain Management	0	*	*	5	1	*
Anesth: Pediatric	5	1	*	1	1	*
Cardiology: Electrophysiology	13	10	2,572,600	3	3	*
Cardiology: Invasive	57	15	1,752,848	22	7	2,231,937
Cardiology: Inv-Intervntnl	125	25	2,282,596	14	6	1,921,804
Cardiology: Noninvasive	57	19	2,003,245	26	11	976,584
Critical Care: Intensivist	0	*	*	1	1	*
Dentistry	0	*	*	9	1	*
Dermatology	0	*	*	4	3	*
Dermatology: MOHS Surgery	0	*	*	0	*	*
Emergency Medicine	0	*	*	0	*	*
Endocrinology/Metabolism	0	*	*	5	3	*
Family Practice (w/ OB)	55	9	432,941	81	16	571,100
Family Practice (w/o OB)	55	9	587,000	159	24	513,476
Family Practice: Sports Med	1	1	*	2	1	*
Gastroenterology	9	1	*	20	9	1,335,918
Gastroenterology: Hepatology	14	2	*	0	*	*
Geriatrics	0	*	*	1	1	*
Hematology/Oncology	5	3	*	2	2	*
Hem/Onc: Oncology (only)	0	*	*	1	1	*
Infectious Disease	0	*	*	3	1	*
Internal Medicine: General	18	3	625,323	257	36	654,094
Internal Med: Hospitalist	0	*	*	20	5	326,990
Internal Med: Pediatric	0	*	*	1	1	*
Nephrology	4	1	*	3	1	*
Neurology	18	3	1,295,989	16	7	678,103
OBGYN: General	37	9	934,465	22	14	675,286
OBGYN: Gynecology (only)	3	2	*	2	1	*
OBGYN: Gyn Oncology	0	*	*	0	*	*
OBGYN: Maternal & Fetal Med	0	*	*	1	1	*
OBGYN: Repro Endocrinology	1	1	*	2	1	*
Occupational Medicine	0	*	*	0	*	*
Ophthalmology	5	2	*	5	4	*
Ophthalmology: Pediatric	0	*	*	0	*	*
Ophthalmology: Retina	7	2	*	1	1	*
Orthopedic (Non-surgical)	3	1	*	2	1	*
Orthopedic Surgery: General	32	9	1,333,412	9	6	*
Ortho Surg: Foot & Ankle	4	4	*	0	*	*
Ortho Surg: Hand	6	6	*	0	*	*
Ortho Surg: Hip & Joint	4	3	*	0	*	*
Ortho Surg: Oncology	0	*	*	0	*	*
Ortho Surg: Pediatric	2	2	*	0	*	*
Ortho Surg: Spine	2	2	*	1	1	*
Ortho Surg: Trauma	1	1	*	0	*	*
Ortho Surg: Sports Med	15	7	1,818,000	0	*	*
Otorhinolaryngology	9	3	*	1	1	*
Otorhinolaryngology: Pediatric	0	*	*	0	*	*
Pathology: Anatomic & Clinical	0	*	*	0	*	*
Pathology: Anatomic	0	*	*	0	*	*
Pathology: Clinical	0	*	*	0	*	*

Table 35: Physician Gross Charges with over 10% Technical Component by Group Type (continued)

	Single-specialty			Multispecialty		
	Physicians	Medical Practices	Median	Physicians	Medical Practices	Median
Pediatrics: General	22	4	554,221	66	16	496,844
Ped: Adolescent Medicine	0	*	*	0	*	*
Ped: Allergy/Immunology	0	*	*	1	1	*
Ped: Cardiology	9	3	*	0	*	*
Ped: Child Development	*	*	*	0	*	*
Ped: Critical Care/Intensivist	0	*	*	0	*	*
Ped: Emergency Medicine	0	*	*	0	*	*
Ped: Endocrinology	0	*	*	0	*	*
Ped: Gastroenterology	0	*	*	0	*	*
Ped: Genetics	*	*	*	0	*	*
Ped: Hematology/Oncology	0	*	*	0	*	*
Ped: Hospitalist	0	*	*	0	*	*
Ped: Infectious Disease	0	*	*	0	*	*
Ped: Neonatal Medicine	0	*	*	0	*	*
Ped: Nephrology	0	*	*	0	*	*
Ped: Neurology	0	*	*	1	1	*
Ped: Pulmonology	0	*	*	0	*	*
Ped: Rheumatology	0	*	*	0	*	*
Ped: Sports Medicine	*	*	*	0	*	*
Physiatry (Phys Med & Rehab)	3	3	*	3	1	*
Podiatry: General	0	*	*	2	2	*
Podiatry: Surg-Foot & Ankle	8	1	*	0	*	*
Podiatry: Surg-Forefoot Only	0	*	*	0	*	*
Psychiatry: General	0	*	*	4	3	*
Psychiatry: Child & Adolescent	0	*	*	0	*	*
Psychiatry: Geriatric	*	*	*	0	*	*
Pulmonary Medicine	0	*	*	9	8	*
Pulmonary Med: Critical Care	5	1	*	12	4	686,243
Radiation Oncology	4	1	*	0	*	*
Radiology: Diagnostic-Inv	18	4	941,109	12	2	*
Radiology: Diagnostic-Noninv	19	3	1,544,317	38	10	3,094,635
Radiology: Nuclear Medicine	10	2	*	1	1	*
Rheumatology	0	*	*	13	9	747,624
Sleep Medicine	0	*	*	0	*	*
Surgery: General	14	2	*	19	13	904,742
Surg: Cardiovascular	5	1	*	0	*	*
Surg: Cardiovascular-Pediatric	0	*	*	0	*	*
Surg: Colon and Rectal	0	*	*	0	*	*
Surg: Neurological	10	2	*	4	3	*
Surg: Oncology	0	*	*	1	1	*
Surg: Oral	0	*	*	0	*	*
Surg: Pediatric	0	*	*	0	*	*
Surg: Plastic & Reconstruction	0	*	*	0	*	*
Surg: Plastic & Recon-Hand	1	1	*	0	*	*
Surg: Plastic & Recon-Pediatric	0	*	*	0	*	*
Surg: Thoracic (primary)	0	*	*	0	*	*
Surg: Transplant	0	*	*	0	*	*
Surg: Trauma	0	*	*	0	*	*
Surg: Trauma-Burn	0	*	*	0	*	*
Surg: Vascular (primary)	4	1	*	1	1	*
Urgent Care	15	1	*	4	3	*
Urology	11	1	*	4	3	*
Urology: Pediatric	0	*	*	0	*	*

　　MEDICAL GROUP MANAGEMENT ASSOCIATION™

Table 36: Physician Compensation to Gross Charges Ratio (TC Excluded)

	Physicians	Medical Practices	Mean	Std. Dev.	25th %tile	Median	75th %tile	90th %tile
Allergy/Immunology	71	50	.358	.104	.288	.358	.417	.491
Anesthesiology	335	40	.433	.140	.320	.424	.532	.623
Anesth: Pain Management	28	13	.251	.063	.198	.222	.310	.341
Anesth: Pediatric	0	*	*	*	*	*	*	*
Cardiology: Electrophysiology	19	14	.295	.097	.213	.245	.396	.433
Cardiology: Invasive	98	40	.301	.109	.214	.279	.364	.429
Cardiology: Inv-Intervntnl	124	42	.309	.120	.221	.279	.372	.471
Cardiology: Noninvasive	89	44	.347	.141	.247	.302	.414	.515
Critical Care: Intensivist	15	8	.429	.189	.307	.375	.508	.796
Dentistry	10	4	.368	.063	.311	.372	.415	.471
Dermatology	135	71	.317	.096	.249	.297	.365	.433
Dermatology: MOHS Surgery	11	10	.324	.072	.254	.326	.375	.443
Emergency Medicine	175	18	.399	.137	.310	.387	.473	.542
Endocrinology/Metabolism	89	55	.402	.134	.311	.393	.485	.588
Family Practice (w/ OB)	621	91	.371	.092	.306	.369	.426	.482
Family Practice (w/o OB)	1,709	185	.369	.115	.290	.370	.430	.504
Family Practice: Sports Med	3	3	*	*	*	*	*	*
Gastroenterology	289	98	.272	.085	.216	.258	.305	.375
Gastroenterology: Hepatology	19	3	.223	.035	.200	.219	.244	.286
Geriatrics	18	12	.455	.116	.344	.465	.577	.603
Hematology/Oncology	132	51	.523	.193	.387	.472	.648	.831
Hem/Onc: Oncology (only)	42	20	.541	.164	.441	.518	.597	.809
Infectious Disease	75	37	.426	.178	.297	.372	.520	.734
Internal Medicine: General	1,511	180	.380	.116	.302	.370	.442	.514
Internal Med: Hospitalist	151	37	.505	.154	.395	.484	.603	.728
Internal Med: Pediatric	31	13	.419	.158	.312	.399	.447	.743
Nephrology	131	46	.359	.163	.259	.322	.406	.613
Neurology	222	74	.346	.133	.260	.319	.392	.555
OBGYN: General	526	114	.311	.092	.244	.302	.363	.422
OBGYN: Gynecology (only)	89	33	.317	.155	.218	.256	.359	.515
OBGYN: Gyn Oncology	12	8	.399	.165	.276	.355	.417	.739
OBGYN: Maternal & Fetal Med	28	10	.380	.137	.282	.355	.417	.611
OBGYN: Repro Endocrinology	11	4	.303	.065	.273	.300	.358	.403
Occupational Medicine	46	25	.427	.146	.340	.383	.521	.661
Ophthalmology	133	60	.273	.093	.201	.257	.316	.406
Ophthalmology: Pediatric	3	3	*	*	*	*	*	*
Ophthalmology: Retina	4	4	*	*	*	*	*	*
Orthopedic (Non-surgical)	11	9	.264	.080	.210	.226	.277	.446
Orthopedic Surgery: General	236	69	.286	.092	.226	.274	.311	.417
Ortho Surg: Foot & Ankle	10	8	.317	.134	.213	.304	.343	.626
Ortho Surg: Hand	27	19	.319	.108	.256	.297	.360	.528
Ortho Surg: Hip & Joint	25	12	.314	.107	.242	.271	.384	.514
Ortho Surg: Oncology	0	*	*	*	*	*	*	*
Ortho Surg: Pediatric	7	7	*	*	*	*	*	*
Ortho Surg: Spine	23	15	.268	.060	.226	.269	.289	.339
Ortho Surg: Trauma	12	7	.264	.133	.169	.211	.322	.541
Ortho Surg: Sports Med	50	26	.272	.079	.215	.257	.304	.379
Otorhinolaryngology	183	74	.270	.075	.210	.258	.317	.364
Otorhinolaryngology: Pediatric	1	1	*	*	*	*	*	*
Pathology: Anatomic & Clinical	46	15	.389	.179	.262	.346	.466	.622
Pathology: Anatomic	8	3	*	*	*	*	*	*
Pathology: Clinical	15	6	.295	.060	.253	.286	.312	.406

Table 36: Physician Compensation to Gross Charges Ratio (TC Excluded) (continued)

	Physicians	Medical Practices	Mean	Std. Dev.	25th %tile	Median	75th %tile	90th %tile
Pediatrics: General	917	147	.352	.108	.272	.338	.399	.489
Ped: Adolescent Medicine	37	7	.336	.069	.295	.371	.385	.403
Ped: Allergy/Immunology	6	5	*	*	*	*	*	*
Ped: Cardiology	19	10	.315	.102	.242	.279	.368	.541
Ped: Child Development	11	5	.477	.232	.321	.340	.638	.889
Ped: Critical Care/Intensivist	27	10	.590	.221	.367	.576	.791	.886
Ped: Emergency Medicine	6	1	*	*	*	*	*	*
Ped: Endocrinology	8	7	*	*	*	*	*	*
Ped: Gastroenterology	10	6	.394	.123	.290	.366	.477	.643
Ped: Genetics	7	3	*	*	*	*	*	*
Ped: Hematology/Oncology	17	11	.393	.168	.239	.378	.533	.651
Ped: Hospitalist	13	5	.568	.149	.473	.534	.686	.815
Ped: Infectious Disease	0	*	*	*	*	*	*	*
Ped: Neonatal Medicine	53	15	.406	.191	.252	.357	.514	.751
Ped: Nephrology	6	4	*	*	*	*	*	*
Ped: Neurology	25	14	.469	.147	.347	.455	.595	.663
Ped: Pulmonology	8	7	*	*	*	*	*	*
Ped: Rheumatology	3	2	*	*	*	*	*	*
Ped: Sports Medicine	0	*	*	*	*	*	*	*
Physiatry (Phys Med & Rehab)	50	27	.390	.149	.280	.361	.482	.576
Podiatry: General	67	38	.268	.059	.230	.259	.302	.349
Podiatry: Surg-Foot & Ankle	16	9	.241	.043	.208	.226	.270	.326
Podiatry: Surg-Forefoot Only	4	2	*	*	*	*	*	*
Psychiatry: General	119	36	.459	.156	.363	.425	.506	.664
Psychiatry: Child & Adolescent	19	11	.492	.158	.361	.482	.610	.744
Psychiatry: Geriatric	10	6	.405	.150	.285	.350	.518	.687
Pulmonary Medicine	110	57	.324	.096	.254	.311	.361	.443
Pulmonary Med: Critical Care	60	22	.360	.091	.288	.376	.412	.460
Radiation Oncology	52	19	.295	.090	.213	.296	.352	.418
Radiology: Diagnostic-Inv	164	25	.333	.132	.247	.301	.387	.508
Radiology: Diagnostic-Noninv	183	34	.335	.106	.240	.326	.423	.467
Radiology: Nuclear Medicine	14	10	.382	.133	.290	.405	.458	.571
Rheumatology	113	57	.382	.156	.259	.349	.480	.587
Sleep Medicine	3	2	*	*	*	*	*	*
Surgery: General	434	125	.289	.108	.212	.265	.335	.413
Surg: Cardiovascular	94	30	.287	.096	.208	.262	.340	.441
Surg: Cardiovascular-Pediatric	4	4	*	*	*	*	*	*
Surg: Colon and Rectal	18	11	.297	.119	.203	.268	.394	.460
Surg: Neurological	77	31	.252	.077	.192	.229	.294	.377
Surg: Oncology	5	2	*	*	*	*	*	*
Surg: Oral	21	8	.243	.060	.197	.245	.271	.333
Surg: Pediatric	9	4	*	*	*	*	*	*
Surg: Plastic & Reconstruction	44	26	.283	.085	.217	.266	.323	.428
Surg: Plastic & Recon-Hand	3	2	*	*	*	*	*	*
Surg: Plastic & Recon-Pediatric	1	1	*	*	*	*	*	*
Surg: Thoracic (primary)	17	6	.243	.046	.204	.227	.288	.317
Surg: Transplant	8	4	*	*	*	*	*	*
Surg: Trauma	11	4	.340	.143	.215	.310	.471	.610
Surg: Trauma-Burn	7	2	*	*	*	*	*	*
Surg: Vascular (primary)	44	25	.305	.139	.199	.265	.398	.505
Urgent Care	193	47	.356	.105	.279	.340	.412	.495
Urology	147	63	.277	.088	.217	.258	.318	.407
Urology: Pediatric	2	1	*	*	*	*	*	*

MEDICAL GROUP MANAGEMENT ASSOCIATION™

Table 37: Physician Compensation to Gross Charges Ratio (TC Excluded) by Group Type

	Single-specialty			Multispecialty		
	Physicians	Medical Practices	Median	Physicians	Medical Practices	Median
Allergy/Immunology	8	4	*	63	46	.363
Anesthesiology	149	12	.440	186	28	.417
Anesth: Pain Management	18	5	.221	10	8	.250
Anesth: Pediatric	0	*	*	0	*	*
Cardiology: Electrophysiology	10	6	.276	9	8	*
Cardiology: Invasive	30	11	.285	68	29	.276
Cardiology: Inv-Intervntnl	60	16	.277	64	26	.282
Cardiology: Noninvasive	25	10	.331	64	34	.294
Critical Care: Intensivist	0	*	*	15	8	.375
Dentistry	2	1	*	8	3	*
Dermatology	6	4	*	129	67	.297
Dermatology: MOHS Surgery	2	2	*	9	8	*
Emergency Medicine	68	5	.345	107	13	.400
Endocrinology/Metabolism	1	1	*	88	54	.388
Family Practice (w/ OB)	85	24	.416	536	67	.367
Family Practice (w/o OB)	178	43	.373	1,531	142	.368
Family Practice: Sports Med	1	1	*	2	2	*
Gastroenterology	100	16	.283	189	82	.242
Gastroenterology: Hepatology	19	3	.219	0	*	*
Geriatrics	0	*	*	18	12	.465
Hematology/Oncology	35	8	.433	97	43	.482
Hem/Onc: Oncology (only)	11	2	*	31	18	.480
Infectious Disease	34	9	.346	41	28	.395
Internal Medicine: General	53	20	.344	1,458	160	.370
Internal Med: Hospitalist	0	*	*	151	37	.484
Internal Med: Pediatric	0	*	*	31	13	.399
Nephrology	44	6	.274	87	40	.343
Neurology	60	9	.318	162	65	.320
OBGYN: General	102	23	.282	424	91	.307
OBGYN: Gynecology (only)	9	5	*	80	28	.245
OBGYN: Gyn Oncology	0	*	*	12	8	.355
OBGYN: Maternal & Fetal Med	5	3	*	23	7	.354
OBGYN: Repro Endocrinology	0	*	*	11	4	.300
Occupational Medicine	0	*	*	46	25	.383
Ophthalmology	11	4	.372	122	56	.252
Ophthalmology: Pediatric	1	1	*	2	2	*
Ophthalmology: Retina	1	1	*	3	3	*
Orthopedic (Non-surgical)	0	*	*	11	9	.226
Orthopedic Surgery: General	38	12	.285	198	57	.273
Ortho Surg: Foot & Ankle	6	5	*	4	3	*
Ortho Surg: Hand	15	10	.319	12	9	.275
Ortho Surg: Hip & Joint	12	7	.303	13	5	.269
Ortho Surg: Oncology	0	*	*	0	*	*
Ortho Surg: Pediatric	3	3	*	4	4	*
Ortho Surg: Spine	11	6	.269	12	9	.264
Ortho Surg: Trauma	7	5	*	5	2	*
Ortho Surg: Sports Med	29	12	.254	21	14	.258
Otorhinolaryngology	39	6	.216	144	68	.262
Otorhinolaryngology: Pediatric	0	*	*	1	1	*
Pathology: Anatomic & Clinical	6	1	*	40	14	.330
Pathology: Anatomic	5	1	*	3	2	*
Pathology: Clinical	0	*	*	15	6	.286

Table 37: Physician Compensation to Gross Charges Ratio (TC Excluded) by Group Type (continued)

	Single-specialty			Multispecialty		
	Physicians	Medical Practices	Median	Physicians	Medical Practices	Median
Pediatrics: General	225	28	.321	692	119	.346
Ped: Adolescent Medicine	4	1	*	33	6	.377
Ped: Allergy/Immunology	2	1	*	4	4	*
Ped: Cardiology	1	1	*	18	9	.276
Ped: Child Development	*	*	*	11	5	.340
Ped: Critical Care/Intensivist	13	3	.648	14	7	.506
Ped: Emergency Medicine	0	*	*	6	1	*
Ped: Endocrinology	1	1	*	7	6	*
Ped: Gastroenterology	1	1	*	9	5	*
Ped: Genetics	*	*	*	7	3	*
Ped: Hematology/Oncology	4	2	*	13	9	.440
Ped: Hospitalist	0	*	*	13	5	.534
Ped: Infectious Disease	0	*	*	0	*	*
Ped: Neonatal Medicine	17	3	.600	36	12	.326
Ped: Nephrology	0	*	*	6	4	*
Ped: Neurology	5	3	*	20	11	.450
Ped: Pulmonology	1	1	*	7	6	*
Ped: Rheumatology	0	*	*	3	2	*
Ped: Sports Medicine	*	*	*	0	*	*
Physiatry (Phys Med & Rehab)	3	2	*	47	25	.367
Podiatry: General	0	*	*	67	38	.259
Podiatry: Surg-Foot & Ankle	2	1	*	14	8	.230
Podiatry: Surg-Forefoot Only	0	*	*	4	2	*
Psychiatry: General	3	1	*	116	35	.426
Psychiatry: Child & Adolescent	6	2	*	13	9	.435
Psychiatry: Geriatric	*	*	*	10	6	.350
Pulmonary Medicine	1	1	*	109	56	.311
Pulmonary Med: Critical Care	17	3	.312	43	19	.387
Radiation Oncology	29	8	.306	23	11	.220
Radiology: Diagnostic-Inv	98	10	.353	66	15	.260
Radiology: Diagnostic-Noninv	93	10	.364	90	24	.292
Radiology: Nuclear Medicine	4	3	*	10	7	.405
Rheumatology	14	3	.257	99	54	.382
Sleep Medicine	2	1	*	1	1	*
Surgery: General	75	16	.216	359	109	.277
Surg: Cardiovascular	61	14	.250	33	16	.323
Surg: Cardiovascular-Pediatric	3	3	*	1	1	*
Surg: Colon and Rectal	7	4	*	11	7	.306
Surg: Neurological	31	9	.205	46	22	.249
Surg: Oncology	0	*	*	5	2	*
Surg: Oral	13	3	.246	8	5	*
Surg: Pediatric	2	1	*	7	3	*
Surg: Plastic & Reconstruction	5	2	*	39	24	.281
Surg: Plastic & Recon-Hand	0	*	*	3	2	*
Surg: Plastic & Recon-Pediatric	1	1	*	0	*	*
Surg: Thoracic (primary)	12	2	*	5	4	*
Surg: Transplant	4	1	*	4	3	*
Surg: Trauma	3	1	*	8	3	*
Surg: Trauma-Burn	7	2	*	0	*	*
Surg: Vascular (primary)	7	3	*	37	22	.233
Urgent Care	22	2	*	171	45	.352
Urology	23	7	.231	124	56	.259
Urology: Pediatric	0	*	*	2	1	*

　　MEDICAL GROUP MANAGEMENT ASSOCIATION™

Table 38A: Physician Compensation to Gross Charges Ratio (TC Excluded) by Geographic Section for All Practices

	Eastern		Midwest		Southern		Western	
	Physicians	Median	Physicians	Median	Physicians	Median	Physicians	Median
Allergy/Immunology	8	*	29	.363	13	.389	21	.313
Anesthesiology	31	.342	153	.449	67	.418	84	.419
Anesth: Pain Management	2	*	8	*	18	.215	0	*
Anesth: Pediatric	*	*	0	*	0	*	0	*
Cardiology: Electrophysiology	2	*	8	*	6	*	3	*
Cardiology: Invasive	11	.274	37	.300	37	.246	13	.251
Cardiology: Inv-Intervntnl	18	.236	46	.304	47	.288	13	.259
Cardiology: Noninvasive	20	.273	24	.275	28	.307	17	.379
Critical Care: Intensivist	6	*	7	*	0	*	2	*
Dentistry	5	*	*	*	5	*	0	*
Dermatology	19	.274	64	.315	17	.317	35	.288
Dermatology: MOHS Surgery	0	*	4	*	4	*	3	*
Emergency Medicine	46	.420	56	.407	25	*	48	.324
Endocrinology/Metabolism	15	.342	34	.404	23	.440	17	.326
Family Practice (w/ OB)	49	.364	419	.380	41	.337	112	.304
Family Practice (w/o OB)	347	.382	843	.367	198	.391	321	.348
Family Practice: Sports Med	0	*	1	*	0	*	2	*
Gastroenterology	36	.208	120	.254	77	.259	56	.277
Gastroenterology: Hepatology	0	*	0	*	19	.219	0	*
Geriatrics	1	*	13	.443	0	*	4	*
Hematology/Oncology	18	.633	46	.444	44	.429	24	.510
Hem/Onc: Oncology (only)	15	.584	19	.467	5	*	3	*
Infectious Disease	20	.393	25	.395	15	.346	15	.341
Internal Medicine: General	315	.346	638	.385	227	.394	331	.332
Internal Med: Hospitalist	20	.382	86	.477	20	.499	25	.564
Internal Med: Pediatric	5	*	10	.298	10	*	6	*
Nephrology	43	.296	38	.355	36	.346	14	.295
Neurology	38	.291	126	.324	26	.309	32	.344
OBGYN: General	104	.265	205	.330	89	.263	128	.307
OBGYN: Gynecology (only)	9	*	57	.231	15	.301	8	*
OBGYN: Gyn Oncology	3	*	5	*	3	*	1	*
OBGYN: Maternal & Fetal Med	3	*	21	.356	2	*	2	*
OBGYN: Repro Endocrinology	3	*	8	*	0	*	0	*
Occupational Medicine	2	*	29	.421	3	*	12	.359
Ophthalmology	26	.228	65	.269	18	.234	24	.273
Ophthalmology: Pediatric	1	*	1	*	0	*	1	*
Ophthalmology: Retina	0	*	2	*	1	*	1	*
Orthopedic (Non-surgical)	0	*	6	*	1	*	4	*
Orthopedic Surgery: General	24	.212	132	.275	36	.282	44	.284
Ortho Surg: Foot & Ankle	2	*	6	*	0	*	2	*
Ortho Surg: Hand	5	*	15	.279	0	*	7	*
Ortho Surg: Hip & Joint	6	*	15	.269	0	*	4	*
Ortho Surg: Oncology	0	*	*	*	0	*	*	*
Ortho Surg: Pediatric	1	*	6	*	0	*	0	*
Ortho Surg: Spine	1	*	18	.269	0	*	4	*
Ortho Surg: Trauma	7	*	3	*	2	*	0	*
Ortho Surg: Sports Med	8	*	23	.300	9	*	10	.262
Otorhinolaryngology	26	.263	95	.253	26	.273	36	.245
Otorhinolaryngology: Pediatric	0	*	1	*	0	*	*	*
Pathology: Anatomic & Clinical	16	.236	14	.462	13	.447	3	*
Pathology: Anatomic	0	*	1	*	5	*	2	*
Pathology: Clinical	4	*	6	*	5	*	0	*

Table 38A: Physician Compensation to Gross Charges Ratio (TC Excluded) by Geographic Section for All Practices (continued)

	Eastern		Midwest		Southern		Western	
	Physicians	Median	Physicians	Median	Physicians	Median	Physicians	Median
Pediatrics: General	178	.337	426	.347	120	.336	193	.312
Ped: Adolescent Medicine	2	*	25	*	10	.336	0	*
Ped: Allergy/Immunology	1	*	3	*	0	*	2	*
Ped: Cardiology	4	*	6	*	1	*	8	*
Ped: Child Development	1	*	7	*	1	*	2	*
Ped: Critical Care/Intensivist	2	*	18	.577	7	*	0	*
Ped: Emergency Medicine	0	*	6	*	*	*	*	*
Ped: Endocrinology	1	*	3	*	1	*	3	*
Ped: Gastroenterology	3	*	3	*	1	*	3	*
Ped: Genetics	0	*	2	*	0	*	5	*
Ped: Hematology/Oncology	2	*	6	*	3	*	6	*
Ped: Hospitalist	0	*	3	*	1	*	9	*
Ped: Infectious Disease	*	*	0	*	0	*	0	*
Ped: Neonatal Medicine	7	*	28	.312	17	.600	1	*
Ped: Nephrology	1	*	2	*	*	*	3	*
Ped: Neurology	3	*	17	.455	2	*	3	*
Ped: Pulmonology	3	*	3	*	1	*	1	*
Ped: Rheumatology	1	*	*	*	*	*	2	*
Ped: Sports Medicine	0	*	*	*	*	*	*	*
Physiatry (Phys Med & Rehab)	5	*	35	.376	2	*	8	*
Podiatry: General	3	*	39	.273	10	.275	15	.220
Podiatry: Surg-Foot & Ankle	4	*	8	*	0	*	4	*
Podiatry: Surg-Forefoot Only	3	*	1	*	0	*	0	*
Psychiatry: General	16	.462	76	.426	10	.395	17	.409
Psychiatry: Child & Adolescent	0	*	11	.447	8	*	0	*
Psychiatry: Geriatric	4	*	2	*	4	*	0	*
Pulmonary Medicine	18	.267	42	.314	32	.314	18	.331
Pulmonary Med: Critical Care	15	.395	19	.376	20	.312	6	*
Radiation Oncology	2	*	23	.310	18	.310	9	*
Radiology: Diagnostic-Inv	20	.264	79	.319	36	.306	29	*
Radiology: Diagnostic-Noninv	47	.333	68	.300	64	.352	4	*
Radiology: Nuclear Medicine	5	*	5	*	4	*	0	*
Rheumatology	18	.293	50	.420	28	.299	17	.300
Sleep Medicine	0	*	2	*	0	*	1	*
Surgery: General	71	.201	188	.297	96	.241	79	.297
Surg: Cardiovascular	9	*	26	.311	39	.249	20	.269
Surg: Cardiovascular-Pediatric	*	*	1	*	2	*	1	*
Surg: Colon and Rectal	8	*	7	*	1	*	2	*
Surg: Neurological	26	.222	31	.262	12	.215	8	*
Surg: Oncology	1	*	4	*	*	*	0	*
Surg: Oral	8	*	6	*	3	*	4	*
Surg: Pediatric	3	*	2	*	0	*	4	*
Surg: Plastic & Reconstruction	7	*	15	.288	8	*	14	.287
Surg: Plastic & Recon-Hand	0	*	3	*	0	*	*	*
Surg: Plastic & Recon-Pediatric	0	*	*	*	1	*	*	*
Surg: Thoracic (primary)	3	*	14	.234	0	*	0	*
Surg: Transplant	2	*	1	*	4	*	1	*
Surg: Trauma	3	*	5	*	3	*	*	*
Surg: Trauma-Burn	0	*	0	*	6	*	1	*
Surg: Vascular (primary)	13	.417	19	.233	3	*	9	*
Urgent Care	2	*	77	.405	40	.292	74	.316
Urology	27	.236	70	.268	25	.260	25	.248
Urology: Pediatric	*	*	0	*	0	*	2	*

Table 38B: Physician Compensation to Gross Charges Ratio (TC Excluded) by Geographic Section for Single-specialty Practices

	Eastern		Midwest		Southern		Western	
	Physicians	Median	Physicians	Median	Physicians	Median	Physicians	Median
Allergy/Immunology	1	*	*	*	2	*	5	*
Anesthesiology	0	*	55	.510	44	.406	50	.394
Anesth: Pain Management	0	*	3	*	15	.209	0	*
Anesth: Pediatric	*	*	*	*	0	*	0	*
Cardiology: Electrophysiology	1	*	4	*	5	*	0	*
Cardiology: Invasive	2	*	9	*	14	.276	5	*
Cardiology: Inv-Intervntnl	10	.269	21	.400	24	.226	5	*
Cardiology: Noninvasive	9	*	1	*	14	.407	1	*
Critical Care: Intensivist	0	*	*	*	0	*	*	*
Dentistry	2	*	*	*	*	*	0	*
Dermatology	3	*	0	*	1	*	2	*
Dermatology: MOHS Surgery	0	*	1	*	1	*	*	*
Emergency Medicine	0	*	*	*	25	*	43	.326
Endocrinology/Metabolism	0	*	1	*	0	*	*	*
Family Practice (w/ OB)	11	.442	28	.444	10	*	36	.366
Family Practice (w/o OB)	71	.385	44	.394	15	.305	48	.298
Family Practice: Sports Med	0	*	0	*	0	*	1	*
Gastroenterology	4	*	43	.284	30	.287	23	.281
Gastroenterology: Hepatology	0	*	0	*	19	.219	0	*
Geriatrics	*	*	*	*	*	*	0	*
Hematology/Oncology	0	*	6	*	22	.398	7	*
Hem/Onc: Oncology (only)	9	*	0	*	*	*	2	*
Infectious Disease	11	*	5	*	9	*	9	*
Internal Medicine: General	12	.500	17	.413	7	*	17	.294
Internal Med: Hospitalist	*	*	*	*	0	*	0	*
Internal Med: Pediatric	*	*	0	*	*	*	*	*
Nephrology	27	.287	1	*	11	*	5	*
Neurology	4	*	45	.315	3	*	8	*
OBGYN: General	20	.297	10	.329	33	.235	39	.297
OBGYN: Gynecology (only)	2	*	0	*	6	*	1	*
OBGYN: Gyn Oncology	0	*	*	*	*	*	*	*
OBGYN: Maternal & Fetal Med	0	*	3	*	2	*	0	*
OBGYN: Repro Endocrinology	*	*	0	*	0	*	0	*
Occupational Medicine	0	*	0	*	0	*	*	*
Ophthalmology	9	*	0	*	1	*	1	*
Ophthalmology: Pediatric	0	*	0	*	0	*	1	*
Ophthalmology: Retina	0	*	0	*	1	*	0	*
Orthopedic (Non-surgical)	0	*	0	*	0	*	0	*
Orthopedic Surgery: General	5	*	15	.281	1	*	17	.292
Ortho Surg: Foot & Ankle	2	*	2	*	0	*	2	*
Ortho Surg: Hand	4	*	6	*	0	*	5	*
Ortho Surg: Hip & Joint	6	*	5	*	0	*	1	*
Ortho Surg: Oncology	0	*	*	*	0	*	*	*
Ortho Surg: Pediatric	0	*	3	*	0	*	0	*
Ortho Surg: Spine	1	*	9	*	0	*	1	*
Ortho Surg: Trauma	3	*	2	*	2	*	0	*
Ortho Surg: Sports Med	7	*	9	*	9	*	4	*
Otorhinolaryngology	11	*	14	*	7	*	7	*
Otorhinolaryngology: Pediatric	*	*	0	*	0	*	*	*
Pathology: Anatomic & Clinical	0	*	0	*	6	*	0	*
Pathology: Anatomic	*	*	*	*	5	*	0	*
Pathology: Clinical	*	*	0	*	0	*	0	*

Table 38B: Physician Compensation to Gross Charges Ratio (TC Excluded) by Geographic Section for Single-specialty Practices (continued)

	Eastern		Midwest		Southern		Western	
	Physicians	Median	Physicians	Median	Physicians	Median	Physicians	Median
Pediatrics: General	45	.266	117	.334	27	.310	36	.318
Ped: Adolescent Medicine	*	*	*	*	4	*	0	*
Ped: Allergy/Immunology	*	*	*	*	*	*	2	*
Ped: Cardiology	0	*	1	*	0	*	0	*
Ped: Critical Care/Intensivist	*	*	7	*	6	*	0	*
Ped: Emergency Medicine	0	*	*	*	*	*	*	*
Ped: Endocrinology	*	*	*	*	0	*	1	*
Ped: Gastroenterology	*	*	0	*	1	*	0	*
Ped: Hematology/Oncology	*	*	0	*	2	*	2	*
Ped: Hospitalist	*	*	*	*	*	*	0	*
Ped: Infectious Disease	*	*	*	*	*	*	0	*
Ped: Neonatal Medicine	*	*	*	*	16	*	1	*
Ped: Nephrology	*	*	*	*	*	*	0	*
Ped: Neurology	0	*	4	*	1	*	0	*
Ped: Pulmonology	*	*	0	*	*	*	1	*
Ped: Rheumatology	*	*	*	*	*	*	0	*
Physiatry (Phys Med & Rehab)	2	*	1	*	0	*	0	*
Podiatry: General	*	*	0	*	0	*	*	*
Podiatry: Surg-Foot & Ankle	0	*	2	*	*	*	0	*
Podiatry: Surg-Forefoot Only	*	*	*	*	*	*	0	*
Psychiatry: General	0	*	3	*	*	*	*	*
Psychiatry: Child & Adolescent	0	*	*	*	6	*	*	*
Pulmonary Medicine	0	*	0	*	1	*	0	*
Pulmonary Med: Critical Care	1	*	0	*	10	*	6	*
Radiation Oncology	0	*	7	*	16	.313	6	*
Radiology: Diagnostic-Inv	6	*	43	.421	26	.339	23	*
Radiology: Diagnostic-Noninv	23	*	19	.360	50	.349	1	*
Radiology: Nuclear Medicine	0	*	2	*	2	*	0	*
Rheumatology	0	*	2	*	8	*	4	*
Sleep Medicine	0	*	2	*	0	*	*	*
Surgery: General	17	*	6	*	39	.217	13	.659
Surg: Cardiovascular	5	*	7	*	34	.249	15	.262
Surg: Cardiovascular-Pediatric	*	*	*	*	2	*	1	*
Surg: Colon and Rectal	5	*	0	*	*	*	2	*
Surg: Neurological	13	*	11	.184	7	*	0	*
Surg: Oncology	*	*	0	*	*	*	*	*
Surg: Oral	6	*	*	*	3	*	4	*
Surg: Pediatric	*	*	2	*	0	*	0	*
Surg: Plastic & Reconstruction	*	*	*	*	4	*	1	*
Surg: Plastic & Recon-Hand	0	*	*	*	0	*	*	*
Surg: Plastic & Recon-Pediatric	*	*	*	*	1	*	*	*
Surg: Thoracic (primary)	2	*	10	*	0	*	*	*
Surg: Transplant	*	*	*	*	4	*	*	*
Surg: Trauma	*	*	0	*	3	*	*	*
Surg: Trauma-Burn	*	*	0	*	6	*	1	*
Surg: Vascular (primary)	3	*	0	*	0	*	4	*
Urgent Care	0	*	3	*	19	*	0	*
Urology	10	*	7	*	3	*	3	*
Urology: Pediatric	*	*	*	*	0	*	0	*

Table 38C: Physician Compensation to Gross Charges Ratio (TC Excluded) by Geographic Section for Multispecialty Practices

	Eastern		Midwest		Southern		Western	
	Physicians	Median	Physicians	Median	Physicians	Median	Physicians	Median
Allergy/Immunology	7	*	29	.363	11	.390	16	.348
Anesthesiology	31	.342	98	.429	23	.424	34	.444
Anesth: Pain Management	2	*	5	*	3	*	0	*
Anesth: Pediatric	*	*	0	*	0	*	*	*
Cardiology: Electrophysiology	1	*	4	*	1	*	3	*
Cardiology: Invasive	9	*	28	.301	23	.245	8	*
Cardiology: Inv-Intervntnl	8	*	25	.281	23	.340	8	*
Cardiology: Noninvasive	11	.257	23	.273	14	.294	16	.381
Critical Care: Intensivist	6	*	7	*	*	*	2	*
Dentistry	3	*	*	*	5	*	0	*
Dermatology	16	.250	64	.315	16	.315	33	.288
Dermatology: MOHS Surgery	0	*	3	*	3	*	3	*
Emergency Medicine	46	.420	56	.407	0	*	5	*
Endocrinology/Metabolism	15	.342	33	.403	23	.440	17	.326
Family Practice (w/ OB)	38	.337	391	.378	31	.359	76	.297
Family Practice (w/o OB)	276	.381	799	.362	183	.394	273	.362
Family Practice: Sports Med	0	*	1	*	0	*	1	*
Gastroenterology	32	.207	77	.241	47	.245	33	.268
Gastroenterology: Hepatology	0	*	*	*	0	*	0	*
Geriatrics	1	*	13	.443	0	*	4	*
Hematology/Oncology	18	.633	40	.445	22	.454	17	.471
Hem/Onc: Oncology (only)	6	*	19	.467	5	*	1	*
Infectious Disease	9	*	20	.380	6	*	6	*
Internal Medicine: General	303	.343	621	.384	220	.399	314	.336
Internal Med: Hospitalist	20	.382	86	.477	20	.499	25	.564
Internal Med: Pediatric	5	*	10	.298	10	*	6	*
Nephrology	16	.309	37	.354	25	.462	9	*
Neurology	34	.286	81	.327	23	.321	24	.318
OBGYN: General	84	.261	195	.330	56	.295	89	.310
OBGYN: Gynecology (only)	7	*	57	.231	9	*	7	*
OBGYN: Gyn Oncology	3	*	5	*	3	*	1	*
OBGYN: Maternal & Fetal Med	3	*	18	.351	0	*	2	*
OBGYN: Repro Endocrinology	3	*	8	*	*	*	0	*
Occupational Medicine	2	*	29	.421	3	*	12	.359
Ophthalmology	17	.196	65	.269	17	.247	23	.272
Ophthalmology: Pediatric	1	*	1	*	0	*	0	*
Ophthalmology: Retina	0	*	2	*	0	*	1	*
Orthopedic (Non-surgical)	0	*	6	*	1	*	4	*
Orthopedic Surgery: General	19	.202	117	.275	35	.283	27	.270
Ortho Surg: Foot & Ankle	0	*	4	*	0	*	*	*
Ortho Surg: Hand	1	*	9	*	0	*	2	*
Ortho Surg: Hip & Joint	*	*	10	.263	0	*	3	*
Ortho Surg: Oncology	*	*	*	*	0	*	*	*
Ortho Surg: Pediatric	1	*	3	*	0	*	0	*
Ortho Surg: Spine	0	*	9	*	0	*	3	*
Ortho Surg: Trauma	4	*	1	*	*	*	0	*
Ortho Surg: Sports Med	1	*	14	.302	0	*	6	*
Otorhinolaryngology	15	.229	81	.269	19	.270	29	.258
Otorhinolaryngology: Pediatric	0	*	1	*	*	*	*	*
Pathology: Anatomic & Clinical	16	.236	14	.462	7	*	3	*
Pathology: Anatomic	0	*	1	*	0	*	2	*
Pathology: Clinical	4	*	6	*	5	*	0	*

Table 38C: Physician Compensation to Gross Charges Ratio (TC Excluded) by Geographic Section for Multispecialty Practices (continued)

	Eastern		Midwest		Southern		Western	
	Physicians	Median	Physicians	Median	Physicians	Median	Physicians	Median
Pediatrics: General	133	.354	309	.350	93	.363	157	.309
Ped: Adolescent Medicine	2	*	25	*	6	*	*	*
Ped: Allergy/Immunology	1	*	3	*	0	*	*	*
Ped: Cardiology	4	*	5	*	1	*	8	*
Ped: Child Development	1	*	7	*	1	*	2	*
Ped: Critical Care/Intensivist	2	*	11	.558	1	*	0	*
Ped: Emergency Medicine	*	*	6	*	*	*	*	*
Ped: Endocrinology	1	*	3	*	1	*	2	*
Ped: Gastroenterology	3	*	3	*	*	*	3	*
Ped: Genetics	0	*	2	*	0	*	5	*
Ped: Hematology/Oncology	2	*	6	*	1	*	4	*
Ped: Hospitalist	0	*	3	*	1	*	9	*
Ped: Infectious Disease	*	*	0	*	0	*	0	*
Ped: Neonatal Medicine	7	*	28	.312	1	*	0	*
Ped: Nephrology	1	*	2	*	*	*	3	*
Ped: Neurology	3	*	13	.451	1	*	3	*
Ped: Pulmonology	3	*	3	*	1	*	0	*
Ped: Rheumatology	1	*	*	*	*	*	2	*
Ped: Sports Medicine	0	*	*	*	*	*	*	*
Physiatry (Phys Med & Rehab)	3	*	34	.375	2	*	8	*
Podiatry: General	3	*	39	.273	10	.275	15	.220
Podiatry: Surg-Foot & Ankle	4	*	6	*	0	*	4	*
Podiatry: Surg-Forefoot Only	3	*	1	*	0	*	0	*
Psychiatry: General	16	.462	73	.431	10	.395	17	.409
Psychiatry: Child & Adolescent	0	*	11	.447	2	*	0	*
Psychiatry: Geriatric	4	*	2	*	4	*	0	*
Pulmonary Medicine	18	.267	42	.314	31	.317	18	.331
Pulmonary Med: Critical Care	14	.391	19	.376	10	.400	0	*
Radiation Oncology	2	*	16	.252	2	*	3	*
Radiology: Diagnostic-Inv	14	.242	36	.265	10	.267	6	*
Radiology: Diagnostic-Noninv	24	*	49	.292	14	.363	3	*
Radiology: Nuclear Medicine	5	*	3	*	2	*	0	*
Rheumatology	18	.293	48	.410	20	.483	13	.318
Sleep Medicine	0	*	0	*	0	*	1	*
Surgery: General	54	.212	182	.296	57	.254	66	.296
Surg: Cardiovascular	4	*	19	.335	5	*	5	*
Surg: Cardiovascular-Pediatric	*	*	1	*	*	*	*	*
Surg: Colon and Rectal	3	*	7	*	1	*	0	*
Surg: Neurological	13	.232	20	.299	5	*	8	*
Surg: Oncology	1	*	4	*	*	*	0	*
Surg: Oral	2	*	6	*	0	*	0	*
Surg: Pediatric	3	*	*	*	0	*	4	*
Surg: Plastic & Reconstruction	7	*	15	.288	4	*	13	.307
Surg: Plastic & Recon-Hand	0	*	3	*	*	*	*	*
Surg: Plastic & Recon-Pediatric	0	*	*	*	*	*	*	*
Surg: Thoracic (primary)	1	*	4	*	*	*	0	*
Surg: Transplant	2	*	1	*	0	*	1	*
Surg: Trauma	3	*	5	*	0	*	*	*
Surg: Trauma-Burn	0	*	0	*	*	*	*	*
Surg: Vascular (primary)	10	.328	19	.233	3	*	5	*
Urgent Care	2	*	74	.408	21	.367	74	.316
Urology	17	.244	63	.264	22	.271	22	.242
Urology: Pediatric	*	*	0	*	*	*	2	*

Table 39: Physician Compensation to Gross Charges Ratio (TC Excluded) by Percent of Capitation Revenue

	No capitation		10% or less		11% to 50%		51% or more	
	Physicians	Median	Physicians	Median	Physicians	Median	Physicians	Median
Allergy/Immunology	32	.345	20	.362	13	.359	6	*
Anesthesiology	240	.458	40	.414	48	.280	7	*
Anesth: Pain Management	23	.277	2	*	3	*	0	*
Anesth: Pediatric	0	*	*	*	0	*	*	*
Cardiology: Electrophysiology	11	.232	5	*	2	*	1	*
Cardiology: Invasive	52	.272	42	.308	1	*	3	*
Cardiology: Inv-Intervntnl	72	.297	44	.239	4	*	3	*
Cardiology: Noninvasive	46	.302	23	.399	14	.244	6	*
Critical Care: Intensivist	0	*	5	*	8	*	2	*
Dentistry	2	*	3	*	4	*	0	*
Dermatology	65	.347	39	.298	25	.226	6	*
Dermatology: MOHS Surgery	5	*	6	*	0	*	0	*
Emergency Medicine	83	.335	39	.404	53	.438	0	*
Endocrinology/Metabolism	40	.349	28	.426	17	.393	3	*
Family Practice (w/ OB)	268	.367	184	.382	164	.335	4	*
Family Practice (w/o OB)	873	.358	410	.386	356	.358	55	.372
Family Practice: Sports Med	1	*	1	*	0	*	*	*
Gastroenterology	196	.270	53	.242	32	.215	7	*
Gastroenterology: Hepatology	16	*	0	*	3	*	0	*
Geriatrics	2	*	8	*	8	*	0	*
Hematology/Oncology	57	.471	36	.449	27	.551	3	*
Hem/Onc: Oncology (only)	31	.559	3	*	8	*	0	*
Infectious Disease	41	.370	18	.375	14	.369	2	*
Internal Medicine: General	642	.371	427	.381	353	.347	69	.425
Internal Med: Hospitalist	94	.449	45	.573	10	.428	2	*
Internal Med: Pediatric	14	.381	13	.404	4	*	0	*
Nephrology	82	.317	22	.374	25	.320	1	*
Neurology	113	.320	61	.347	38	.279	10	.391
OBGYN: General	262	.297	115	.339	126	.266	23	.314
OBGYN: Gynecology (only)	60	.233	17	.330	7	*	5	*
OBGYN: Gyn Oncology	5	*	3	*	4	*	*	*
OBGYN: Maternal & Fetal Med	19	.381	4	*	5	*	*	*
OBGYN: Repro Endocrinology	1	*	8	*	2	*	0	*
Occupational Medicine	21	.364	12	.372	10	.444	3	*
Ophthalmology	71	.257	28	.243	22	.210	12	.320
Ophthalmology: Pediatric	1	*	0	*	2	*	0	*
Ophthalmology: Retina	2	*	0	*	2	*	0	*
Orthopedic (Non-surgical)	5	*	3	*	1	*	2	*
Orthopedic Surgery: General	129	.283	47	.280	56	.225	4	*
Ortho Surg: Foot & Ankle	7	*	1	*	2	*	*	*
Ortho Surg: Hand	20	.304	2	*	4	*	1	*
Ortho Surg: Hip & Joint	20	.284	2	*	2	*	1	*
Ortho Surg: Oncology	0	*	*	*	*	*	*	*
Ortho Surg: Pediatric	4	*	1	*	2	*	0	*
Ortho Surg: Spine	18	.269	0	*	3	*	2	*
Ortho Surg: Trauma	7	*	*	*	5	*	*	*
Ortho Surg: Sports Med	34	.250	8	*	4	*	3	*
Otorhinolaryngology	90	.266	43	.295	46	.208	4	*
Otorhinolaryngology: Pediatric	1	*	*	*	*	*	*	*
Pathology: Anatomic & Clinical	22	.373	13	.388	9	*	2	*
Pathology: Anatomic	7	*	0	*	1	*	*	*
Pathology: Clinical	5	*	8	*	2	*	*	*

Table 39: Physician Compensation to Gross Charges Ratio (TC Excluded) by Percent of Capitation Revenue (continued)

	No capitation		10% or less		11% to 50%		51% or more	
	Physicians	Median	Physicians	Median	Physicians	Median	Physicians	Median
Pediatrics: General	469	.342	208	.366	203	.308	27	.348
Ped: Adolescent Medicine	17	.381	0	*	16	.313	*	*
Ped: Allergy/Immunology	0	*	1	*	5	*	*	*
Ped: Cardiology	6	*	7	*	6	*	0	*
Ped: Child Development	0	*	5	*	6	*	*	*
Ped: Critical Care/Intensivist	19	.657	1	*	7	*	*	*
Ped: Emergency Medicine	6	*	*	*	*	*	*	*
Ped: Endocrinology	1	*	3	*	4	*	*	*
Ped: Gastroenterology	2	*	4	*	4	*	*	*
Ped: Genetics	2	*	5	*	*	*	*	*
Ped: Hematology/Oncology	5	*	7	*	5	*	0	*
Ped: Hospitalist	3	*	9	*	1	*	0	*
Ped: Infectious Disease	*	*	0	*	*	*	*	*
Ped: Neonatal Medicine	16	.255	28	.425	9	*	0	*
Ped: Nephrology	0	*	4	*	2	*	*	*
Ped: Neurology	12	.575	7	*	6	*	*	*
Ped: Pulmonology	1	*	1	*	6	*	*	*
Ped: Rheumatology	*	*	2	*	1	*	*	*
Ped: Sports Medicine	0	*	*	*	*	*	*	*
Physiatry (Phys Med & Rehab)	29	.340	10	.440	9	*	2	*
Podiatry: General	34	.247	13	.273	14	.247	6	*
Podiatry: Surg-Foot & Ankle	6	*	5	*	2	*	3	*
Podiatry: Surg-Forefoot Only	3	*	1	*	*	*	0	*
Psychiatry: General	39	.409	33	.491	45	.379	2	*
Psychiatry: Child & Adolescent	11	.570	4	*	3	*	1	*
Psychiatry: Geriatric	5	*	3	*	1	*	*	*
Pulmonary Medicine	47	.336	36	.285	24	.286	3	*
Pulmonary Med: Critical Care	43	.389	9	*	8	*	0	*
Radiation Oncology	34	.305	3	*	14	.211	1	*
Radiology: Diagnostic-Inv	83	.309	23	.274	52	.314	6	*
Radiology: Diagnostic-Noninv	133	.363	17	.374	33	.242	0	*
Radiology: Nuclear Medicine	8	*	1	*	4	*	0	*
Rheumatology	53	.301	44	.384	13	.399	2	*
Sleep Medicine	2	*	0	*	1	*	*	*
Surgery: General	263	.253	91	.296	70	.254	10	.449
Surg: Cardiovascular	70	.254	9	*	13	.260	2	*
Surg: Cardiovascular-Pediatric	3	*	1	*	0	*	*	*
Surg: Colon and Rectal	9	*	2	*	6	*	0	*
Surg: Neurological	56	.218	11	.293	10	.249	0	*
Surg: Oncology	1	*	*	*	4	*	*	*
Surg: Oral	16	.247	1	*	4	*	0	*
Surg: Pediatric	2	*	4	*	3	*	*	*
Surg: Plastic & Reconstruction	11	.307	18	.253	14	.272	1	*
Surg: Plastic & Recon-Hand	1	*	*	*	2	*	*	*
Surg: Plastic & Recon-Pediatric	0	*	1	*	*	*	*	*
Surg: Thoracic (primary)	15	.226	2	*	0	*	0	*
Surg: Transplant	5	*	1	*	2	*	*	*
Surg: Trauma	3	*	3	*	5	*	*	*
Surg: Trauma-Burn	6	*	1	*	0	*	*	*
Surg: Vascular (primary)	24	.316	5	*	15	.233	0	*
Urgent Care	99	.305	51	.427	25	.363	16	.365
Urology	79	.255	37	.281	27	.232	4	*
Urology: Pediatric	0	*	2	*	0	*	*	*

Table 40: Physician Compensation to Gross Charges Ratio (TC Excluded) by Years in Specialty

	1 to 2 years		3 to 7 years		8 to 17 years		18 years or more	
	Physicians	Median	Physicians	Median	Physicians	Median	Physicians	Median
Allergy/Immunology	3	*	9	*	25	.359	26	.348
Anesthesiology	17	.385	58	.463	121	.417	82	.425
Anesth: Pain Management	4	*	9	*	7	*	4	*
Anesth: Pediatric	0	*	0	*	0	*	0	*
Cardiology: Electrophysiology	2	*	7	*	9	*	1	*
Cardiology: Invasive	0	*	22	.274	38	.266	29	.291
Cardiology: Inv-Intervntnl	5	*	20	.296	47	.281	39	.305
Cardiology: Noninvasive	1	*	13	.379	24	.326	41	.292
Critical Care: Intensivist	0	*	1	*	11	.375	3	*
Dentistry	0	*	0	*	6	*	4	*
Dermatology	5	*	19	.285	44	.309	48	.317
Dermatology: MOHS Surgery	0	*	4	*	4	*	2	*
Emergency Medicine	13	.277	51	.348	64	.422	37	.422
Endocrinology/Metabolism	1	*	10	.397	32	.381	32	.376
Family Practice (w/ OB)	58	.339	153	.370	188	.369	141	.385
Family Practice (w/o OB)	67	.380	327	.368	481	.372	565	.364
Family Practice: Sports Med	0	*	0	*	2	*	1	*
Gastroenterology	13	.222	45	.276	103	.261	97	.262
Gastroenterology: Hepatology	1	*	3	*	5	*	10	.216
Geriatrics	0	*	3	*	6	*	3	*
Hematology/Oncology	5	*	20	.435	44	.487	49	.488
Hem/Onc: Oncology (only)	0	*	4	*	13	.589	11	.584
Infectious Disease	5	*	15	.344	22	.400	20	.374
Internal Medicine: General	80	.347	318	.360	442	.358	442	.363
Internal Med: Hospitalist	24	.505	46	.480	32	.490	19	.437
Internal Med: Pediatric	6	*	10	.406	10	.381	1	*
Nephrology	8	*	22	.322	33	.295	42	.329
Neurology	10	.280	34	.322	78	.316	68	.291
OBGYN: General	26	.254	125	.310	166	.302	123	.305
OBGYN: Gynecology (only)	1	*	5	*	25	.236	55	.292
OBGYN: Gyn Oncology	1	*	1	*	4	*	2	*
OBGYN: Maternal & Fetal Med	1	*	6	*	10	.351	5	*
OBGYN: Repro Endocrinology	0	*	0	*	3	*	1	*
Occupational Medicine	2	*	9	*	13	.431	13	.403
Ophthalmology	5	*	18	.233	53	.247	36	.284
Ophthalmology: Pediatric	*	*	0	*	2	*	1	*
Ophthalmology: Retina	0	*	3	*	1	*	0	*
Orthopedic (Non-surgical)	0	*	3	*	2	*	5	*
Orthopedic Surgery: General	7	*	26	.279	70	.280	91	.270
Ortho Surg: Foot & Ankle	1	*	4	*	3	*	2	*
Ortho Surg: Hand	1	*	4	*	12	.304	9	*
Ortho Surg: Hip & Joint	1	*	2	*	13	.269	9	*
Ortho Surg: Oncology	0	*	*	*	0	*	0	*
Ortho Surg: Pediatric	0	*	2	*	2	*	3	*
Ortho Surg: Spine	2	*	3	*	11	.270	7	*
Ortho Surg: Trauma	0	*	6	*	4	*	2	*
Ortho Surg: Sports Med	3	*	9	*	28	.244	9	*
Otorhinolaryngology	6	*	36	.264	45	.211	70	.270
Otorhinolaryngology: Pediatric	0	*	0	*	0	*	0	*
Pathology: Anatomic & Clinical	3	*	4	*	18	.395	19	.311
Pathology: Anatomic	*	*	1	*	0	*	7	*
Pathology: Clinical	2	*	4	*	4	*	5	*

Table 40: Physician Compensation to Gross Charges Ratio (TC Excluded) by Years in Specialty (continued)

	1 to 2 years		3 to 7 years		8 to 17 years		18 years or more	
	Physicians	Median	Physicians	Median	Physicians	Median	Physicians	Median
Pediatrics: General	50	.325	200	.330	277	.334	275	.344
Ped: Adolescent Medicine	2	*	6	*	10	.379	14	.323
Ped: Allergy/Immunology	*	*	1	*	1	*	4	*
Ped: Cardiology	0	*	6	*	5	*	6	*
Ped: Child Development	0	*	3	*	0	*	1	*
Ped: Critical Care/Intensivist	1	*	7	*	15	.513	3	*
Ped: Emergency Medicine	*	*	0	*	4	*	2	*
Ped: Endocrinology	1	*	2	*	0	*	3	*
Ped: Gastroenterology	0	*	4	*	1	*	4	*
Ped: Genetics	0	*	3	*	1	*	3	*
Ped: Hematology/Oncology	0	*	5	*	5	*	6	*
Ped: Hospitalist	1	*	5	*	3	*	1	*
Ped: Infectious Disease	0	*	0	*	0	*	0	*
Ped: Neonatal Medicine	1	*	9	*	19	.484	13	.373
Ped: Nephrology	*	*	1	*	3	*	1	*
Ped: Neurology	1	*	8	*	9	*	5	*
Ped: Pulmonology	0	*	3	*	5	*	0	*
Ped: Rheumatology	*	*	2	*	1	*	*	*
Ped: Sports Medicine	*	*	*	*	0	*	*	*
Physiatry (Phys Med & Rehab)	1	*	19	.355	21	.354	6	*
Podiatry: General	2	*	12	.235	23	.276	15	.280
Podiatry: Surg-Foot & Ankle	0	*	2	*	7	*	4	*
Podiatry: Surg-Forefoot Only	0	*	0	*	2	*	2	*
Psychiatry: General	6	*	16	.481	34	.429	35	.400
Psychiatry: Child & Adolescent	1	*	3	*	6	*	4	*
Psychiatry: Geriatric	*	*	0	*	5	*	5	*
Pulmonary Medicine	2	*	11	.306	47	.301	34	.291
Pulmonary Med: Critical Care	4	*	13	.370	21	.370	14	.403
Radiation Oncology	1	*	11	.291	19	.303	13	.278
Radiology: Diagnostic-Inv	3	*	32	.316	55	.319	54	.275
Radiology: Diagnostic-Noninv	8	*	34	.291	66	.351	68	.343
Radiology: Nuclear Medicine	0	*	3	*	4	*	7	*
Rheumatology	5	*	15	.426	31	.336	41	.300
Sleep Medicine	1	*	0	*	1	*	1	*
Surgery: General	21	.221	64	.255	133	.252	151	.281
Surg: Cardiovascular	2	*	20	.244	38	.262	21	.253
Surg: Cardiovascular-Pediatric	1	*	1	*	2	*	*	*
Surg: Colon and Rectal	1	*	2	*	7	*	5	*
Surg: Neurological	4	*	15	.219	25	.241	28	.227
Surg: Oncology	*	*	0	*	1	*	*	*
Surg: Oral	1	*	3	*	8	*	8	*
Surg: Pediatric	2	*	3	*	1	*	3	*
Surg: Plastic & Reconstruction	4	*	7	*	12	.247	15	.264
Surg: Plastic & Recon-Hand	*	*	0	*	0	*	0	*
Surg: Plastic & Recon-Pediatric	*	*	0	*	1	*	*	*
Surg: Thoracic (primary)	0	*	2	*	9	*	5	*
Surg: Transplant	2	*	1	*	4	*	1	*
Surg: Trauma	1	*	2	*	5	*	3	*
Surg: Trauma-Burn	0	*	1	*	1	*	5	*
Surg: Vascular (primary)	3	*	7	*	15	.227	12	.249
Urgent Care	6	*	42	.318	64	.336	50	.350
Urology	3	*	27	.271	46	.266	50	.243
Urology: Pediatric	*	*	1	*	1	*	*	*

Table 41: Physician Ambulatory Encounters

	Physicians	Medical Practices	Mean	Std. Dev.	25th %tile	Median	75th %tile	90th %tile
Allergy/Immunology	78	47	3,727	2,424	2,102	3,030	4,721	6,786
Anesthesiology	39	5	2,946	3,577	777	1,384	2,547	10,584
Anesth: Pain Management	14	7	1,886	1,180	1,030	1,468	2,945	4,110
Anesth: Pediatric	0	*	*	*	*	*	*	*
Cardiology: Electrophysiology	33	24	2,020	1,174	1,018	1,770	2,999	3,840
Cardiology: Invasive	219	65	2,419	1,549	1,334	1,861	3,034	5,043
Cardiology: Inv-Intervntnl	277	73	2,578	1,939	1,304	1,971	3,403	4,931
Cardiology: Noninvasive	209	76	2,688	1,728	1,460	2,234	3,353	5,342
Critical Care: Intensivist	4	3	*	*	*	*	*	*
Dentistry	19	5	3,316	2,542	1,806	2,198	3,735	7,691
Dermatology	170	88	5,468	2,102	4,123	5,222	6,478	8,303
Dermatology: MOHS Surgery	13	11	5,631	2,326	3,325	5,727	7,615	8,916
Emergency Medicine	127	14	3,062	1,027	2,417	3,115	3,670	4,410
Endocrinology/Metabolism	105	67	3,062	1,106	2,223	2,877	3,760	4,438
Family Practice (w/ OB)	841	143	4,245	1,734	3,132	3,878	4,975	6,281
Family Practice (w/o OB)	2,764	359	4,508	1,552	3,487	4,318	5,335	6,433
Family Practice: Sports Med	15	12	5,509	3,653	2,599	5,049	8,071	12,164
Gastroenterology	351	117	1,766	815	1,205	1,603	2,169	2,852
Gastroenterology: Hepatology	43	9	1,517	458	1,219	1,445	1,830	2,142
Geriatrics	31	14	2,865	1,611	1,887	2,210	4,319	5,371
Hematology/Oncology	170	68	3,512	1,693	2,335	3,136	4,352	5,696
Hem/Onc: Oncology (only)	45	19	3,621	1,947	2,276	3,365	4,277	6,287
Infectious Disease	66	34	1,251	716	656	1,083	1,745	2,272
Internal Medicine: General	2,186	283	3,637	1,419	2,752	3,503	4,332	5,334
Internal Med: Hospitalist	88	25	2,095	1,393	910	2,119	2,642	4,034
Internal Med: Pediatric	42	17	3,423	1,788	2,174	3,248	5,152	5,780
Nephrology	111	46	2,697	2,025	980	2,095	3,531	5,951
Neurology	259	90	2,544	1,473	1,746	2,269	2,904	3,717
OBGYN: General	760	164	3,349	1,586	2,246	3,115	4,200	5,262
OBGYN: Gynecology (only)	91	36	3,065	1,246	2,155	2,935	3,980	4,786
OBGYN: Gyn Oncology	11	7	1,665	932	932	1,280	2,511	3,277
OBGYN: Maternal & Fetal Med	18	9	2,059	939	1,535	1,996	2,547	2,906
OBGYN: Repro Endocrinology	11	6	3,829	1,173	2,906	3,733	4,582	5,790
Occupational Medicine	49	26	3,611	1,376	2,697	3,300	4,453	5,622
Ophthalmology	221	81	5,214	2,137	4,010	5,016	5,940	8,558
Ophthalmology: Pediatric	10	7	4,714	1,765	3,514	5,074	5,990	7,382
Ophthalmology: Retina	43	14	4,839	1,698	3,593	4,458	5,690	7,449
Orthopedic (Non-surgical)	34	17	4,292	1,767	3,062	4,224	5,628	6,754
Orthopedic Surgery: General	410	120	3,620	1,519	2,591	3,364	4,434	5,429
Ortho Surg: Foot & Ankle	30	26	3,921	1,589	2,859	3,464	4,637	5,787
Ortho Surg: Hand	64	39	4,106	1,452	3,246	3,782	4,958	6,110
Ortho Surg: Hip & Joint	59	31	3,045	1,440	1,906	2,819	3,878	4,927
Ortho Surg: Oncology	0	*	*	*	*	*	*	*
Ortho Surg: Pediatric	14	13	3,910	1,449	2,715	3,609	4,954	6,289
Ortho Surg: Spine	63	42	2,816	1,307	1,871	2,605	3,410	4,712
Ortho Surg: Trauma	15	10	2,840	903	2,300	2,497	3,820	4,413
Ortho Surg: Sports Med	126	58	3,640	1,557	2,629	3,479	4,607	5,583
Otorhinolaryngology	199	83	3,516	1,168	2,598	3,360	4,280	5,138
Otorhinolaryngology: Pediatric	2	2	*	*	*	*	*	*
Pathology: Anatomic & Clinical	12	4	3,763	1,961	3,164	3,720	4,377	7,443
Pathology: Anatomic	7	3	*	*	*	*	*	*
Pathology: Clinical	28	4	5,132	1,089	4,603	4,834	5,455	7,157

Table 41: Physician Ambulatory Encounters (continued)

	Physicians	Medical Practices	Mean	Std. Dev.	25th %tile	Median	75th %tile	90th %tile
Pediatrics: General	1,181	211	4,842	1,876	3,630	4,510	5,761	7,234
Ped: Adolescent Medicine	43	6	4,845	1,465	3,915	4,669	5,632	6,946
Ped: Allergy/Immunology	6	5	*	*	*	*	*	*
Ped: Cardiology	25	13	2,410	1,402	1,430	1,829	3,288	4,981
Ped: Child Development	8	5	*	*	*	*	*	*
Ped: Critical Care/Intensivist	12	2	*	*	*	*	*	*
Ped: Emergency Medicine	6	1	*	*	*	*	*	*
Ped: Endocrinology	10	8	1,985	969	1,327	1,800	2,319	4,078
Ped: Gastroenterology	7	5	*	*	*	*	*	*
Ped: Genetics	10	4	1,740	1,291	914	1,155	2,856	4,222
Ped: Hematology/Oncology	16	10	1,676	983	898	1,384	2,805	3,231
Ped: Hospitalist	2	2	*	*	*	*	*	*
Ped: Infectious Disease	0	*	*	*	*	*	*	*
Ped: Neonatal Medicine	7	6	*	*	*	*	*	*
Ped: Nephrology	5	3	*	*	*	*	*	*
Ped: Neurology	23	13	1,786	739	1,226	1,665	2,153	2,981
Ped: Pulmonology	10	6	1,359	807	748	1,138	1,821	3,158
Ped: Rheumatology	2	1	*	*	*	*	*	*
Ped: Sports Medicine	0	*	*	*	*	*	*	*
Physiatry (Phys Med & Rehab)	77	47	2,066	1,472	996	1,684	2,814	3,910
Podiatry: General	71	42	3,714	1,161	3,097	3,706	4,447	5,311
Podiatry: Surg-Foot & Ankle	28	16	3,983	937	3,495	4,089	4,578	5,087
Podiatry: Surg-Forefoot Only	4	3	*	*	*	*	*	*
Psychiatry: General	129	40	2,394	1,418	1,541	2,260	2,849	3,861
Psychiatry: Child & Adolescent	15	10	2,150	757	1,654	1,992	2,593	3,404
Psychiatry: Geriatric	9	5	*	*	*	*	*	*
Pulmonary Medicine	144	71	2,185	1,208	1,306	1,856	2,872	3,843
Pulmonary Med: Critical Care	75	27	1,621	927	995	1,427	2,109	2,963
Radiation Oncology	32	13	1,710	1,319	752	1,080	2,777	4,168
Radiology: Diagnostic-Inv	79	12	10,260	4,943	5,149	10,364	15,200	16,596
Radiology: Diagnostic-Noninv	94	19	10,100	4,783	5,200	9,432	14,211	16,917
Radiology: Nuclear Medicine	15	7	4,468	486	4,200	4,200	4,644	5,502
Rheumatology	137	72	3,449	1,604	2,276	3,337	4,386	5,449
Sleep Medicine	2	2	*	*	*	*	*	*
Surgery: General	476	148	1,790	810	1,210	1,696	2,200	2,835
Surg: Cardiovascular	70	24	638	334	409	574	752	997
Surg: Cardiovascular-Pediatric	2	2	*	*	*	*	*	*
Surg: Colon and Rectal	17	8	1,601	468	1,214	1,644	1,907	2,369
Surg: Neurological	111	35	1,740	1,140	1,129	1,479	1,974	2,759
Surg: Oncology	7	3	*	*	*	*	*	*
Surg: Oral	15	8	2,633	1,530	1,500	1,800	3,621	5,377
Surg: Pediatric	12	6	1,110	624	609	949	1,696	2,203
Surg: Plastic & Reconstruction	45	27	2,445	1,109	1,806	2,130	2,990	3,844
Surg: Plastic & Recon-Hand	2	2	*	*	*	*	*	*
Surg: Plastic & Recon-Pediatric	2	1	*	*	*	*	*	*
Surg: Thoracic (primary)	7	6	*	*	*	*	*	*
Surg: Transplant	8	4	*	*	*	*	*	*
Surg: Trauma	11	4	872	357	646	784	1,025	1,654
Surg: Trauma-Burn	8	3	*	*	*	*	*	*
Surg: Vascular (primary)	51	27	1,632	748	1,128	1,573	2,042	2,816
Urgent Care	230	59	5,305	2,071	4,123	4,993	6,049	8,057
Urology	200	83	3,320	1,735	2,299	2,861	3,799	5,090
Urology: Pediatric	3	2	*	*	*	*	*	*

Table 42: Physician Ambulatory Encounters by Group Type

	Single-specialty			Multispecialty		
	Physicians	Medical Practices	Median	Physicians	Medical Practices	Median
Allergy/Immunology	17	4	3,036	61	43	3,023
Anesthesiology	15	1	*	24	4	1,192
Anesth: Pain Management	11	4	1,512	3	3	*
Anesth: Pediatric	0	*	*	0	*	*
Cardiology: Electrophysiology	20	14	2,371	13	10	1,502
Cardiology: Invasive	112	27	1,748	107	38	2,261
Cardiology: Inv-Intervntnl	177	37	1,920	100	36	2,192
Cardiology: Noninvasive	117	35	2,143	92	41	2,495
Critical Care: Intensivist	0	*	*	4	3	*
Dentistry	2	1	*	17	4	2,390
Dermatology	19	9	6,118	151	79	5,165
Dermatology: MOHS Surgery	5	4	*	8	7	*
Emergency Medicine	50	4	3,486	77	10	2,839
Endocrinology/Metabolism	8	6	*	97	61	2,856
Family Practice (w/ OB)	183	48	3,538	658	95	4,015
Family Practice (w/o OB)	552	141	4,594	2,212	218	4,280
Family Practice: Sports Med	7	5	*	8	7	*
Gastroenterology	126	18	1,584	225	99	1,665
Gastroenterology: Hepatology	39	7	1,445	4	2	*
Geriatrics	0	*	*	31	14	2,210
Hematology/Oncology	48	12	2,869	122	56	3,202
Hem/Onc: Oncology (only)	20	3	3,527	25	16	2,675
Infectious Disease	23	8	1,146	43	26	1,001
Internal Medicine: General	216	49	3,452	1,970	234	3,506
Internal Med: Hospitalist	3	1	*	98	28	1,986
Internal Med: Pediatric	3	1	*	39	16	3,203
Nephrology	36	5	1,841	75	41	2,095
Neurology	79	15	2,416	180	75	2,119
OBGYN: General	199	43	3,720	561	121	2,884
OBGYN: Gynecology (only)	12	8	3,097	79	28	2,935
OBGYN: Gyn Oncology	0	*	*	11	7	1,280
OBGYN: Maternal & Fetal Med	6	2	*	12	7	2,188
OBGYN: Repro Endocrinology	2	2	*	9	4	*
Occupational Medicine	4	1	*	45	25	3,287
Ophthalmology	67	13	5,291	154	68	4,748
Ophthalmology: Pediatric	8	5	*	2	2	*
Ophthalmology: Retina	39	10	4,451	4	4	*
Orthopedic (Non-surgical)	11	3	4,346	23	14	3,628
Orthopedic Surgery: General	186	48	3,618	224	72	3,239
Ortho Surg: Foot & Ankle	23	21	3,558	7	5	*
Ortho Surg: Hand	46	29	3,849	18	10	3,632
Ortho Surg: Hip & Joint	40	23	2,861	19	8	2,819
Ortho Surg: Oncology	0	*	*	0	*	*
Ortho Surg: Pediatric	9	8	*	5	5	*
Ortho Surg: Spine	44	28	2,620	19	14	2,405
Ortho Surg: Trauma	14	9	2,509	1	1	*
Ortho Surg: Sports Med	93	40	3,486	33	18	3,370
Otorhinolaryngology	38	8	3,258	161	75	3,375
Otorhinolaryngology: Pediatric	1	1	*	1	1	*
Pathology: Anatomic & Clinical	0	*	*	12	4	3,720
Pathology: Anatomic	0	*	*	7	3	*
Pathology: Clinical	7	2	*	21	2	*

Table 42: Physician Ambulatory Encounters by Group Type (continued)

	Single-specialty			Multispecialty		
	Physicians	Medical Practices	Median	Physicians	Medical Practices	Median
Pediatrics: General	356	54	4,643	825	157	4,460
Ped: Adolescent Medicine	4	1	*	39	5	4,369
Ped: Allergy/Immunology	2	1	*	4	4	*
Ped: Cardiology	9	4	*	16	9	2,876
Ped: Child Development	*	*	*	8	5	*
Ped: Critical Care/Intensivist	0	*	*	12	2	*
Ped: Emergency Medicine	0	*	*	6	1	*
Ped: Endocrinology	1	1	*	9	7	*
Ped: Gastroenterology	1	1	*	6	4	*
Ped: Genetics	*	*	*	10	4	1,155
Ped: Hematology/Oncology	4	2	*	12	8	1,384
Ped: Hospitalist	0	*	*	2	2	*
Ped: Infectious Disease	0	*	*	0	*	*
Ped: Neonatal Medicine	2	2	*	5	4	*
Ped: Nephrology	0	*	*	5	3	*
Ped: Neurology	6	4	*	17	9	1,565
Ped: Pulmonology	6	2	*	4	4	*
Ped: Rheumatology	0	*	*	2	1	*
Ped: Sports Medicine	*	*	*	0	*	*
Physiatry (Phys Med & Rehab)	23	17	1,981	54	30	1,617
Podiatry: General	1	1	*	70	41	3,707
Podiatry: Surg-Foot & Ankle	5	3	*	23	13	4,036
Podiatry: Surg-Forefoot Only	1	1	*	3	2	*
Psychiatry: General	3	1	*	126	39	2,272
Psychiatry: Child & Adolescent	5	2	*	10	8	2,062
Psychiatry: Geriatric	*	*	*	9	5	*
Pulmonary Medicine	21	6	1,274	123	65	2,022
Pulmonary Med: Critical Care	27	6	867	48	21	1,741
Radiation Oncology	19	5	812	13	8	2,662
Radiology: Diagnostic-Inv	57	6	7,583	22	6	16,596
Radiology: Diagnostic-Noninv	62	8	9,014	32	11	11,708
Radiology: Nuclear Medicine	11	3	4,200	4	4	*
Rheumatology	20	6	1,637	117	66	3,579
Sleep Medicine	0	*	*	2	2	*
Surgery: General	92	20	1,873	384	128	1,678
Surg: Cardiovascular	38	10	560	32	14	583
Surg: Cardiovascular-Pediatric	2	2	*	0	*	*
Surg: Colon and Rectal	6	2	*	11	6	1,763
Surg: Neurological	54	10	1,503	57	25	1,415
Surg: Oncology	0	*	*	7	3	*
Surg: Oral	7	2	*	8	6	*
Surg: Pediatric	3	2	*	9	4	*
Surg: Plastic & Reconstruction	10	4	1,857	35	23	2,242
Surg: Plastic & Recon-Hand	1	1	*	1	1	*
Surg: Plastic & Recon-Pediatric	2	1	*	0	*	*
Surg: Thoracic (primary)	2	2	*	5	4	*
Surg: Transplant	4	1	*	4	3	*
Surg: Trauma	0	*	*	11	4	784
Surg: Trauma-Burn	7	2	*	1	1	*
Surg: Vascular (primary)	8	3	*	43	24	1,625
Urgent Care	36	3	4,754	194	56	5,013
Urology	55	14	3,158	145	69	2,812
Urology: Pediatric	1	1	*	2	1	*

Table 43: Physician Ambulatory Encounters by Hospital Ownership

	Hospital Owned			Non-hospital Owned		
	Physicians	Medical Practices	Median	Physicians	Medical Practices	Median
Allergy/Immunology	11	9	3,062	67	38	3,023
Anesthesiology	0	*	*	39	5	1,384
Anesth: Pain Management	2	2	*	12	5	1,546
Anesth: Pediatric	*	*	*	0	*	*
Cardiology: Electrophysiology	3	2	*	30	22	1,676
Cardiology: Invasive	33	9	1,675	186	56	1,896
Cardiology: Inv-Intervntnl	26	7	1,595	251	66	2,015
Cardiology: Noninvasive	30	10	2,847	172	65	2,168
Critical Care: Intensivist	3	2	*	1	1	*
Dentistry	0	*	*	18	4	2,078
Dermatology	32	18	4,531	136	69	5,491
Dermatology: MOHS Surgery	5	4	*	8	7	*
Emergency Medicine	53	6	2,891	74	8	3,369
Endocrinology/Metabolism	41	24	2,766	64	43	3,102
Family Practice (w/ OB)	295	58	3,767	545	84	4,033
Family Practice (w/o OB)	1,364	180	4,329	1,387	177	4,296
Family Practice: Sports Med	7	6	*	8	6	*
Gastroenterology	48	22	1,780	300	94	1,589
Gastroenterology: Hepatology	*	*	*	43	9	1,445
Geriatrics	13	7	2,138	18	7	3,663
Hematology/Oncology	27	12	2,752	141	55	3,349
Hem/Onc: Oncology (only)	4	4	*	41	15	3,372
Infectious Disease	17	12	733	49	22	1,107
Internal Medicine: General	792	112	3,594	1,340	169	3,492
Internal Med: Hospitalist	63	11	2,152	38	18	997
Internal Med: Pediatric	17	8	4,778	25	9	2,911
Nephrology	25	10	2,096	86	36	2,037
Neurology	40	19	1,701	217	70	2,324
OBGYN: General	222	57	3,033	514	105	3,259
OBGYN: Gynecology (only)	56	12	3,217	35	24	2,527
OBGYN: Gyn Oncology	5	3	*	6	4	*
OBGYN: Maternal & Fetal Med	10	4	1,996	8	5	*
OBGYN: Repro Endocrinology	7	3	*	2	2	*
Occupational Medicine	18	7	3,368	31	19	3,300
Ophthalmology	34	16	4,172	176	63	5,088
Ophthalmology: Pediatric	0	*	*	9	6	*
Ophthalmology: Retina	1	1	*	42	13	4,455
Orthopedic (Non-surgical)	7	6	*	27	11	4,346
Orthopedic Surgery: General	47	19	3,335	359	100	3,369
Ortho Surg: Foot & Ankle	*	*	*	30	26	3,464
Ortho Surg: Hand	1	1	*	63	38	3,784
Ortho Surg: Hip & Joint	0	*	*	58	30	2,828
Ortho Surg: Oncology	*	*	*	0	*	*
Ortho Surg: Pediatric	0	*	*	14	13	3,609
Ortho Surg: Spine	1	1	*	62	41	2,576
Ortho Surg: Trauma	0	*	*	9	8	*
Ortho Surg: Sports Med	6	4	*	113	52	3,486
Otorhinolaryngology	40	20	3,415	157	62	3,360
Otorhinolaryngology: Pediatric	*	*	*	2	2	*
Pathology: Anatomic & Clinical	5	1	*	7	3	*
Pathology: Anatomic	0	*	*	7	3	*
Pathology: Clinical	2	1	*	26	3	4,739

Table 43: Physician Ambulatory Encounters by Hospital Ownership (continued)

	Hospital Owned			Non-hospital Owned		
	Physicians	Medical Practices	Median	Physicians	Medical Practices	Median
Pediatrics: General	447	82	4,569	713	127	4,524
Ped: Adolescent Medicine	11	2	*	32	4	4,291
Ped: Allergy/Immunology	1	1	*	5	4	*
Ped: Cardiology	3	3	*	22	10	1,984
Ped: Child Development	3	2	*	5	3	*
Ped: Critical Care/Intensivist	0	*	*	12	2	*
Ped: Emergency Medicine	6	1	*	*	*	*
Ped: Endocrinology	5	4	*	5	4	*
Ped: Gastroenterology	3	3	*	4	2	*
Ped: Genetics	2	1	*	8	3	*
Ped: Hematology/Oncology	5	3	*	11	7	1,450
Ped: Hospitalist	0	*	*	2	2	*
Ped: Infectious Disease	0	*	*	0	*	*
Ped: Neonatal Medicine	1	1	*	6	5	*
Ped: Nephrology	1	1	*	4	2	*
Ped: Neurology	11	7	1,497	12	6	1,848
Ped: Pulmonology	2	2	*	8	4	*
Ped: Rheumatology	*	*	*	2	1	*
Ped: Sports Medicine	*	*	*	0	*	*
Physiatry (Phys Med & Rehab)	20	9	1,288	57	38	1,879
Podiatry: General	30	13	3,714	39	28	3,681
Podiatry: Surg-Foot & Ankle	6	4	*	22	12	4,089
Podiatry: Surg-Forefoot Only	0	*	*	4	3	*
Psychiatry: General	46	21	1,640	73	18	2,424
Psychiatry: Child & Adolescent	7	5	*	8	5	*
Psychiatry: Geriatric	2	2	*	7	3	*
Pulmonary Medicine	25	14	2,093	119	57	1,821
Pulmonary Med: Critical Care	9	6	*	66	21	1,453
Radiation Oncology	4	3	*	28	10	1,026
Radiology: Diagnostic-Inv	0	*	*	79	12	10,364
Radiology: Diagnostic-Noninv	4	2	*	90	17	9,689
Radiology: Nuclear Medicine	1	1	*	14	6	4,200
Rheumatology	36	18	3,323	100	53	3,487
Sleep Medicine	1	1	*	1	1	*
Surgery: General	96	40	1,515	375	107	1,767
Surg: Cardiovascular	7	4	*	63	20	546
Surg: Cardiovascular-Pediatric	0	*	*	2	2	*
Surg: Colon and Rectal	0	*	*	17	8	1,644
Surg: Neurological	12	8	1,251	99	27	1,523
Surg: Oncology	*	*	*	7	3	*
Surg: Oral	1	1	*	14	7	2,277
Surg: Pediatric	7	4	*	5	2	*
Surg: Plastic & Reconstruction	5	4	*	40	23	2,071
Surg: Plastic & Recon-Hand	1	1	*	1	1	*
Surg: Plastic & Recon-Pediatric	*	*	*	2	1	*
Surg: Thoracic (primary)	3	3	*	4	3	*
Surg: Transplant	3	2	*	5	2	*
Surg: Trauma	9	3	*	2	1	*
Surg: Trauma-Burn	1	1	*	7	2	*
Surg: Vascular (primary)	8	7	*	43	20	1,573
Urgent Care	60	21	4,322	170	38	5,138
Urology	28	15	2,398	170	67	3,059
Urology: Pediatric	0	*	*	3	2	*

MEDICAL GROUP MANAGEMENT ASSOCIATION™

Table 44: Physician Ambulatory Encounters by Geographic Section

	Eastern		Midwest		Southern		Western	
	Physicians	Median	Physicians	Median	Physicians	Median	Physicians	Median
Allergy/Immunology	7	*	25	3,796	27	2,456	19	3,341
Anesthesiology	10	*	8	*	15	*	6	*
Anesth: Pain Management	0	*	5	*	9	*	0	*
Anesth: Pediatric	*	*	0	*	0	*	0	*
Cardiology: Electrophysiology	3	*	9	*	13	1,822	8	*
Cardiology: Invasive	19	1,551	76	1,811	88	2,025	36	2,252
Cardiology: Inv-Intervntnl	24	1,453	76	2,060	140	2,129	37	1,589
Cardiology: Noninvasive	81	2,228	59	2,510	45	2,159	24	2,177
Critical Care: Intensivist	0	*	2	*	0	*	2	*
Dentistry	14	2,420	*	*	5	*	0	*
Dermatology	26	5,891	65	5,408	26	5,260	53	4,947
Dermatology: MOHS Surgery	1	*	4	*	5	*	3	*
Emergency Medicine	36	2,901	40	2,774	33	*	18	2,633
Endocrinology/Metabolism	17	3,145	35	2,948	29	2,766	24	2,843
Family Practice (w/ OB)	74	3,418	523	4,012	93	4,452	151	3,526
Family Practice (w/o OB)	501	4,525	1,125	4,211	625	4,714	513	3,973
Family Practice: Sports Med	1	*	6	*	3	*	5	*
Gastroenterology	49	1,866	130	1,500	111	1,625	61	1,583
Gastroenterology: Hepatology	1	*	17	*	20	1,525	5	*
Geriatrics	11	*	11	2,057	3	*	6	*
Hematology/Oncology	28	3,018	76	3,504	38	2,978	28	2,723
Hem/Onc: Oncology (only)	18	4,273	12	2,286	3	*	12	3,352
Infectious Disease	8	*	26	1,048	15	1,292	17	1,001
Internal Medicine: General	547	3,502	700	3,441	465	3,449	474	3,580
Internal Med: Hospitalist	10	2,631	47	2,232	27	472	17	2,111
Internal Med: Pediatric	1	*	17	3,424	17	2,952	7	*
Nephrology	33	4,137	31	2,760	29	1,487	18	1,108
Neurology	67	2,342	113	2,212	35	2,324	44	2,084
OBGYN: General	154	2,968	288	3,123	135	3,696	183	2,813
OBGYN: Gynecology (only)	13	2,034	56	3,330	15	2,892	7	*
OBGYN: Gyn Oncology	2	*	5	*	3	*	1	*
OBGYN: Maternal & Fetal Med	3	*	9	*	1	*	5	*
OBGYN: Repro Endocrinology	4	*	4	*	1	*	2	*
Occupational Medicine	3	*	24	3,205	7	*	15	4,401
Ophthalmology	39	6,460	90	4,946	41	4,744	51	4,433
Ophthalmology: Pediatric	2	*	3	*	0	*	5	*
Ophthalmology: Retina	11	*	19	5,690	8	*	5	*
Orthopedic (Non-surgical)	5	*	7	*	4	*	18	4,598
Orthopedic Surgery: General	59	3,400	181	3,510	73	3,369	97	2,999
Ortho Surg: Foot & Ankle	6	*	11	3,333	8	*	5	*
Ortho Surg: Hand	11	4,323	24	3,578	15	3,749	14	3,935
Ortho Surg: Hip & Joint	14	2,612	27	2,837	7	*	11	1,906
Ortho Surg: Oncology	0	*	*	*	0	*	*	*
Ortho Surg: Pediatric	1	*	11	4,230	2	*	0	*
Ortho Surg: Spine	9	*	34	2,466	7	*	13	2,312
Ortho Surg: Trauma	5	*	3	*	3	*	4	*
Ortho Surg: Sports Med	17	4,008	43	3,839	37	3,629	29	2,760
Otorhinolaryngology	35	3,156	79	3,375	41	3,843	44	2,978
Otorhinolaryngology: Pediatric	0	*	1	*	1	*	*	*
Pathology: Anatomic & Clinical	3	*	6	*	3	*	0	*
Pathology: Anatomic	0	*	3	*	2	*	2	*
Pathology: Clinical	21	*	0	*	2	*	5	*

Table 44: Physician Ambulatory Encounters by Geographic Section (continued)

	Eastern		Midwest		Southern		Western	
	Physicians	Median	Physicians	Median	Physicians	Median	Physicians	Median
Pediatrics: General	256	4,500	475	4,281	209	5,183	241	4,484
Ped: Adolescent Medicine	1	*	33	4,217	9	*	0	*
Ped: Allergy/Immunology	0	*	3	*	1	*	2	*
Ped: Cardiology	5	*	10	1,997	1	*	9	*
Ped: Child Development	0	*	5	*	0	*	3	*
Ped: Critical Care/Intensivist	0	*	4	*	8	*	0	*
Ped: Emergency Medicine	0	*	6	*	*	*	*	*
Ped: Endocrinology	0	*	6	*	1	*	3	*
Ped: Gastroenterology	0	*	4	*	0	*	3	*
Ped: Genetics	3	*	2	*	0	*	5	*
Ped: Hematology/Oncology	0	*	9	*	1	*	6	*
Ped: Hospitalist	0	*	1	*	1	*	0	*
Ped: Infectious Disease	*	*	0	*	0	*	0	*
Ped: Neonatal Medicine	0	*	3	*	3	*	1	*
Ped: Nephrology	0	*	2	*	*	*	3	*
Ped: Neurology	1	*	17	1,797	2	*	3	*
Ped: Pulmonology	0	*	8	*	1	*	1	*
Ped: Rheumatology	0	*	*	*	*	*	2	*
Ped: Sports Medicine	0	*	*	*	*	*	*	*
Physiatry (Phys Med & Rehab)	7	*	50	1,720	5	*	15	1,454
Podiatry: General	5	*	33	3,753	10	3,209	23	3,363
Podiatry: Surg-Foot & Ankle	5	*	11	4,154	2	*	10	4,127
Podiatry: Surg-Forefoot Only	0	*	3	*	0	*	1	*
Psychiatry: General	23	2,260	73	2,216	6	*	27	2,284
Psychiatry: Child & Adolescent	1	*	9	*	5	*	0	*
Psychiatry: Geriatric	3	*	2	*	4	*	0	*
Pulmonary Medicine	31	1,736	46	1,904	36	1,782	31	2,124
Pulmonary Med: Critical Care	9	*	26	1,636	26	1,146	14	1,310
Radiation Oncology	0	*	9	*	16	815	7	*
Radiology: Diagnostic-Inv	15	3,840	17	16,596	12	6,308	35	11,697
Radiology: Diagnostic-Noninv	5	*	23	7,844	36	11,524	30	4,783
Radiology: Nuclear Medicine	3	*	0	*	1	*	11	4,200
Rheumatology	25	3,108	55	3,526	30	3,097	27	3,377
Sleep Medicine	0	*	0	*	1	*	1	*
Surgery: General	79	2,001	195	1,645	115	1,765	87	1,546
Surg: Cardiovascular	8	*	28	620	16	634	18	479
Surg: Cardiovascular-Pediatric	*	*	0	*	1	*	1	*
Surg: Colon and Rectal	7	*	9	*	0	*	1	*
Surg: Neurological	31	1,430	50	1,344	22	1,860	8	*
Surg: Oncology	1	*	5	*	*	*	1	*
Surg: Oral	0	*	7	*	4	*	4	*
Surg: Pediatric	1	*	2	*	2	*	7	*
Surg: Plastic & Reconstruction	7	*	13	2,432	10	1,996	15	1,961
Surg: Plastic & Recon-Hand	1	*	1	*	0	*	*	*
Surg: Plastic & Recon-Pediatric	0	*	*	*	2	*	*	*
Surg: Thoracic (primary)	2	*	5	*	0	*	0	*
Surg: Transplant	2	*	1	*	4	*	1	*
Surg: Trauma	3	*	3	*	5	*	*	*
Surg: Trauma-Burn	1	*	0	*	6	*	1	*
Surg: Vascular (primary)	13	1,667	24	1,572	5	*	9	*
Urgent Care	23	6,613	88	4,554	39	4,954	80	5,199
Urology	38	3,238	72	2,881	47	2,991	43	2,652
Urology: Pediatric	*	*	0	*	0	*	3	*

Table 45: Physician Ambulatory Encounters by Percent of Capitation Revenue

	No capitation		10% or less		11% to 50%		51% or more	
	Physicians	Median	Physicians	Median	Physicians	Median	Physicians	Median
Allergy/Immunology	29	3,062	28	2,645	12	3,831	9	*
Anesthesiology	15	*	17	*	1	*	6	*
Anesth: Pain Management	12	1,468	1	*	1	*	0	*
Anesth: Pediatric	0	*	*	*	0	*	*	*
Cardiology: Electrophysiology	21	1,582	7	*	4	*	1	*
Cardiology: Invasive	143	1,865	56	1,795	16	2,177	4	*
Cardiology: Inv-Intervntnl	183	2,020	71	1,920	19	1,800	3	*
Cardiology: Noninvasive	119	2,143	38	2,574	36	2,099	16	3,182
Critical Care: Intensivist	0	*	1	*	1	*	2	*
Dentistry	2	*	3	*	13	*	0	*
Dermatology	76	5,129	45	5,408	34	5,683	15	4,858
Dermatology: MOHS Surgery	9	*	4	*	0	*	0	*
Emergency Medicine	54	3,428	40	3,248	33	2,417	0	*
Endocrinology/Metabolism	41	2,766	34	3,215	24	2,602	5	*
Family Practice (w/ OB)	366	3,825	272	4,089	195	3,679	4	*
Family Practice (w/o OB)	1,263	4,331	622	4,111	675	4,355	134	4,965
Family Practice: Sports Med	8	*	5	*	1	*	*	*
Gastroenterology	216	1,598	62	1,824	54	1,216	18	1,973
Gastroenterology: Hepatology	40	1,497	0	*	3	*	0	*
Geriatrics	2	*	11	2,210	18	2,106	0	*
Hematology/Oncology	80	3,504	48	3,296	28	2,482	5	*
Hem/Onc: Oncology (only)	33	3,525	2	*	6	*	4	*
Infectious Disease	33	998	17	1,146	14	1,030	2	*
Internal Medicine: General	900	3,462	503	3,517	564	3,431	197	4,136
Internal Med: Hospitalist	54	2,128	25	554	1	*	11	1,936
Internal Med: Pediatric	14	3,447	21	2,906	7	*	0	*
Nephrology	63	2,760	22	1,441	24	2,423	1	*
Neurology	143	2,281	51	2,033	48	2,309	17	1,952
OBGYN: General	377	3,305	152	3,132	162	2,901	68	2,441
OBGYN: Gynecology (only)	64	3,308	14	2,559	8	*	5	*
OBGYN: Gyn Oncology	4	*	3	*	4	*	*	*
OBGYN: Maternal & Fetal Med	8	*	5	*	5	*	*	*
OBGYN: Repro Endocrinology	4	*	3	*	2	*	2	*
Occupational Medicine	25	3,185	10	4,701	11	3,070	3	*
Ophthalmology	129	5,166	34	4,784	34	4,748	24	4,192
Ophthalmology: Pediatric	9	*	0	*	1	*	0	*
Ophthalmology: Retina	40	4,455	0	*	3	*	0	*
Orthopedic (Non-surgical)	21	4,226	5	*	1	*	7	*
Orthopedic Surgery: General	272	3,336	63	3,431	62	3,312	13	3,384
Ortho Surg: Foot & Ankle	25	3,428	2	*	3	*	*	*
Ortho Surg: Hand	48	3,721	8	*	7	*	1	*
Ortho Surg: Hip & Joint	54	2,965	2	*	2	*	1	*
Ortho Surg: Oncology	0	*	*	*	*	*	*	*
Ortho Surg: Pediatric	11	3,496	2	*	1	*	0	*
Ortho Surg: Spine	53	2,543	3	*	5	*	2	*
Ortho Surg: Trauma	14	2,509	*	*	1	*	*	*
Ortho Surg: Sports Med	110	3,479	8	*	4	*	3	*
Otorhinolaryngology	103	3,329	46	3,805	37	2,901	13	3,166
Otorhinolaryngology: Pediatric	2	*	*	*	*	*	*	*
Pathology: Anatomic & Clinical	4	*	8	*	0	*	0	*
Pathology: Anatomic	4	*	0	*	3	*	*	*
Pathology: Clinical	5	*	3	*	20	*	*	*

Table 45: Physician Ambulatory Encounters by Percent of Capitation Revenue (continued)

	No capitation		10% or less		11% to 50%		51% or more	
	Physicians	Median	Physicians	Median	Physicians	Median	Physicians	Median
Pediatrics: General	541	4,549	221	4,208	322	4,555	76	5,177
Ped: Adolescent Medicine	19	4,346	6	*	14	*	*	*
Ped: Allergy/Immunology	1	*	1	*	4	*	*	*
Ped: Cardiology	8	*	14	1,783	3	*	0	*
Ped: Child Development	2	*	4	*	2	*	*	*
Ped: Critical Care/Intensivist	0	*	0	*	4	*	*	*
Ped: Emergency Medicine	6	*	*	*	*	*	*	*
Ped: Endocrinology	4	*	3	*	3	*	*	*
Ped: Gastroenterology	2	*	4	*	1	*	*	*
Ped: Genetics	2	*	8	*	*	*	*	*
Ped: Hematology/Oncology	5	*	8	*	3	*	0	*
Ped: Hospitalist	0	*	0	*	1	*	0	*
Ped: Infectious Disease	*	*	0	*	*	*	*	*
Ped: Neonatal Medicine	4	*	1	*	2	*	0	*
Ped: Nephrology	0	*	4	*	1	*	*	*
Ped: Neurology	12	1,892	7	*	4	*	*	*
Ped: Pulmonology	6	*	1	*	3	*	*	*
Ped: Rheumatology	*	*	2	*	0	*	*	*
Ped: Sports Medicine	0	*	*	*	*	*	*	*
Physiatry (Phys Med & Rehab)	51	1,831	11	1,425	13	1,495	2	*
Podiatry: General	29	3,680	12	3,739	18	3,694	12	3,768
Podiatry: Surg-Foot & Ankle	10	3,742	7	*	5	*	6	*
Podiatry: Surg-Forefoot Only	1	*	3	*	*	*	0	*
Psychiatry: General	49	2,487	24	1,678	40	2,129	16	2,638
Psychiatry: Child & Adolescent	8	*	2	*	4	*	1	*
Psychiatry: Geriatric	4	*	3	*	1	*	*	*
Pulmonary Medicine	71	1,860	33	2,093	30	1,678	10	2,992
Pulmonary Med: Critical Care	54	1,313	12	1,605	9	*	0	*
Radiation Oncology	25	847	2	*	4	*	1	*
Radiology: Diagnostic-Inv	59	8,142	13	16,596	2	*	5	*
Radiology: Diagnostic-Noninv	73	8,843	7	*	9	*	1	*
Radiology: Nuclear Medicine	13	4,200	0	*	1	*	1	*
Rheumatology	63	3,309	46	3,650	20	3,694	7	*
Sleep Medicine	1	*	0	*	1	*	*	*
Surgery: General	260	1,764	117	1,762	73	1,471	23	1,934
Surg: Cardiovascular	41	638	9	*	18	535	2	*
Surg: Cardiovascular-Pediatric	1	*	1	*	0	*	*	*
Surg: Colon and Rectal	8	*	1	*	7	*	0	*
Surg: Neurological	82	1,492	18	1,655	11	1,318	0	*
Surg: Oncology	2	*	*	*	5	*	*	*
Surg: Oral	11	1,650	2	*	2	*	0	*
Surg: Pediatric	4	*	5	*	3	*	*	*
Surg: Plastic & Reconstruction	11	2,378	17	2,242	16	1,942	1	*
Surg: Plastic & Recon-Hand	2	*	*	*	0	*	*	*
Surg: Plastic & Recon-Pediatric	0	*	2	*	*	*	*	*
Surg: Thoracic (primary)	5	*	2	*	0	*	0	*
Surg: Transplant	5	*	1	*	2	*	*	*
Surg: Trauma	5	*	1	*	5	*	*	*
Surg: Trauma-Burn	6	*	1	*	1	*	*	*
Surg: Vascular (primary)	32	1,586	5	*	14	1,405	0	*
Urgent Care	114	5,227	58	4,528	39	5,016	17	5,052
Urology	115	2,850	47	2,830	27	3,099	11	2,464
Urology: Pediatric	1	*	2	*	0	*	*	*

Table 46: Physician Ambulatory Encounters by Years in Specialty

	1 to 2 years		3 to 7 years		8 to 17 years		18 years or more	
	Physicians	Median	Physicians	Median	Physicians	Median	Physicians	Median
Allergy/Immunology	5	*	9	*	26	3,040	28	3,429
Anesthesiology	0	*	2	*	10	1,192	9	*
Anesth: Pain Management	1	*	4	*	6	*	2	*
Anesth: Pediatric	0	*	0	*	0	*	0	*
Cardiology: Electrophysiology	2	*	7	*	19	1,582	5	*
Cardiology: Invasive	7	*	52	1,697	74	1,920	67	1,873
Cardiology: Inv-Intervntnl	7	*	44	1,580	119	1,920	96	2,437
Cardiology: Noninvasive	2	*	34	1,487	51	2,122	97	2,228
Critical Care: Intensivist	0	*	1	*	2	*	1	*
Dentistry	0	*	0	*	6	*	4	*
Dermatology	10	4,992	28	5,710	54	5,036	54	5,123
Dermatology: MOHS Surgery	1	*	3	*	4	*	3	*
Emergency Medicine	11	3,252	39	3,100	47	3,069	22	2,982
Endocrinology/Metabolism	2	*	15	2,425	40	3,416	29	2,856
Family Practice (w/ OB)	82	3,254	228	3,749	266	4,059	187	4,056
Family Practice (w/o OB)	141	3,482	497	4,044	750	4,298	813	4,564
Family Practice: Sports Med	2	*	2	*	8	*	2	*
Gastroenterology	19	1,337	54	1,631	125	1,584	119	1,705
Gastroenterology: Hepatology	1	*	8	*	15	1,486	19	1,576
Geriatrics	1	*	2	*	10	2,240	6	*
Hematology/Oncology	7	*	32	2,656	57	2,933	66	3,545
Hem/Onc: Oncology (only)	0	*	2	*	16	3,445	17	3,532
Infectious Disease	4	*	13	986	21	1,146	18	1,299
Internal Medicine: General	139	2,810	428	3,369	589	3,678	573	3,668
Internal Med: Hospitalist	14	538	25	1,119	30	2,148	21	2,301
Internal Med: Pediatric	10	2,952	12	2,909	9	*	2	*
Nephrology	8	*	18	2,762	28	1,917	36	1,911
Neurology	14	1,905	48	2,220	93	2,285	67	2,382
OBGYN: General	31	2,229	168	3,087	243	3,361	159	3,080
OBGYN: Gynecology (only)	1	*	4	*	26	3,206	58	2,799
OBGYN: Gyn Oncology	0	*	1	*	4	*	2	*
OBGYN: Maternal & Fetal Med	2	*	4	*	8	*	3	*
OBGYN: Repro Endocrinology	0	*	0	*	7	*	1	*
Occupational Medicine	3	*	8	*	13	4,244	17	3,300
Ophthalmology	9	*	39	4,363	78	5,076	58	5,181
Ophthalmology: Pediatric	*	*	3	*	3	*	1	*
Ophthalmology: Retina	2	*	12	5,097	19	4,458	8	*
Orthopedic (Non-surgical)	0	*	6	*	9	*	15	3,479
Orthopedic Surgery: General	19	3,017	63	3,522	118	3,408	167	3,307
Ortho Surg: Foot & Ankle	6	*	9	*	12	3,772	3	*
Ortho Surg: Hand	4	*	15	4,940	28	3,646	16	3,678
Ortho Surg: Hip & Joint	2	*	7	*	27	2,819	21	2,674
Ortho Surg: Oncology	0	*	*	*	0	*	0	*
Ortho Surg: Pediatric	1	*	4	*	6	*	3	*
Ortho Surg: Spine	6	*	10	3,001	29	2,838	17	1,921
Ortho Surg: Trauma	0	*	8	*	3	*	3	*
Ortho Surg: Sports Med	9	*	26	3,621	68	3,472	20	2,691
Otorhinolaryngology	8	*	40	3,203	50	3,631	69	3,299
Otorhinolaryngology: Pediatric	0	*	0	*	1	*	0	*
Pathology: Anatomic & Clinical	1	*	1	*	5	*	5	*
Pathology: Anatomic	*	*	2	*	0	*	5	*
Pathology: Clinical	2	*	1	*	10	4,689	11	5,285

Table 46: Physician Ambulatory Encounters by Years in Specialty (continued)

	1 to 2 years		3 to 7 years		8 to 17 years		18 years or more	
	Physicians	Median	Physicians	Median	Physicians	Median	Physicians	Median
Pediatrics: General	64	3,758	238	4,243	313	4,684	322	4,801
Ped: Adolescent Medicine	3	*	10	4,502	12	4,202	13	4,669
Ped: Allergy/Immunology	*	*	1	*	1	*	4	*
Ped: Cardiology	0	*	6	*	7	*	9	*
Ped: Child Development	0	*	1	*	2	*	1	*
Ped: Critical Care/Intensivist	1	*	2	*	8	*	1	*
Ped: Emergency Medicine	*	*	0	*	4	*	2	*
Ped: Endocrinology	2	*	2	*	1	*	3	*
Ped: Gastroenterology	0	*	3	*	0	*	2	*
Ped: Genetics	1	*	4	*	2	*	3	*
Ped: Hematology/Oncology	0	*	3	*	3	*	7	*
Ped: Hospitalist	0	*	0	*	0	*	0	*
Ped: Infectious Disease	0	*	0	*	0	*	0	*
Ped: Neonatal Medicine	0	*	2	*	1	*	3	*
Ped: Nephrology	*	*	1	*	3	*	0	*
Ped: Neurology	1	*	8	*	7	*	5	*
Ped: Pulmonology	0	*	3	*	7	*	0	*
Ped: Rheumatology	*	*	2	*	0	*	*	*
Ped: Sports Medicine	*	*	*	*	0	*	*	*
Physiatry (Phys Med & Rehab)	8	*	25	1,553	30	1,885	5	*
Podiatry: General	3	*	15	3,302	23	3,363	16	4,521
Podiatry: Surg-Foot & Ankle	0	*	8	*	10	4,369	6	*
Podiatry: Surg-Forefoot Only	0	*	2	*	0	*	1	*
Psychiatry: General	5	*	20	1,653	33	2,295	33	2,208
Psychiatry: Child & Adolescent	1	*	1	*	5	*	3	*
Psychiatry: Geriatric	*	*	0	*	4	*	5	*
Pulmonary Medicine	3	*	16	1,762	50	1,986	53	1,736
Pulmonary Med: Critical Care	5	*	18	1,221	26	1,474	22	1,519
Radiation Oncology	0	*	7	*	15	1,063	8	*
Radiology: Diagnostic-Inv	3	*	13	11,429	30	11,358	31	9,993
Radiology: Diagnostic-Noninv	2	*	19	9,184	30	8,422	30	9,223
Radiology: Nuclear Medicine	0	*	2	*	5	*	8	*
Rheumatology	4	*	17	2,555	45	3,633	49	3,459
Sleep Medicine	0	*	0	*	0	*	1	*
Surgery: General	24	1,231	83	1,690	142	1,837	153	1,798
Surg: Cardiovascular	3	*	10	660	35	619	10	560
Surg: Cardiovascular-Pediatric	0	*	1	*	1	*	*	*
Surg: Colon and Rectal	1	*	3	*	5	*	5	*
Surg: Neurological	8	*	22	1,299	38	1,526	33	1,590
Surg: Oncology	*	*	0	*	2	*	*	*
Surg: Oral	1	*	2	*	4	*	6	*
Surg: Pediatric	3	*	3	*	1	*	5	*
Surg: Plastic & Reconstruction	3	*	11	2,242	12	2,329	13	2,130
Surg: Plastic & Recon-Hand	*	*	0	*	1	*	0	*
Surg: Plastic & Recon-Pediatric	*	*	1	*	1	*	*	*
Surg: Thoracic (primary)	0	*	1	*	3	*	2	*
Surg: Transplant	2	*	1	*	4	*	1	*
Surg: Trauma	2	*	0	*	9	*	0	*
Surg: Trauma-Burn	0	*	1	*	2	*	5	*
Surg: Vascular (primary)	2	*	12	1,462	17	1,684	12	1,200
Urgent Care	11	5,428	51	5,129	72	4,728	52	4,798
Urology	4	*	39	2,556	62	3,085	70	2,882
Urology: Pediatric	*	*	1	*	2	*	*	*

Table 47: Physician Ambulatory Encounters by Gender

	Male			Female		
	Physicians	Medical Practices	Median	Physicians	Medical Practices	Median
Allergy/Immunology	65	41	3,062	10	9	2,049
Anesthesiology	29	5	1,929	6	4	*
Anesth: Pain Management	9	4	*	4	2	*
Anesth: Pediatric	0	*	*	0	*	*
Cardiology: Electrophysiology	28	21	1,655	4	4	*
Cardiology: Invasive	199	62	1,865	14	13	1,610
Cardiology: Inv-Intervntnl	264	70	2,004	7	7	*
Cardiology: Noninvasive	184	72	2,390	23	15	1,561
Critical Care: Intensivist	3	3	*	1	1	*
Dentistry	13	4	2,198	6	4	*
Dermatology	118	69	5,491	44	32	4,431
Dermatology: MOHS Surgery	8	6	*	4	4	*
Emergency Medicine	111	14	3,100	15	6	3,213
Endocrinology/Metabolism	74	54	2,962	25	23	2,632
Family Practice (w/ OB)	598	122	4,091	226	99	3,391
Family Practice (w/o OB)	2,019	342	4,493	523	205	3,724
Family Practice: Sports Med	12	9	5,994	3	3	*
Gastroenterology	314	110	1,618	28	25	1,532
Gastroenterology: Hepatology	40	9	1,444	3	2	*
Geriatrics	20	11	2,140	10	5	2,325
Hematology/Oncology	140	64	3,280	25	20	2,434
Hem/Onc: Oncology (only)	35	16	3,312	8	7	*
Infectious Disease	54	30	1,123	11	8	790
Internal Medicine: General	1,612	272	3,605	482	173	3,151
Internal Med: Hospitalist	53	24	982	17	12	839
Internal Med: Pediatric	28	15	3,548	14	7	2,358
Nephrology	90	43	2,096	18	13	1,842
Neurology	196	81	2,229	56	33	2,332
OBGYN: General	459	148	3,252	286	117	2,881
OBGYN: Gynecology (only)	41	32	2,527	9	8	*
OBGYN: Gyn Oncology	10	6	1,464	1	1	*
OBGYN: Maternal & Fetal Med	14	7	1,996	3	3	*
OBGYN: Repro Endocrinology	7	6	*	4	3	*
Occupational Medicine	32	21	3,300	10	7	4,372
Ophthalmology	188	74	5,076	27	24	4,227
Ophthalmology: Pediatric	9	6	*	0	*	*
Ophthalmology: Retina	41	13	4,451	1	1	*
Orthopedic (Non-surgical)	31	15	4,226	2	2	*
Orthopedic Surgery: General	380	115	3,371	6	5	*
Ortho Surg: Foot & Ankle	28	24	3,417	1	1	*
Ortho Surg: Hand	60	37	3,765	2	2	*
Ortho Surg: Hip & Joint	57	30	2,768	*	*	*
Ortho Surg: Oncology	0	*	*	*	*	*
Ortho Surg: Pediatric	13	12	3,721	1	1	*
Ortho Surg: Spine	62	41	2,576	*	*	*
Ortho Surg: Trauma	14	9	2,509	1	1	*
Ortho Surg: Sports Med	111	54	3,486	7	5	*
Otorhinolaryngology	172	79	3,378	15	13	2,901
Otorhinolaryngology: Pediatric	2	2	*	0	*	*
Pathology: Anatomic & Clinical	6	2	*	6	3	*
Pathology: Anatomic	7	3	*	0	*	*
Pathology: Clinical	17	4	5,163	11	3	4,617

Table 47: Physician Ambulatory Encounters by Gender (continued)

	Male			Female		
	Physicians	Medical Practices	Median	Physicians	Medical Practices	Median
Pediatrics: General	666	184	4,870	481	171	4,151
Ped: Adolescent Medicine	21	5	4,786	8	4	*
Ped: Allergy/Immunology	4	3	*	1	1	*
Ped: Cardiology	23	13	1,736	2	1	*
Ped: Child Development	4	3	*	4	3	*
Ped: Critical Care/Intensivist	9	2	*	3	2	*
Ped: Emergency Medicine	4	1	*	2	1	*
Ped: Endocrinology	7	7	*	3	3	*
Ped: Gastroenterology	7	5	*	0	*	*
Ped: Genetics	3	2	*	7	3	*
Ped: Hematology/Oncology	11	8	1,363	5	4	*
Ped: Hospitalist	2	2	*	0	*	*
Ped: Infectious Disease	0	*	*	0	*	*
Ped: Neonatal Medicine	5	4	*	2	2	*
Ped: Nephrology	4	2	*	0	*	*
Ped: Neurology	17	11	1,781	3	3	*
Ped: Pulmonology	8	4	*	1	1	*
Ped: Rheumatology	2	1	*	0	*	*
Ped: Sports Medicine	*	*	*	0	*	*
Physiatry (Phys Med & Rehab)	52	35	1,787	20	15	1,504
Podiatry: General	58	37	3,707	7	7	*
Podiatry: Surg-Foot & Ankle	27	16	4,142	1	1	*
Podiatry: Surg-Forefoot Only	3	2	*	1	1	*
Psychiatry: General	84	34	2,308	28	16	2,017
Psychiatry: Child & Adolescent	11	6	1,992	3	3	*
Psychiatry: Geriatric	9	5	*	0	*	*
Pulmonary Medicine	120	62	1,803	15	13	1,860
Pulmonary Med: Critical Care	65	25	1,443	6	5	*
Radiation Oncology	27	13	1,339	5	4	*
Radiology: Diagnostic-Inv	69	12	10,271	10	2	*
Radiology: Diagnostic-Noninv	75	15	9,698	15	7	8,506
Radiology: Nuclear Medicine	11	5	4,200	4	3	*
Rheumatology	106	61	3,639	25	20	2,671
Sleep Medicine	2	2	*	0	*	*
Surgery: General	423	141	1,686	34	30	1,521
Surg: Cardiovascular	61	21	517	2	2	*
Surg: Cardiovascular-Pediatric	2	2	*	*	*	*
Surg: Colon and Rectal	15	7	1,563	0	*	*
Surg: Neurological	97	31	1,479	6	5	*
Surg: Oncology	5	3	*	2	1	*
Surg: Oral	12	7	1,800	1	1	*
Surg: Pediatric	10	5	949	2	2	*
Surg: Plastic & Reconstruction	39	25	2,226	5	5	*
Surg: Plastic & Recon-Hand	2	2	*	0	*	*
Surg: Plastic & Recon-Pediatric	2	1	*	*	*	*
Surg: Thoracic (primary)	6	6	*	1	1	*
Surg: Transplant	8	4	*	*	*	*
Surg: Trauma	8	3	*	1	1	*
Surg: Trauma-Burn	8	3	*	0	*	*
Surg: Vascular (primary)	45	26	1,598	4	3	*
Urgent Care	179	54	5,016	47	28	4,613
Urology	185	79	2,862	6	6	*
Urology: Pediatric	3	2	*	0	*	*

　　　MEDICAL GROUP MANAGEMENT ASSOCIATION™

Table 48: Physician Hospital Encounters

	Physicians	Medical Practices	Mean	Std. Dev.	25th %tile	Median	75th %tile	90th %tile
Allergy/Immunology	14	11	171	264	48	65	142	744
Anesthesiology	192	19	480	457	72	384	744	1,002
Anesth: Pain Management	17	7	378	512	95	126	461	1,449
Anesth: Pediatric	15	3	745	574	556	580	664	1,625
Cardiology: Electrophysiology	84	48	1,335	691	860	1,286	1,785	2,414
Cardiology: Invasive	295	77	1,335	690	857	1,210	1,656	2,274
Cardiology: Inv-Intervntnl	417	98	1,505	754	945	1,426	1,990	2,561
Cardiology: Noninvasive	296	94	1,329	760	721	1,283	1,754	2,323
Critical Care: Intensivist	10	7	1,284	561	866	1,162	1,644	2,297
Dentistry	0	*	*	*	*	*	*	*
Dermatology	54	31	109	138	30	53	108	310
Dermatology: MOHS Surgery	5	5	*	*	*	*	*	*
Emergency Medicine	21	6	2,421	1,147	2,307	2,910	3,233	3,348
Endocrinology/Metabolism	95	61	842	732	331	580	1,203	2,032
Family Practice (w/ OB)	825	142	450	356	223	381	569	857
Family Practice (w/o OB)	1,713	283	480	430	193	374	650	975
Family Practice: Sports Med	7	6	*	*	*	*	*	*
Gastroenterology	381	118	854	599	433	747	1,045	1,726
Gastroenterology: Hepatology	56	14	1,075	454	724	966	1,367	1,616
Geriatrics	24	12	508	455	209	305	671	1,342
Hematology/Oncology	210	70	1,055	644	616	981	1,383	1,935
Hem/Onc: Oncology (only)	62	22	901	520	541	794	1,266	1,696
Infectious Disease	48	34	1,664	762	1,084	1,718	2,291	2,807
Internal Medicine: General	1,940	265	802	647	327	649	1,083	1,673
Internal Med: Hospitalist	177	46	1,790	877	1,016	1,818	2,405	3,023
Internal Med: Pediatric	72	25	678	521	279	587	912	1,670
Nephrology	103	47	1,540	837	831	1,401	2,182	2,824
Neurology	273	87	728	677	213	550	986	1,686
OBGYN: General	647	156	247	333	69	135	289	535
OBGYN: Gynecology (only)	33	16	123	102	40	93	206	293
OBGYN: Gyn Oncology	10	6	183	136	106	135	231	463
OBGYN: Maternal & Fetal Med	23	11	895	784	248	803	1,333	2,004
OBGYN: Repro Endocrinology	0	*	*	*	*	*	*	*
Occupational Medicine	3	2	*	*	*	*	*	*
Ophthalmology	57	29	194	208	46	125	269	526
Ophthalmology: Pediatric	7	6	*	*	*	*	*	*
Ophthalmology: Retina	20	9	210	172	54	221	293	386
Orthopedic (Non-surgical)	11	6	151	88	76	132	248	276
Orthopedic Surgery: General	367	112	175	214	62	114	194	389
Ortho Surg: Foot & Ankle	26	22	117	74	66	108	151	189
Ortho Surg: Hand	43	29	78	70	38	60	76	169
Ortho Surg: Hip & Joint	49	27	104	107	53	68	103	204
Ortho Surg: Oncology	2	2	*	*	*	*	*	*
Ortho Surg: Pediatric	10	9	182	148	51	128	310	470
Ortho Surg: Spine	40	31	236	273	82	145	311	606
Ortho Surg: Trauma	14	8	124	88	51	80	225	259
Ortho Surg: Sports Med	86	45	228	376	58	91	180	529
Otorhinolaryngology	165	72	217	403	52	86	167	494
Otorhinolaryngology: Pediatric	2	2	*	*	*	*	*	*
Pathology: Anatomic & Clinical	0	*	*	*	*	*	*	*
Pathology: Anatomic	0	*	*	*	*	*	*	*
Pathology: Clinical	0	*	*	*	*	*	*	*

Table 48: Physician Hospital Encounters (continued)

	Physicians	Medical Practices	Mean	Std. Dev.	25th %tile	Median	75th %tile	90th %tile
Pediatrics: General	1,174	211	384	324	177	325	497	707
Ped: Adolescent Medicine	37	7	364	290	176	262	570	829
Ped: Allergy/Immunology	3	2	*	*	*	*	*	*
Ped: Cardiology	27	11	948	737	533	701	1,236	2,100
Ped: Child Development	0	*	*	*	*	*	*	*
Ped: Critical Care/Intensivist	30	7	1,222	632	700	1,110	1,683	2,224
Ped: Emergency Medicine	0	*	*	*	*	*	*	*
Ped: Endocrinology	10	7	217	177	76	200	294	600
Ped: Gastroenterology	10	4	1,459	710	866	1,670	2,096	2,096
Ped: Genetics	10	4	204	161	119	145	212	603
Ped: Hematology/Oncology	25	11	1,086	365	772	1,084	1,493	1,515
Ped: Hospitalist	17	5	1,504	763	1,138	1,575	2,034	2,689
Ped: Infectious Disease	3	2	*	*	*	*	*	*
Ped: Neonatal Medicine	39	12	1,967	731	1,470	2,224	2,224	3,026
Ped: Nephrology	8	5	*	*	*	*	*	*
Ped: Neurology	22	12	613	543	236	478	955	1,519
Ped: Pulmonology	11	6	1,411	813	616	1,196	2,224	2,813
Ped: Rheumatology	3	2	*	*	*	*	*	*
Ped: Sports Medicine	0	*	*	*	*	*	*	*
Physiatry (Phys Med & Rehab)	46	33	1,050	936	183	843	1,609	2,597
Podiatry: General	27	20	70	62	33	49	90	129
Podiatry: Surg-Foot & Ankle	9	7	*	*	*	*	*	*
Podiatry: Surg-Forefoot Only	4	1	*	*	*	*	*	*
Psychiatry: General	87	30	715	695	221	514	983	1,840
Psychiatry: Child & Adolescent	12	9	815	713	140	737	1,221	2,132
Psychiatry: Geriatric	10	5	1,391	1,141	194	1,503	2,443	3,038
Pulmonary Medicine	126	59	1,763	884	892	1,882	2,453	2,852
Pulmonary Med: Critical Care	98	28	2,013	856	1,294	2,171	2,682	3,102
Radiation Oncology	27	12	313	485	44	94	248	1,263
Radiology: Diagnostic-Inv	0	*	*	*	*	*	*	*
Radiology: Diagnostic-Noninv	0	*	*	*	*	*	*	*
Radiology: Nuclear Medicine	0	*	*	*	*	*	*	*
Rheumatology	126	66	255	318	94	172	312	512
Sleep Medicine	8	2	*	*	*	*	*	*
Surgery: General	466	144	448	406	175	320	569	961
Surg: Cardiovascular	105	28	300	173	197	270	372	472
Surg: Cardiovascular-Pediatric	2	2	*	*	*	*	*	*
Surg: Colon and Rectal	12	7	377	300	167	286	566	992
Surg: Neurological	110	36	457	409	186	357	571	992
Surg: Oncology	5	1	*	*	*	*	*	*
Surg: Oral	6	4	*	*	*	*	*	*
Surg: Pediatric	10	5	438	358	111	467	640	1,136
Surg: Plastic & Reconstruction	22	14	143	135	51	88	186	397
Surg: Plastic & Recon-Hand	7	3	*	*	*	*	*	*
Surg: Plastic & Recon-Pediatric	2	1	*	*	*	*	*	*
Surg: Thoracic (primary)	31	9	360	288	195	244	404	767
Surg: Transplant	8	4	*	*	*	*	*	*
Surg: Trauma	13	4	1,630	972	1,113	1,414	2,256	3,377
Surg: Trauma-Burn	6	2	*	*	*	*	*	*
Surg: Vascular (primary)	61	30	472	379	209	360	676	875
Urgent Care	10	9	185	160	66	132	320	469
Urology	182	71	294	298	112	212	355	564
Urology: Pediatric	4	3	*	*	*	*	*	*

Table 49: Physician Hospital Encounters by Group Type

	Single-specialty			Multispecialty		
	Physicians	Medical Practices	Median	Physicians	Medical Practices	Median
Allergy/Immunology	3	2	*	11	9	86
Anesthesiology	145	8	427	47	11	369
Anesth: Pain Management	15	5	109	2	2	*
Anesth: Pediatric	0	*	*	15	3	580
Cardiology: Electrophysiology	58	32	1,338	26	16	1,244
Cardiology: Invasive	165	41	1,219	130	36	1,172
Cardiology: Inv-Intervntnl	269	57	1,405	148	41	1,454
Cardiology: Noninvasive	177	48	1,359	119	46	1,130
Critical Care: Intensivist	1	1	*	9	6	*
Dentistry	0	*	*	0	*	*
Dermatology	5	2	*	49	29	52
Dermatology: MOHS Surgery	1	1	*	4	4	*
Emergency Medicine	7	1	*	14	5	2,472
Endocrinology/Metabolism	8	6	*	87	55	600
Family Practice (w/ OB)	185	48	455	640	94	354
Family Practice (w/o OB)	376	103	420	1,337	180	361
Family Practice: Sports Med	3	3	*	4	3	*
Gastroenterology	147	21	902	234	97	643
Gastroenterology: Hepatology	40	8	944	16	6	1,170
Geriatrics	0	*	*	24	12	305
Hematology/Oncology	94	20	1,097	116	50	835
Hem/Onc: Oncology (only)	32	4	799	30	18	778
Infectious Disease	7	6	*	41	28	1,749
Internal Medicine: General	149	39	763	1,791	226	640
Internal Med: Hospitalist	6	2	*	171	44	1,824
Internal Med: Pediatric	4	2	*	68	23	636
Nephrology	33	7	2,205	70	40	1,213
Neurology	101	17	796	172	70	492
OBGYN: General	233	55	142	414	101	125
OBGYN: Gynecology (only)	6	4	*	27	12	88
OBGYN: Gyn Oncology	0	*	*	10	6	135
OBGYN: Maternal & Fetal Med	8	3	*	15	8	453
OBGYN: Repro Endocrinology	0	*	*	0	*	*
Occupational Medicine	0	*	*	3	2	*
Ophthalmology	33	9	156	24	20	51
Ophthalmology: Pediatric	5	4	*	2	2	*
Ophthalmology: Retina	18	7	221	2	2	*
Orthopedic (Non-surgical)	1	1	*	10	5	135
Orthopedic Surgery: General	176	50	114	191	62	112
Ortho Surg: Foot & Ankle	20	17	97	6	5	*
Ortho Surg: Hand	32	21	59	11	8	65
Ortho Surg: Hip & Joint	34	19	68	15	8	87
Ortho Surg: Oncology	1	1	*	1	1	*
Ortho Surg: Pediatric	7	6	*	3	3	*
Ortho Surg: Spine	27	21	151	13	10	127
Ortho Surg: Trauma	14	8	80	0	*	*
Ortho Surg: Sports Med	57	30	78	29	15	178
Otorhinolaryngology	53	13	97	112	59	77
Otorhinolaryngology: Pediatric	1	1	*	1	1	*
Pathology: Anatomic & Clinical	0	*	*	0	*	*
Pathology: Anatomic	0	*	*	0	*	*
Pathology: Clinical	0	*	*	0	*	*

Table 49: Physician Hospital Encounters by Group Type (continued)

	Single-specialty			Multispecialty		
	Physicians	Medical Practices	Median	Physicians	Medical Practices	Median
Pediatrics: General	413	64	318	761	147	328
Ped: Adolescent Medicine	4	1	*	33	6	262
Ped: Allergy/Immunology	2	1	*	1	1	*
Ped: Cardiology	14	5	613	13	6	1,022
Ped: Child Development	*	*	*	0	*	*
Ped: Critical Care/Intensivist	20	3	1,209	10	4	1,032
Ped: Emergency Medicine	0	*	*	0	*	*
Ped: Endocrinology	3	2	*	7	5	*
Ped: Gastroenterology	6	2	*	4	2	*
Ped: Genetics	*	*	*	10	4	145
Ped: Hematology/Oncology	11	3	1,191	14	8	942
Ped: Hospitalist	3	1	*	14	4	1,500
Ped: Infectious Disease	2	1	*	1	1	*
Ped: Neonatal Medicine	13	2	*	26	10	1,698
Ped: Nephrology	2	1	*	6	4	*
Ped: Neurology	7	4	*	15	8	577
Ped: Pulmonology	8	3	*	3	3	*
Ped: Rheumatology	1	1	*	2	1	*
Ped: Sports Medicine	*	*	*	0	*	*
Physiatry (Phys Med & Rehab)	14	10	545	32	23	980
Podiatry: General	0	*	*	27	20	49
Podiatry: Surg-Foot & Ankle	2	2	*	7	5	*
Podiatry: Surg-Forefoot Only	0	*	*	4	1	*
Psychiatry: General	6	2	*	81	28	491
Psychiatry: Child & Adolescent	3	1	*	9	8	*
Psychiatry: Geriatric	*	*	*	10	5	1,503
Pulmonary Medicine	29	9	2,273	97	50	1,701
Pulmonary Med: Critical Care	37	7	2,495	61	21	1,749
Radiation Oncology	9	3	*	18	9	84
Radiology: Diagnostic-Inv	0	*	*	0	*	*
Radiology: Diagnostic-Noninv	0	*	*	0	*	*
Radiology: Nuclear Medicine	0	*	*	0	*	*
Rheumatology	26	7	197	100	59	167
Sleep Medicine	4	1	*	4	1	*
Surgery: General	117	26	471	349	118	287
Surg: Cardiovascular	56	13	304	49	15	233
Surg: Cardiovascular-Pediatric	2	2	*	0	*	*
Surg: Colon and Rectal	5	2	*	7	5	*
Surg: Neurological	57	12	375	53	24	295
Surg: Oncology	0	*	*	5	1	*
Surg: Oral	3	1	*	3	3	*
Surg: Pediatric	3	2	*	7	3	*
Surg: Plastic & Reconstruction	5	2	*	17	12	92
Surg: Plastic & Recon-Hand	6	2	*	1	1	*
Surg: Plastic & Recon-Pediatric	2	1	*	0	*	*
Surg: Thoracic (primary)	18	2	*	13	7	417
Surg: Transplant	1	1	*	7	3	*
Surg: Trauma	0	*	*	13	4	1,414
Surg: Trauma-Burn	6	2	*	0	*	*
Surg: Vascular (primary)	16	5	376	45	25	356
Urgent Care	0	*	*	10	9	132
Urology	65	17	256	117	54	175
Urology: Pediatric	2	2	*	2	1	*

MEDICAL GROUP MANAGEMENT ASSOCIATION™

Table 50: Physician Surgery/Anesthesia Cases

	Physicians	Medical Practices	Mean	Std. Dev.	25th %tile	Median	75th %tile	90th %tile
Allergy/Immunology	8	7	*	*	*	*	*	*
Anesthesiology	251	28	970	383	711	900	1,147	1,411
Anesth: Pain Management	16	5	960	684	205	891	1,371	2,063
Anesth: Pediatric	0	*	*	*	*	*	*	*
Cardiology: Electrophysiology	16	13	442	593	162	236	302	1,857
Cardiology: Invasive	45	22	287	505	44	76	257	899
Cardiology: Inv-Intervntnl	101	37	453	811	56	143	362	1,846
Cardiology: Noninvasive	32	18	433	454	122	188	821	1,280
Critical Care: Intensivist	4	3	*	*	*	*	*	*
Dentistry	0	*	*	*	*	*	*	*
Dermatology	54	28	2,156	990	1,532	2,288	3,074	3,354
Dermatology: MOHS Surgery	2	2	*	*	*	*	*	*
Emergency Medicine	19	3	248	150	133	199	334	537
Endocrinology/Metabolism	16	14	586	865	48	107	1,148	2,209
Family Practice (w/ OB)	438	70	429	459	157	273	536	963
Family Practice (w/o OB)	1,097	144	387	445	126	229	422	963
Family Practice: Sports Med	4	4	*	*	*	*	*	*
Gastroenterology	232	71	1,491	577	1,144	1,415	1,772	2,301
Gastroenterology: Hepatology	37	7	1,476	479	1,150	1,331	1,735	2,229
Geriatrics	6	3	*	*	*	*	*	*
Hematology/Oncology	60	29	313	525	54	117	265	1,293
Hem/Onc: Oncology (only)	10	7	1,167	1,305	50	499	2,581	3,075
Infectious Disease	13	11	93	50	56	68	143	170
Internal Medicine: General	762	119	313	490	66	134	269	867
Internal Med: Hospitalist	19	13	301	494	44	65	204	1,230
Internal Med: Pediatric	24	11	290	526	74	134	264	676
Nephrology	21	16	115	126	41	67	109	336
Neurology	54	28	214	199	52	165	289	532
OBGYN: General	498	114	640	568	251	466	797	1,404
OBGYN: Gynecology (only)	39	27	592	699	174	421	606	1,415
OBGYN: Gyn Oncology	6	4	*	*	*	*	*	*
OBGYN: Maternal & Fetal Med	13	7	452	540	70	198	769	1,556
OBGYN: Repro Endocrinology	1	1	*	*	*	*	*	*
Occupational Medicine	14	9	304	274	95	190	545	778
Ophthalmology	145	50	576	348	335	504	758	1,036
Ophthalmology: Pediatric	8	5	*	*	*	*	*	*
Ophthalmology: Retina	31	11	269	295	138	175	248	669
Orthopedic (Non-surgical)	17	8	682	365	429	605	825	1,294
Orthopedic Surgery: General	281	85	830	601	441	686	1,045	1,477
Ortho Surg: Foot & Ankle	27	24	766	551	390	612	882	1,514
Ortho Surg: Hand	54	32	785	527	444	591	943	1,498
Ortho Surg: Hip & Joint	48	27	672	371	352	559	1,005	1,302
Ortho Surg: Oncology	0	*	*	*	*	*	*	*
Ortho Surg: Pediatric	11	10	706	457	352	689	928	1,656
Ortho Surg: Spine	52	32	540	388	226	443	740	1,125
Ortho Surg: Trauma	14	9	551	241	369	450	744	984
Ortho Surg: Sports Med	109	47	656	504	308	468	925	1,415
Otorhinolaryngology	127	51	959	629	446	855	1,339	1,867
Otorhinolaryngology: Pediatric	1	1	*	*	*	*	*	*
Pathology: Anatomic & Clinical	0	*	*	*	*	*	*	*
Pathology: Anatomic	0	*	*	*	*	*	*	*
Pathology: Clinical	0	*	*	*	*	*	*	*

Table 50: Physician Surgery/Anesthesia Cases (continued)

	Physicians	Medical Practices	Mean	Std. Dev.	25th %tile	Median	75th %tile	90th %tile
Pediatrics: General	469	93	230	404	58	108	195	478
Ped: Adolescent Medicine	10	2	*	*	*	*	*	*
Ped: Allergy/Immunology	0	*	*	*	*	*	*	*
Ped: Cardiology	8	4	*	*	*	*	*	*
Ped: Child Development	0	*	*	*	*	*	*	*
Ped: Critical Care/Intensivist	12	2	*	*	*	*	*	*
Ped: Emergency Medicine	0	*	*	*	*	*	*	*
Ped: Endocrinology	0	*	*	*	*	*	*	*
Ped: Gastroenterology	3	3	*	*	*	*	*	*
Ped: Genetics	5	2	*	*	*	*	*	*
Ped: Hematology/Oncology	3	2	*	*	*	*	*	*
Ped: Hospitalist	1	1	*	*	*	*	*	*
Ped: Infectious Disease	0	*	*	*	*	*	*	*
Ped: Neonatal Medicine	6	6	*	*	*	*	*	*
Ped: Nephrology	0	*	*	*	*	*	*	*
Ped: Neurology	1	1	*	*	*	*	*	*
Ped: Pulmonology	5	1	*	*	*	*	*	*
Ped: Rheumatology	0	*	*	*	*	*	*	*
Ped: Sports Medicine	0	*	*	*	*	*	*	*
Physiatry (Phys Med & Rehab)	15	13	487	484	77	329	803	1,377
Podiatry: General	33	23	1,686	1,045	887	1,746	2,576	3,132
Podiatry: Surg-Foot & Ankle	18	9	1,866	722	1,282	1,835	2,383	2,963
Podiatry: Surg-Forefoot Only	3	2	*	*	*	*	*	*
Psychiatry: General	4	3	*	*	*	*	*	*
Psychiatry: Child & Adolescent	1	1	*	*	*	*	*	*
Psychiatry: Geriatric	4	3	*	*	*	*	*	*
Pulmonary Medicine	66	35	250	206	115	196	318	513
Pulmonary Med: Critical Care	41	18	189	146	80	137	282	442
Radiation Oncology	10	5	825	751	72	587	1,648	1,796
Radiology: Diagnostic-Inv	0	*	*	*	*	*	*	*
Radiology: Diagnostic-Noninv	0	*	*	*	*	*	*	*
Radiology: Nuclear Medicine	0	*	*	*	*	*	*	*
Rheumatology	66	33	559	551	262	399	605	1,354
Sleep Medicine	0	*	*	*	*	*	*	*
Surgery: General	303	101	823	427	535	769	1,048	1,331
Surg: Cardiovascular	69	19	348	150	239	308	424	601
Surg: Cardiovascular-Pediatric	3	3	*	*	*	*	*	*
Surg: Colon and Rectal	15	7	695	579	216	416	962	1,699
Surg: Neurological	85	23	513	450	246	355	594	1,054
Surg: Oncology	4	2	*	*	*	*	*	*
Surg: Oral	8	3	*	*	*	*	*	*
Surg: Pediatric	5	3	*	*	*	*	*	*
Surg: Plastic & Reconstruction	30	14	988	572	444	997	1,265	1,860
Surg: Plastic & Recon-Hand	8	2	*	*	*	*	*	*
Surg: Plastic & Recon-Pediatric	4	2	*	*	*	*	*	*
Surg: Thoracic (primary)	24	6	356	323	212	273	378	749
Surg: Transplant	4	1	*	*	*	*	*	*
Surg: Trauma	5	1	*	*	*	*	*	*
Surg: Trauma-Burn	8	3	*	*	*	*	*	*
Surg: Vascular (primary)	39	20	540	349	268	470	673	1,072
Urgent Care	106	31	402	315	179	284	526	986
Urology	138	54	969	701	496	876	1,276	1,831
Urology: Pediatric	1	1	*	*	*	*	*	*

Table 51: Physician Surgery/Anesthesia Cases by Group Type

	Single-specialty			Multispecialty		
	Physicians	Medical Practices	Median	Physicians	Medical Practices	Median
Allergy/Immunology	0	*	*	8	7	*
Anesthesiology	171	13	900	80	15	899
Anesth: Pain Management	11	4	1,232	5	1	*
Anesth: Pediatric	0	*	*	0	*	*
Cardiology: Electrophysiology	9	7	*	7	6	*
Cardiology: Invasive	18	11	64	27	11	78
Cardiology: Inv-Intervntnl	59	19	114	42	18	247
Cardiology: Noninvasive	10	4	158	22	14	370
Critical Care: Intensivist	0	*	*	4	3	*
Dentistry	0	*	*	0	*	*
Dermatology	4	2	*	50	26	2,231
Dermatology: MOHS Surgery	0	*	*	2	2	*
Emergency Medicine	0	*	*	19	3	199
Endocrinology/Metabolism	1	1	*	15	13	103
Family Practice (w/ OB)	58	18	295	380	52	270
Family Practice (w/o OB)	190	47	275	907	97	226
Family Practice: Sports Med	3	3	*	1	1	*
Gastroenterology	108	16	1,425	124	55	1,401
Gastroenterology: Hepatology	36	6	1,349	1	1	*
Geriatrics	0	*	*	6	3	*
Hematology/Oncology	9	4	*	51	25	138
Hem/Onc: Oncology (only)	0	*	*	10	7	499
Infectious Disease	3	3	*	10	8	68
Internal Medicine: General	63	19	130	699	100	134
Internal Med: Hospitalist	0	*	*	19	13	65
Internal Med: Pediatric	3	1	*	21	10	131
Nephrology	0	*	*	21	16	67
Neurology	4	1	*	50	27	167
OBGYN: General	174	39	313	324	75	564
OBGYN: Gynecology (only)	10	6	146	29	21	450
OBGYN: Gyn Oncology	0	*	*	6	4	*
OBGYN: Maternal & Fetal Med	7	3	*	6	4	*
OBGYN: Repro Endocrinology	1	1	*	0	*	*
Occupational Medicine	4	1	*	10	8	141
Ophthalmology	58	11	540	87	39	458
Ophthalmology: Pediatric	7	4	*	1	1	*
Ophthalmology: Retina	28	8	163	3	3	*
Orthopedic (Non-surgical)	10	2	*	7	6	*
Orthopedic Surgery: General	147	39	573	134	46	818
Ortho Surg: Foot & Ankle	20	19	596	7	5	*
Ortho Surg: Hand	38	24	571	16	8	703
Ortho Surg: Hip & Joint	29	19	478	19	8	770
Ortho Surg: Oncology	0	*	*	0	*	*
Ortho Surg: Pediatric	7	6	*	4	4	*
Ortho Surg: Spine	37	22	354	15	10	478
Ortho Surg: Trauma	13	8	452	1	1	*
Ortho Surg: Sports Med	85	35	487	24	12	312
Otorhinolaryngology	42	10	466	85	41	959
Otorhinolaryngology: Pediatric	1	1	*	0	*	*
Pathology: Anatomic & Clinical	0	*	*	0	*	*
Pathology: Anatomic	0	*	*	0	*	*
Pathology: Clinical	0	*	*	0	*	*

Table 51: Physician Surgery/Anesthesia Cases by Group Type (continued)

	Single-specialty			Multispecialty		
	Physicians	Medical Practices	Median	Physicians	Medical Practices	Median
Pediatrics: General	91	23	98	378	70	111
Ped: Adolescent Medicine	4	1	*	6	1	*
Ped: Allergy/Immunology	0	*	*	0	*	*
Ped: Cardiology	5	3	*	3	1	*
Ped: Child Development	*	*	*	0	*	*
Ped: Critical Care/Intensivist	8	1	*	4	1	*
Ped: Emergency Medicine	0	*	*	0	*	*
Ped: Endocrinology	0	*	*	0	*	*
Ped: Gastroenterology	1	1	*	2	2	*
Ped: Genetics	*	*	*	5	2	*
Ped: Hematology/Oncology	2	1	*	1	1	*
Ped: Hospitalist	0	*	*	1	1	*
Ped: Infectious Disease	0	*	*	0	*	*
Ped: Neonatal Medicine	2	2	*	4	4	*
Ped: Nephrology	0	*	*	0	*	*
Ped: Neurology	1	1	*	0	*	*
Ped: Pulmonology	5	1	*	0	*	*
Ped: Rheumatology	0	*	*	0	*	*
Ped: Sports Medicine	*	*	*	0	*	*
Physiatry (Phys Med & Rehab)	5	5	*	10	8	269
Podiatry: General	1	1	*	32	22	1,782
Podiatry: Surg-Foot & Ankle	5	3	*	13	6	1,940
Podiatry: Surg-Forefoot Only	1	1	*	2	1	*
Psychiatry: General	0	*	*	4	3	*
Psychiatry: Child & Adolescent	0	*	*	1	1	*
Psychiatry: Geriatric	*	*	*	4	3	*
Pulmonary Medicine	2	2	*	64	33	201
Pulmonary Med: Critical Care	13	4	137	28	14	139
Radiation Oncology	7	2	*	3	3	*
Radiology: Diagnostic-Inv	0	*	*	0	*	*
Radiology: Diagnostic-Noninv	0	*	*	0	*	*
Radiology: Nuclear Medicine	0	*	*	0	*	*
Rheumatology	15	3	538	51	30	351
Sleep Medicine	0	*	*	0	*	*
Surgery: General	75	19	783	228	82	764
Surg: Cardiovascular	47	11	325	22	8	275
Surg: Cardiovascular-Pediatric	2	2	*	1	1	*
Surg: Colon and Rectal	6	2	*	9	5	*
Surg: Neurological	51	10	373	34	13	309
Surg: Oncology	0	*	*	4	2	*
Surg: Oral	7	2	*	1	1	*
Surg: Pediatric	3	2	*	2	1	*
Surg: Plastic & Reconstruction	10	4	845	20	10	1,076
Surg: Plastic & Recon-Hand	8	2	*	0	*	*
Surg: Plastic & Recon-Pediatric	2	1	*	2	1	*
Surg: Thoracic (primary)	19	2	*	5	4	*
Surg: Transplant	4	1	*	0	*	*
Surg: Trauma	0	*	*	5	1	*
Surg: Trauma-Burn	7	2	*	1	1	*
Surg: Vascular (primary)	7	2	*	32	18	494
Urgent Care	3	1	*	103	30	288
Urology	58	14	836	80	40	931
Urology: Pediatric	1	1	*	0	*	*

MEDICAL GROUP MANAGEMENT ASSOCIATION™

Table 52: Total RVUs (CMS RBRVS Method)

	Physicians	Medical Practices	Mean	Std. Dev.	25th %tile	Median	75th %tile	90th %tile
Allergy/Immunology	47	29	12,977	5,960	8,091	11,711	17,056	20,668
Anesthesiology	170	17	11,689	4,223	8,895	11,274	13,149	16,930
Anesth: Pain Management	8	4	*	*	*	*	*	*
Anesth: Pediatric	0	*	*	*	*	*	*	*
Cardiology: Electrophysiology	20	16	16,049	5,534	11,577	16,642	20,713	22,340
Cardiology: Invasive	129	39	16,712	6,695	10,677	15,962	22,230	26,280
Cardiology: Inv-Intervntnl	154	43	17,419	5,580	13,369	16,455	21,761	25,329
Cardiology: Noninvasive	118	46	14,558	6,521	10,042	14,171	18,889	24,219
Critical Care: Intensivist	5	4	*	*	*	*	*	*
Dentistry	2	1	*	*	*	*	*	*
Dermatology	91	44	14,435	5,660	10,249	13,596	18,578	22,228
Dermatology: MOHS Surgery	3	2	*	*	*	*	*	*
Emergency Medicine	46	9	6,845	1,998	5,513	6,632	8,207	9,388
Endocrinology/Metabolism	54	35	7,876	2,874	5,698	7,326	9,114	12,840
Family Practice (w/ OB)	456	66	8,266	2,348	6,542	8,039	9,735	11,428
Family Practice (w/o OB)	1,039	126	7,907	2,437	6,195	7,749	9,341	11,095
Family Practice: Sports Med	7	6	*	*	*	*	*	*
Gastroenterology	199	58	16,675	5,336	13,505	16,320	20,045	23,563
Gastroenterology: Hepatology	21	4	15,171	3,662	12,206	14,752	18,184	20,367
Geriatrics	13	7	5,003	1,172	4,314	4,816	5,423	7,250
Hematology/Oncology	104	33	10,216	3,391	7,706	9,688	12,350	14,700
Hem/Onc: Oncology (only)	25	8	10,180	5,709	6,479	8,005	11,942	21,814
Infectious Disease	42	23	8,643	4,292	5,766	7,111	10,783	14,466
Internal Medicine: General	1,068	121	7,679	2,438	5,912	7,519	9,099	10,987
Internal Med: Hospitalist	109	22	6,604	2,442	4,579	6,187	8,312	10,061
Internal Med: Pediatric	24	9	7,400	2,684	5,571	7,358	9,933	10,596
Nephrology	55	23	13,347	6,334	8,495	11,244	17,454	24,052
Neurology	124	42	9,275	3,976	6,669	8,379	10,929	14,176
OBGYN: General	363	67	12,328	4,003	9,421	12,175	14,438	18,122
OBGYN: Gynecology (only)	24	19	8,290	3,887	5,922	7,090	9,913	14,166
OBGYN: Gyn Oncology	5	4	*	*	*	*	*	*
OBGYN: Maternal & Fetal Med	10	4	15,885	7,159	9,204	15,872	22,979	24,764
OBGYN: Repro Endocrinology	3	2	*	*	*	*	*	*
Occupational Medicine	13	8	6,244	1,569	5,323	6,004	7,590	8,713
Ophthalmology	93	32	17,004	4,903	12,928	17,945	20,040	22,776
Ophthalmology: Pediatric	4	2	*	*	*	*	*	*
Ophthalmology: Retina	14	5	21,861	6,396	17,571	22,538	27,717	28,605
Orthopedic (Non-surgical)	12	7	17,696	5,805	11,868	20,083	21,624	24,688
Orthopedic Surgery: General	231	61	16,081	4,971	12,385	15,699	19,248	22,987
Ortho Surg: Foot & Ankle	18	15	18,663	5,558	13,833	18,308	22,482	26,700
Ortho Surg: Hand	32	23	16,533	5,150	12,366	15,299	19,892	26,046
Ortho Surg: Hip & Joint	29	15	14,915	4,303	12,132	14,607	16,676	20,701
Ortho Surg: Oncology	0	*	*	*	*	*	*	*
Ortho Surg: Pediatric	6	5	*	*	*	*	*	*
Ortho Surg: Spine	27	19	17,338	5,445	13,555	17,102	20,807	25,376
Ortho Surg: Trauma	6	4	*	*	*	*	*	*
Ortho Surg: Sports Med	58	23	15,660	5,807	12,061	15,230	19,770	23,461
Otorhinolaryngology	90	39	13,231	4,765	9,757	12,556	16,531	20,106
Otorhinolaryngology: Pediatric	1	1	*	*	*	*	*	*
Pathology: Anatomic & Clinical	21	7	11,716	6,539	5,888	12,232	18,248	19,124
Pathology: Anatomic	5	2	*	*	*	*	*	*
Pathology: Clinical	13	3	8,344	2,333	7,141	8,171	9,868	11,925

*Please note that the Total RVU information provided by the Anesthesiology practices are ASA units. Anesthesiology practices are not represented in Physician Work RVU tables.

Table 52: Total RVUs (CMS RBRVS Method) (continued)

	Physicians	Medical Practices	Mean	Std. Dev.	25th %tile	Median	75th %tile	90th %tile
Pediatrics: General	515	85	8,556	2,741	6,648	8,125	10,525	12,464
Ped: Adolescent Medicine	1	1	*	*	*	*	*	*
Ped: Allergy/Immunology	3	2	*	*	*	*	*	*
Ped: Cardiology	16	5	7,856	2,604	5,795	7,379	10,637	11,427
Ped: Child Development	5	1	*	*	*	*	*	*
Ped: Critical Care/Intensivist	14	4	7,659	1,997	5,988	7,409	8,944	11,324
Ped: Emergency Medicine	0	*	*	*	*	*	*	*
Ped: Endocrinology	3	3	*	*	*	*	*	*
Ped: Gastroenterology	9	4	*	*	*	*	*	*
Ped: Genetics	5	3	*	*	*	*	*	*
Ped: Hematology/Oncology	10	6	7,434	4,063	4,384	6,459	9,433	15,575
Ped: Hospitalist	6	3	*	*	*	*	*	*
Ped: Infectious Disease	2	1	*	*	*	*	*	*
Ped: Neonatal Medicine	27	5	10,702	3,178	6,455	12,295	12,295	13,450
Ped: Nephrology	4	2	*	*	*	*	*	*
Ped: Neurology	10	5	9,029	5,895	3,906	7,574	12,259	20,705
Ped: Pulmonology	8	4	*	*	*	*	*	*
Ped: Rheumatology	1	1	*	*	*	*	*	*
Ped: Sports Medicine	0	*	*	*	*	*	*	*
Physiatry (Phys Med & Rehab)	47	23	10,504	5,531	6,052	8,694	14,808	17,796
Podiatry: General	42	23	10,067	4,092	7,439	9,717	11,276	16,257
Podiatry: Surg-Foot & Ankle	18	9	10,254	2,819	7,731	9,927	12,514	13,535
Podiatry: Surg-Forefoot Only	3	2	*	*	*	*	*	*
Psychiatry: General	63	20	5,779	2,634	4,003	5,003	6,462	9,836
Psychiatry: Child & Adolescent	7	5	*	*	*	*	*	*
Psychiatry: Geriatric	5	2	*	*	*	*	*	*
Pulmonary Medicine	85	34	10,609	5,052	6,926	9,512	13,181	17,344
Pulmonary Med: Critical Care	29	13	10,378	3,726	7,571	10,763	12,641	13,833
Radiation Oncology	21	7	16,070	4,597	12,027	15,782	19,467	23,498
Radiology: Diagnostic-Inv	71	14	15,099	4,774	11,195	16,050	18,223	21,046
Radiology: Diagnostic-Noninv	80	17	13,617	5,625	9,490	12,981	16,501	22,015
Radiology: Nuclear Medicine	18	8	13,499	4,879	9,553	15,375	15,375	16,499
Rheumatology	67	37	9,174	4,079	5,870	9,147	11,068	14,040
Sleep Medicine	2	2	*	*	*	*	*	*
Surgery: General	237	65	12,725	3,812	10,177	12,054	14,885	18,160
Surg: Cardiovascular	44	16	15,679	5,558	10,937	14,544	20,764	23,560
Surg: Cardiovascular-Pediatric	2	2	*	*	*	*	*	*
Surg: Colon and Rectal	5	4	*	*	*	*	*	*
Surg: Neurological	62	18	15,487	4,807	12,275	15,224	18,147	21,917
Surg: Oncology	1	1	*	*	*	*	*	*
Surg: Oral	4	2	*	*	*	*	*	*
Surg: Pediatric	8	4	*	*	*	*	*	*
Surg: Plastic & Reconstruction	31	16	12,739	3,852	10,531	12,502	14,854	18,495
Surg: Plastic & Recon-Hand	0	*	*	*	*	*	*	*
Surg: Plastic & Recon-Pediatric	2	1	*	*	*	*	*	*
Surg: Thoracic (primary)	17	2	*	*	*	*	*	*
Surg: Transplant	5	2	*	*	*	*	*	*
Surg: Trauma	8	2	*	*	*	*	*	*
Surg: Trauma-Burn	7	2	*	*	*	*	*	*
Surg: Vascular (primary)	28	12	12,114	3,777	9,133	12,764	14,719	16,483
Urgent Care	127	36	8,685	2,941	6,437	8,730	10,987	12,134
Urology	87	36	14,198	5,273	11,226	13,980	17,420	20,983
Urology: Pediatric	12	3	8,558	3,496	6,887	7,321	8,938	16,444

Table 53: Total RVU (CMS RBRVS Method) by Group Type

	Single-specialty			Multispecialty		
	Physicians	Medical Practices	Median	Physicians	Medical Practices	Median
Allergy/Immunology	5	2	*	42	27	11,675
Anesthesiology	127	9	12,192	43	8	8,895
Anesth: Pain Management	6	2	*	2	2	*
Anesth: Pediatric	0	*	*	0	*	*
Cardiology: Electrophysiology	12	9	20,425	8	7	*
Cardiology: Invasive	70	18	17,215	59	21	14,275
Cardiology: Inv-Intervntnl	119	29	16,551	35	14	16,192
Cardiology: Noninvasive	69	23	14,443	49	23	12,318
Critical Care: Intensivist	0	*	*	5	4	*
Dentistry	0	*	*	2	1	*
Dermatology	5	2	*	86	42	13,396
Dermatology: MOHS Surgery	2	1	*	1	1	*
Emergency Medicine	0	*	*	46	9	6,632
Endocrinology/Metabolism	2	2	*	52	33	7,369
Family Practice (w/ OB)	81	18	7,103	375	48	8,302
Family Practice (w/o OB)	121	37	7,450	918	89	7,785
Family Practice: Sports Med	3	3	*	4	3	*
Gastroenterology	83	8	17,102	116	50	15,350
Gastroenterology: Hepatology	18	3	14,988	3	1	*
Geriatrics	0	*	*	13	7	4,816
Hematology/Oncology	39	7	10,427	65	26	9,620
Hem/Onc: Oncology (only)	11	2	*	14	6	9,103
Infectious Disease	15	6	8,327	27	17	6,825
Internal Medicine: General	78	16	6,509	990	105	7,556
Internal Med: Hospitalist	0	*	*	109	22	6,187
Internal Med: Pediatric	0	*	*	24	9	7,358
Nephrology	18	4	17,359	37	19	10,029
Neurology	35	6	9,309	89	36	8,269
OBGYN: General	61	6	12,216	302	61	12,050
OBGYN: Gynecology (only)	4	3	*	20	16	6,775
OBGYN: Gyn Oncology	0	*	*	5	4	*
OBGYN: Maternal & Fetal Med	3	1	*	7	3	*
OBGYN: Repro Endocrinology	1	1	*	2	1	*
Occupational Medicine	0	*	*	13	8	6,004
Ophthalmology	20	2	*	73	30	17,776
Ophthalmology: Pediatric	3	1	*	1	1	*
Ophthalmology: Retina	11	2	*	3	3	*
Orthopedic (Non-surgical)	0	*	*	12	7	20,083
Orthopedic Surgery: General	121	28	16,350	110	33	15,017
Ortho Surg: Foot & Ankle	14	12	17,992	4	3	*
Ortho Surg: Hand	24	17	15,725	8	6	*
Ortho Surg: Hip & Joint	22	11	14,415	7	4	*
Ortho Surg: Oncology	0	*	*	0	*	*
Ortho Surg: Pediatric	5	4	*	1	1	*
Ortho Surg: Spine	16	12	16,704	11	7	17,149
Ortho Surg: Trauma	5	3	*	1	1	*
Ortho Surg: Sports Med	45	16	16,149	13	7	13,083
Otorhinolaryngology	5	2	*	85	37	12,528
Otorhinolaryngology: Pediatric	0	*	*	1	1	*
Pathology: Anatomic & Clinical	0	*	*	21	7	12,232
Pathology: Anatomic	0	*	*	5	2	*
Pathology: Clinical	5	1	*	8	2	*

*Please note that the Total RVU conformation provided by the Anesthesiology practices are ASA units. Anesthesiology practices are not represented in Physician Work RVU tables.

Table 53: Total RVU (CMS RBRVS Method) by Group Type (continued)

	Single-specialty			Multispecialty		
	Physicians	Medical Practices	Median	Physicians	Medical Practices	Median
Pediatrics: General	94	15	9,029	421	70	8,012
Ped: Adolescent Medicine	0	*	*	1	1	*
Ped: Allergy/Immunology	2	1	*	1	1	*
Ped: Cardiology	5	1	*	11	4	7,165
Ped: Child Development	*	*	*	5	1	*
Ped: Critical Care/Intensivist	9	2	*	5	2	*
Ped: Emergency Medicine	0	*	*	0	*	*
Ped: Endocrinology	1	1	*	2	2	*
Ped: Gastroenterology	4	1	*	5	3	*
Ped: Genetics	*	*	*	5	3	*
Ped: Hematology/Oncology	2	1	*	8	5	*
Ped: Hospitalist	0	*	*	6	3	*
Ped: Infectious Disease	0	*	*	2	1	*
Ped: Neonatal Medicine	16	2	*	11	3	11,444
Ped: Nephrology	0	*	*	4	2	*
Ped: Neurology	4	2	*	6	3	*
Ped: Pulmonology	6	2	*	2	2	*
Ped: Rheumatology	0	*	*	1	1	*
Ped: Sports Medicine	*	*	*	0	*	*
Physiatry (Phys Med & Rehab)	14	6	16,237	33	17	7,785
Podiatry: General	0	*	*	42	23	9,717
Podiatry: Surg-Foot & Ankle	2	1	*	16	8	10,182
Podiatry: Surg-Forefoot Only	1	1	*	2	1	*
Psychiatry: General	0	*	*	63	20	5,003
Psychiatry: Child & Adolescent	0	*	*	7	5	*
Psychiatry: Geriatric	*	*	*	5	2	*
Pulmonary Medicine	6	3	*	79	31	9,607
Pulmonary Med: Critical Care	4	2	*	25	11	11,532
Radiation Oncology	12	2	*	9	5	*
Radiology: Diagnostic-Inv	48	7	16,429	23	7	13,093
Radiology: Diagnostic-Noninv	38	7	12,886	42	10	13,246
Radiology: Nuclear Medicine	13	4	15,375	5	4	*
Rheumatology	15	4	6,044	52	33	9,489
Sleep Medicine	0	*	*	2	2	*
Surgery: General	45	10	12,149	192	55	12,049
Surg: Cardiovascular	12	4	21,720	32	12	12,463
Surg: Cardiovascular-Pediatric	2	2	*	0	*	*
Surg: Colon and Rectal	1	1	*	4	3	*
Surg: Neurological	28	6	16,546	34	12	13,796
Surg: Oncology	0	*	*	1	1	*
Surg: Oral	3	1	*	1	1	*
Surg: Pediatric	1	1	*	7	3	*
Surg: Plastic & Reconstruction	9	3	*	22	13	12,025
Surg: Plastic & Recon-Hand	0	*	*	0	*	*
Surg: Plastic & Recon-Pediatric	2	1	*	0	*	*
Surg: Thoracic (primary)	16	1	*	1	1	*
Surg: Transplant	4	1	*	1	1	*
Surg: Trauma	0	*	*	8	2	*
Surg: Trauma-Burn	7	2	*	0	*	*
Surg: Vascular (primary)	4	2	*	24	10	13,152
Urgent Care	3	1	*	124	35	8,890
Urology	15	3	12,270	72	33	14,310
Urology: Pediatric	1	1	*	11	2	*

Table 54: Total RVUs (CMS RBRVS Method) by Hospital Ownership

	Hospital Owned			Non-hospital Owned		
	Physicians	Medical Practices	Median	Physicians	Medical Practices	Median
Allergy/Immunology	9	7	*	38	22	11,675
Anesthesiology	15	3	9,961	155	14	11,395
Anesth: Pain Management	2	2	*	6	2	*
Anesth: Pediatric	*	*	*	0	*	*
Cardiology: Electrophysiology	1	1	*	19	15	15,571
Cardiology: Invasive	25	7	15,542	104	32	16,232
Cardiology: Inv-Intervntnl	15	4	19,928	139	39	16,192
Cardiology: Noninvasive	12	5	13,138	106	41	14,207
Critical Care: Intensivist	4	3	*	1	1	*
Dentistry	0	*	*	2	1	*
Dermatology	21	12	12,439	70	32	14,870
Dermatology: MOHS Surgery	0	*	*	3	2	*
Emergency Medicine	22	4	6,847	24	5	5,901
Endocrinology/Metabolism	19	11	7,289	35	24	7,374
Family Practice (w/ OB)	168	24	7,593	288	42	8,292
Family Practice (w/o OB)	419	49	7,074	614	76	8,191
Family Practice: Sports Med	4	3	*	3	3	*
Gastroenterology	19	12	15,240	180	46	16,588
Gastroenterology: Hepatology	*	*	*	21	4	14,752
Geriatrics	7	3	*	6	4	*
Hematology/Oncology	17	6	8,497	87	27	10,475
Hem/Onc: Oncology (only)	1	1	*	24	7	7,749
Infectious Disease	12	8	6,226	30	15	8,202
Internal Medicine: General	327	41	7,214	741	80	7,609
Internal Med: Hospitalist	55	11	5,613	54	11	8,028
Internal Med: Pediatric	9	4	*	15	5	7,486
Nephrology	12	5	8,929	43	18	12,857
Neurology	23	11	8,269	101	31	8,494
OBGYN: General	90	23	10,511	273	44	12,427
OBGYN: Gynecology (only)	6	5	*	18	14	7,875
OBGYN: Gyn Oncology	3	2	*	2	2	*
OBGYN: Maternal & Fetal Med	7	2	*	3	2	*
OBGYN: Repro Endocrinology	2	1	*	1	1	*
Occupational Medicine	1	1	*	12	7	6,059
Ophthalmology	17	9	15,362	76	23	18,227
Ophthalmology: Pediatric	0	*	*	4	2	*
Ophthalmology: Retina	1	1	*	13	4	20,308
Orthopedic (Non-surgical)	4	3	*	8	4	*
Orthopedic Surgery: General	21	8	14,861	210	53	15,778
Ortho Surg: Foot & Ankle	*	*	*	18	15	18,308
Ortho Surg: Hand	1	1	*	31	22	15,723
Ortho Surg: Hip & Joint	0	*	*	29	15	14,607
Ortho Surg: Oncology	*	*	*	0	*	*
Ortho Surg: Pediatric	0	*	*	6	5	*
Ortho Surg: Spine	1	1	*	26	18	16,916
Ortho Surg: Trauma	0	*	*	4	3	*
Ortho Surg: Sports Med	6	4	*	48	18	15,203
Otorhinolaryngology	19	9	13,875	71	30	11,801
Otorhinolaryngology: Pediatric	*	*	*	1	1	*
Pathology: Anatomic & Clinical	11	3	5,888	10	4	16,765
Pathology: Anatomic	0	*	*	5	2	*
Pathology: Clinical	4	1	*	9	2	*

*Please note that the Total RVU conformation provided by the Anesthesiology practices are ASA units. Anesthesiology practices are not represented in Physician Work RVU tables.

Table 54: Total RVUs (CMS RBRVS Method) by Hospital Ownership (continued)

	Hospital Owned			Non-hospital Owned		
	Physicians	Medical Practices	Median	Physicians	Medical Practices	Median
Pediatrics: General	160	26	7,681	355	59	8,253
Ped: Adolescent Medicine	1	1	*	0	*	*
Ped: Allergy/Immunology	0	*	*	3	2	*
Ped: Cardiology	0	*	*	16	5	7,379
Ped: Child Development	0	*	*	5	1	*
Ped: Critical Care/Intensivist	0	*	*	14	4	7,409
Ped: Emergency Medicine	0	*	*	*	*	*
Ped: Endocrinology	1	1	*	2	2	*
Ped: Gastroenterology	1	1	*	8	3	*
Ped: Genetics	0	*	*	5	3	*
Ped: Hematology/Oncology	2	1	*	8	5	*
Ped: Hospitalist	1	1	*	5	2	*
Ped: Infectious Disease	2	1	*	0	*	*
Ped: Neonatal Medicine	9	2	*	18	3	12,295
Ped: Nephrology	1	1	*	3	1	*
Ped: Neurology	3	2	*	7	3	*
Ped: Pulmonology	1	1	*	7	3	*
Ped: Rheumatology	*	*	*	1	1	*
Ped: Sports Medicine	*	*	*	0	*	*
Physiatry (Phys Med & Rehab)	15	6	7,129	32	17	9,887
Podiatry: General	22	9	8,146	20	14	10,366
Podiatry: Surg-Foot & Ankle	5	3	*	13	6	9,440
Podiatry: Surg-Forefoot Only	0	*	*	3	2	*
Psychiatry: General	27	11	5,418	36	9	4,472
Psychiatry: Child & Adolescent	4	3	*	3	2	*
Psychiatry: Geriatric	1	1	*	4	1	*
Pulmonary Medicine	11	6	9,710	74	28	9,473
Pulmonary Med: Critical Care	2	2	*	27	11	11,484
Radiation Oncology	5	3	*	16	4	16,435
Radiology: Diagnostic-Inv	4	2	*	67	12	16,154
Radiology: Diagnostic-Noninv	14	2	*	66	15	12,981
Radiology: Nuclear Medicine	3	2	*	15	6	15,375
Rheumatology	17	11	8,578	50	26	9,237
Sleep Medicine	0	*	*	2	2	*
Surgery: General	44	16	10,386	193	49	12,352
Surg: Cardiovascular	8	3	*	36	13	15,323
Surg: Cardiovascular-Pediatric	0	*	*	2	2	*
Surg: Colon and Rectal	0	*	*	5	4	*
Surg: Neurological	6	3	*	56	15	15,667
Surg: Oncology	*	*	*	1	1	*
Surg: Oral	0	*	*	4	2	*
Surg: Pediatric	3	2	*	5	2	*
Surg: Plastic & Reconstruction	4	3	*	27	13	12,502
Surg: Plastic & Recon-Hand	0	*	*	0	*	*
Surg: Plastic & Recon-Pediatric	*	*	*	2	1	*
Surg: Thoracic (primary)	1	1	*	16	1	*
Surg: Transplant	1	1	*	4	1	*
Surg: Trauma	8	2	*	0	*	*
Surg: Trauma-Burn	0	*	*	7	2	*
Surg: Vascular (primary)	5	4	*	23	8	13,524
Urgent Care	30	11	7,494	97	25	9,070
Urology	11	7	12,602	76	29	14,616
Urology: Pediatric	9	1	*	3	2	*

Table 55: Total RVU (CMS RBRVS Method) by Percent of Capitation Revenue

	No capitation		10% or less		11% to 50%		51% or more	
	Physicians	Median	Physicians	Median	Physicians	Median	Physicians	Median
Allergy/Immunology	14	12,082	14	16,359	11	9,092	8	*
Anesthesiology	143	11,948	5	*	15	*	7	*
Anesth: Pain Management	7	*	1	*	0	*	0	*
Anesth: Pediatric	0	*	*	*	0	*	*	*
Cardiology: Electrophysiology	12	18,335	6	*	2	*	0	*
Cardiology: Invasive	72	17,012	38	18,252	17	11,743	2	*
Cardiology: Inv-Intervntnl	104	16,322	43	17,937	7	*	0	*
Cardiology: Noninvasive	67	15,787	24	13,389	22	6,789	5	*
Critical Care: Intensivist	1	*	2	*	0	*	2	*
Dentistry	0	*	2	*	0	*	0	*
Dermatology	37	12,439	23	13,495	22	14,932	9	*
Dermatology: MOHS Surgery	2	*	1	*	0	*	0	*
Emergency Medicine	6	*	33	7,579	7	*	0	*
Endocrinology/Metabolism	17	7,153	17	7,374	15	6,054	5	*
Family Practice (w/ OB)	133	8,329	156	8,456	162	7,454	4	*
Family Practice (w/o OB)	371	8,366	313	7,200	220	7,362	122	8,694
Family Practice: Sports Med	4	*	1	*	2	*	*	*
Gastroenterology	126	16,741	30	16,014	29	13,772	14	15,394
Gastroenterology: Hepatology	21	14,752	0	*	0	*	0	*
Geriatrics	1	*	7	*	5	*	0	*
Hematology/Oncology	51	11,202	28	9,057	15	8,094	3	*
Hem/Onc: Oncology (only)	16	8,419	0	*	5	*	4	*
Infectious Disease	14	6,385	15	8,803	11	6,191	2	*
Internal Medicine: General	319	7,803	307	7,004	313	7,441	121	7,948
Internal Med: Hospitalist	50	6,750	39	6,161	0	*	15	4,543
Internal Med: Pediatric	11	7,486	11	6,488	2	*	0	*
Nephrology	25	16,940	17	9,098	12	8,034	1	*
Neurology	64	9,271	22	8,220	26	7,514	12	8,294
OBGYN: General	148	12,438	88	11,640	87	11,627	39	12,825
OBGYN: Gynecology (only)	9	*	6	*	5	*	4	*
OBGYN: Gyn Oncology	1	*	3	*	1	*	*	*
OBGYN: Maternal & Fetal Med	5	*	4	*	1	*	*	*
OBGYN: Repro Endocrinology	3	*	0	*	0	*	0	*
Occupational Medicine	6	*	2	*	2	*	3	*
Ophthalmology	44	17,606	16	18,673	17	16,269	16	18,450
Ophthalmology: Pediatric	3	*	0	*	1	*	0	*
Ophthalmology: Retina	12	22,538	0	*	2	*	0	*
Orthopedic (Non-surgical)	1	*	3	*	1	*	7	*
Orthopedic Surgery: General	145	16,129	43	15,172	35	14,186	8	*
Ortho Surg: Foot & Ankle	14	17,992	1	*	3	*	*	*
Ortho Surg: Hand	24	15,176	1	*	6	*	1	*
Ortho Surg: Hip & Joint	24	14,580	2	*	2	*	1	*
Ortho Surg: Oncology	0	*	*	*	*	*	*	*
Ortho Surg: Pediatric	4	*	1	*	1	*	0	*
Ortho Surg: Spine	20	15,625	1	*	4	*	2	*
Ortho Surg: Trauma	5	*	*	*	1	*	*	*
Ortho Surg: Sports Med	49	15,330	2	*	4	*	3	*
Otorhinolaryngology	39	13,955	19	12,372	21	10,850	11	13,544
Otorhinolaryngology: Pediatric	1	*	*	*	*	*	*	*
Pathology: Anatomic & Clinical	2	*	16	6,170	0	*	3	*
Pathology: Anatomic	2	*	0	*	3	*	*	*
Pathology: Clinical	9	*	0	*	4	*	*	*

*Please note that the Total RVU information provided by the Anesthesiology practices are ASA units. Anesthesiology practices are not represented in Physician Work RVU tables.

Table 55: Total RVU (CMS RBRVS Method) by Percent of Capitation Revenue (continued)

	No capitation		10% or less		11% to 50%		51% or more	
	Physicians	Median	Physicians	Median	Physicians	Median	Physicians	Median
Pediatrics: General	151	8,346	132	7,315	178	9,355	53	9,306
Ped: Adolescent Medicine	0	*	1	*	0	*	*	*
Ped: Allergy/Immunology	0	*	0	*	3	*	*	*
Ped: Cardiology	4	*	10	*	2	*	0	*
Ped: Child Development	0	*	0	*	5	*	*	*
Ped: Critical Care/Intensivist	8	*	2	*	4	*	*	*
Ped: Emergency Medicine	0	*	*	*	*	*	*	*
Ped: Endocrinology	0	*	1	*	2	*	*	*
Ped: Gastroenterology	4	*	4	*	1	*	*	*
Ped: Genetics	1	*	4	*	*	*	*	*
Ped: Hematology/Oncology	0	*	6	*	4	*	0	*
Ped: Hospitalist	0	*	5	*	1	*	0	*
Ped: Infectious Disease	*	*	2	*	*	*	*	*
Ped: Neonatal Medicine	1	*	24	12,295	2	*	0	*
Ped: Nephrology	0	*	4	*	0	*	*	*
Ped: Neurology	4	*	6	*	0	*	*	*
Ped: Pulmonology	5	*	1	*	2	*	*	*
Ped: Rheumatology	*	*	0	*	1	*	*	*
Ped: Sports Medicine	0	*	*	*	*	*	*	*
Physiatry (Phys Med & Rehab)	30	9,923	11	7,659	4	*	2	*
Podiatry: General	13	8,406	12	9,526	9	*	8	*
Podiatry: Surg-Foot & Ankle	6	*	1	*	5	*	6	*
Podiatry: Surg-Forefoot Only	1	*	2	*	*	*	0	*
Psychiatry: General	14	6,337	18	4,132	29	4,432	2	*
Psychiatry: Child & Adolescent	2	*	2	*	2	*	1	*
Psychiatry: Geriatric	4	*	1	*	0	*	*	*
Pulmonary Medicine	31	10,734	24	11,171	21	7,175	9	*
Pulmonary Med: Critical Care	16	11,704	7	*	6	*	0	*
Radiation Oncology	14	16,917	3	*	3	*	1	*
Radiology: Diagnostic-Inv	54	16,429	3	*	14	*	0	*
Radiology: Diagnostic-Noninv	54	13,067	13	19,866	13	*	0	*
Radiology: Nuclear Medicine	17	15,375	1	*	0	*	0	*
Rheumatology	27	7,407	24	9,670	10	8,740	6	*
Sleep Medicine	1	*	0	*	1	*	*	*
Surgery: General	116	11,889	56	11,897	47	11,928	17	14,287
Surg: Cardiovascular	15	15,390	10	16,518	17	12,269	2	*
Surg: Cardiovascular-Pediatric	1	*	1	*	0	*	*	*
Surg: Colon and Rectal	1	*	1	*	3	*	0	*
Surg: Neurological	49	15,668	8	*	5	*	0	*
Surg: Oncology	0	*	*	*	1	*	*	*
Surg: Oral	4	*	0	*	0	*	0	*
Surg: Pediatric	2	*	5	*	1	*	*	*
Surg: Plastic & Reconstruction	7	*	14	13,377	9	*	1	*
Surg: Plastic & Recon-Hand	0	*	*	*	0	*	*	*
Surg: Plastic & Recon-Pediatric	0	*	2	*	*	*	*	*
Surg: Thoracic (primary)	17	*	0	*	0	*	0	*
Surg: Transplant	5	*	0	*	0	*	*	*
Surg: Trauma	5	*	3	*	0	*	*	*
Surg: Trauma-Burn	6	*	1	*	0	*	*	*
Surg: Vascular (primary)	17	13,777	1	*	10	11,070	0	*
Urgent Care	39	10,203	39	7,977	30	7,248	19	9,957
Urology	45	14,846	18	14,832	15	12,874	9	*
Urology: Pediatric	1	*	2	*	9	*	*	*

Table 56: Physician Compensation per Total RVU (CMS RBRVS Method)

	Physicians	Medical Practices	Mean	Std. Dev.	25th %tile	Median	75th %tile	90th %tile
Allergy/Immunology	45	27	$24.07	$12.19	$15.48	$20.80	$28.14	$45.69
Anesthesiology	170	17	$30.34	$12.76	$22.53	$27.49	$35.28	$43.67
Anesth: Pain Management	8	4	*	*	*	*	*	*
Anesth: Pediatric	0	*	*	*	*	*	*	*
Cardiology: Electrophysiology	20	16	$21.65	$6.13	$18.12	$19.19	$28.30	$30.46
Cardiology: Invasive	128	39	$25.59	$11.44	$17.40	$23.18	$31.49	$38.98
Cardiology: Inv-Intervntnl	151	41	$25.58	$9.99	$18.63	$24.78	$29.40	$35.75
Cardiology: Noninvasive	108	45	$25.47	$13.47	$16.96	$21.09	$31.13	$45.67
Critical Care: Intensivist	5	4	*	*	*	*	*	*
Dentistry	2	1	*	*	*	*	*	*
Dermatology	87	43	$21.85	$9.85	$16.88	$20.24	$23.91	$27.08
Dermatology: MOHS Surgery	2	2	*	*	*	*	*	*
Emergency Medicine	46	9	$33.94	$8.24	$27.27	$33.12	$39.38	$44.87
Endocrinology/Metabolism	54	35	$24.74	$9.94	$19.05	$22.44	$27.33	$35.73
Family Practice (w/ OB)	454	66	$21.18	$6.40	$17.39	$20.18	$23.49	$27.58
Family Practice (w/o OB)	1,025	125	$21.40	$6.41	$16.89	$20.56	$24.26	$28.68
Family Practice: Sports Med	7	6	*	*	*	*	*	*
Gastroenterology	197	57	$22.22	$10.61	$16.34	$19.33	$25.99	$31.14
Gastroenterology: Hepatology	21	4	$24.06	$5.47	$19.19	$24.09	$28.21	$31.60
Geriatrics	13	7	$27.89	$4.77	$24.33	$26.39	$31.86	$34.76
Hematology/Oncology	100	33	$39.51	$17.91	$25.22	$34.96	$48.92	$68.06
Hem/Onc: Oncology (only)	25	8	$42.25	$16.28	$30.04	$38.29	$56.89	$69.58
Infectious Disease	42	23	$25.78	$10.74	$18.25	$22.79	$33.09	$42.64
Internal Medicine: General	1,054	120	$22.50	$7.16	$17.83	$21.58	$25.07	$30.19
Internal Med: Hospitalist	109	22	$31.86	$10.11	$23.93	$30.10	$39.13	$45.82
Internal Med: Pediatric	24	9	$23.64	$7.33	$19.18	$22.25	$25.43	$38.04
Nephrology	45	21	$21.86	$7.75	$17.57	$22.07	$24.63	$31.20
Neurology	121	41	$25.50	$8.76	$19.31	$23.60	$29.46	$39.02
OBGYN: General	359	66	$22.24	$6.32	$18.11	$21.52	$24.67	$28.66
OBGYN: Gynecology (only)	24	19	$24.52	$9.23	$19.27	$21.72	$28.95	$39.97
OBGYN: Gyn Oncology	5	4	*	*	*	*	*	*
OBGYN: Maternal & Fetal Med	10	4	$32.67	$16.59	$20.34	$24.90	$50.55	$60.09
OBGYN: Repro Endocrinology	3	2	*	*	*	*	*	*
Occupational Medicine	13	8	$28.10	$11.98	$20.17	$23.80	$38.29	$50.43
Ophthalmology	90	30	$17.88	$5.26	$13.60	$16.79	$22.73	$24.96
Ophthalmology: Pediatric	4	2	*	*	*	*	*	*
Ophthalmology: Retina	14	5	$23.45	$6.39	$18.90	$21.88	$24.71	$36.31
Orthopedic (Non-surgical)	12	7	$18.66	$4.76	$16.04	$16.96	$21.07	$28.73
Orthopedic Surgery: General	227	60	$24.89	$10.87	$19.18	$22.89	$26.90	$34.36
Ortho Surg: Foot & Ankle	17	14	$23.62	$12.33	$15.69	$20.18	$26.41	$52.04
Ortho Surg: Hand	32	23	$29.22	$13.68	$18.96	$24.57	$36.94	$54.91
Ortho Surg: Hip & Joint	29	15	$29.57	$18.47	$18.09	$22.81	$34.46	$58.67
Ortho Surg: Oncology	0	*	*	*	*	*	*	*
Ortho Surg: Pediatric	5	4	*	*	*	*	*	*
Ortho Surg: Spine	23	18	$31.75	$15.69	$20.26	$27.59	$37.09	$51.40
Ortho Surg: Trauma	6	4	*	*	*	*	*	*
Ortho Surg: Sports Med	56	23	$28.11	$11.37	$18.84	$24.32	$33.18	$46.86
Otorhinolaryngology	89	38	$24.22	$7.57	$19.01	$22.66	$28.75	$34.65
Otorhinolaryngology: Pediatric	1	1	*	*	*	*	*	*
Pathology: Anatomic & Clinical	20	7	$33.10	$20.37	$15.20	$23.15	$53.19	$56.69
Pathology: Anatomic	5	2	*	*	*	*	*	*
Pathology: Clinical	13	3	$23.95	$5.80	$19.69	$23.33	$27.44	$34.77

*Please note that the Total RVU information provided by the Anesthesiology practices are ASA units. Anesthesiology practices are not represented in Physician Work RVU tables.

Table 56: Physician Compensation per Total RVU (CMS RBRVS Method) (continued)

	Physicians	Medical Practices	Mean	Std. Dev.	25th %tile	Median	75th %tile	90th %tile
Pediatrics: General	501	84	$20.15	$6.16	$16.12	$19.01	$23.51	$27.28
Ped: Adolescent Medicine	1	1	*	*	*	*	*	*
Ped: Allergy/Immunology	3	2	*	*	*	*	*	*
Ped: Cardiology	16	5	$34.82	$14.62	$20.43	$33.71	$46.35	$57.26
Ped: Child Development	5	1	*	*	*	*	*	*
Ped: Critical Care/Intensivist	13	3	$37.67	$17.79	$22.55	$32.64	$55.05	$67.62
Ped: Emergency Medicine	0	*	*	*	*	*	*	*
Ped: Endocrinology	3	3	*	*	*	*	*	*
Ped: Gastroenterology	9	4	*	*	*	*	*	*
Ped: Genetics	5	3	*	*	*	*	*	*
Ped: Hematology/Oncology	10	6	$30.10	$12.07	$18.34	$27.25	$43.17	$47.99
Ped: Hospitalist	6	3	*	*	*	*	*	*
Ped: Infectious Disease	2	1	*	*	*	*	*	*
Ped: Neonatal Medicine	27	5	$38.43	$11.07	$29.46	$38.78	$48.88	$52.83
Ped: Nephrology	4	2	*	*	*	*	*	*
Ped: Neurology	10	5	$32.21	$12.45	$21.13	$31.63	$42.28	$51.83
Ped: Pulmonology	8	4	*	*	*	*	*	*
Ped: Rheumatology	1	1	*	*	*	*	*	*
Ped: Sports Medicine	0	*	*	*	*	*	*	*
Physiatry (Phys Med & Rehab)	44	23	$26.11	$10.43	$17.34	$25.58	$32.85	$41.49
Podiatry: General	41	22	$17.90	$5.12	$14.17	$16.97	$21.20	$24.87
Podiatry: Surg-Foot & Ankle	17	8	$19.40	$7.61	$15.11	$18.95	$20.68	$33.13
Podiatry: Surg-Forefoot Only	3	2	*	*	*	*	*	*
Psychiatry: General	63	20	$32.63	$9.82	$27.61	$31.29	$37.72	$45.37
Psychiatry: Child & Adolescent	7	5	*	*	*	*	*	*
Psychiatry: Geriatric	5	2	*	*	*	*	*	*
Pulmonary Medicine	82	33	$25.33	$11.70	$17.41	$22.38	$27.76	$43.97
Pulmonary Med: Critical Care	26	12	$23.18	$8.48	$17.71	$21.39	$28.46	$38.96
Radiation Oncology	20	6	$30.89	$9.37	$23.73	$31.72	$34.82	$41.86
Radiology: Diagnostic-Inv	69	14	$29.71	$10.33	$23.20	$28.75	$35.35	$45.01
Radiology: Diagnostic-Noninv	80	17	$30.13	$11.80	$21.11	$29.34	$38.69	$46.17
Radiology: Nuclear Medicine	17	7	$32.41	$16.15	$23.65	$24.80	$46.26	$58.06
Rheumatology	63	35	$25.31	$10.49	$17.92	$22.65	$30.04	$38.96
Sleep Medicine	2	2	*	*	*	*	*	*
Surgery: General	234	64	$23.88	$9.08	$17.93	$21.68	$28.02	$34.86
Surg: Cardiovascular	43	16	$32.70	$11.23	$25.22	$31.93	$39.90	$47.91
Surg: Cardiovascular-Pediatric	2	2	*	*	*	*	*	*
Surg: Colon and Rectal	5	4	*	*	*	*	*	*
Surg: Neurological	62	18	$32.08	$12.71	$24.60	$28.35	$38.86	$52.06
Surg: Oncology	1	1	*	*	*	*	*	*
Surg: Oral	3	1	*	*	*	*	*	*
Surg: Pediatric	7	3	*	*	*	*	*	*
Surg: Plastic & Reconstruction	29	16	$27.60	$11.04	$20.28	$25.26	$34.87	$42.78
Surg: Plastic & Recon-Hand	0	*	*	*	*	*	*	*
Surg: Plastic & Recon-Pediatric	1	1	*	*	*	*	*	*
Surg: Thoracic (primary)	17	2	*	*	*	*	*	*
Surg: Transplant	5	2	*	*	*	*	*	*
Surg: Trauma	8	2	*	*	*	*	*	*
Surg: Trauma-Burn	6	2	*	*	*	*	*	*
Surg: Vascular (primary)	28	12	$28.34	$8.51	$21.87	$27.45	$35.08	$39.37
Urgent Care	127	36	$20.48	$5.53	$16.48	$19.83	$22.94	$26.53
Urology	83	35	$25.77	$10.71	$17.59	$22.84	$31.32	$43.94
Urology: Pediatric	12	3	$22.88	$7.02	$19.14	$20.14	$22.59	$38.62

Table 57: Physician Compensation per Total RVU (CMS RBRVS Method) by Group Type

	Single-specialty			Multispecialty		
	Physicians	Medical Practices	Median	Physicians	Medical Practices	Median
Allergy/Immunology	5	2	*	40	25	$21.07
Anesthesiology	127	9	$26.98	43	8	$29.24
Anesth: Pain Management	6	2	*	2	2	*
Anesth: Pediatric	0	*	*	0	*	*
Cardiology: Electrophysiology	12	9	$18.76	8	7	*
Cardiology: Invasive	69	18	$21.44	59	21	$24.82
Cardiology: Inv-Intervntnl	118	28	$24.51	33	13	$25.27
Cardiology: Noninvasive	64	23	$19.61	44	22	$22.42
Critical Care: Intensivist	0	*	*	5	4	*
Dentistry	0	*	*	2	1	*
Dermatology	4	2	*	83	41	$20.24
Dermatology: MOHS Surgery	1	1	*	1	1	*
Emergency Medicine	0	*	*	46	9	$33.12
Endocrinology/Metabolism	2	2	*	52	33	$22.09
Family Practice (w/ OB)	80	18	$19.33	374	48	$20.35
Family Practice (w/o OB)	118	37	$20.03	907	88	$20.63
Family Practice: Sports Med	3	3	*	4	3	*
Gastroenterology	83	8	$19.79	114	49	$19.08
Gastroenterology: Hepatology	18	3	$24.07	3	1	*
Geriatrics	0	*	*	13	7	$26.39
Hematology/Oncology	36	7	$49.68	64	26	$31.72
Hem/Onc: Oncology (only)	11	2	*	14	6	$37.30
Infectious Disease	15	6	$22.58	27	17	$22.98
Internal Medicine: General	78	16	$23.52	976	104	$21.41
Internal Med: Hospitalist	0	*	*	109	22	$30.10
Internal Med: Pediatric	0	*	*	24	9	$22.25
Nephrology	13	4	$18.48	32	17	$22.21
Neurology	35	6	$24.53	86	35	$23.57
OBGYN: General	60	6	$19.06	299	60	$21.79
OBGYN: Gynecology (only)	4	3	*	20	16	$21.72
OBGYN: Gyn Oncology	0	*	*	5	4	*
OBGYN: Maternal & Fetal Med	3	1	*	7	3	*
OBGYN: Repro Endocrinology	1	1	*	2	1	*
Occupational Medicine	0	*	*	13	8	$23.80
Ophthalmology	20	2	*	70	28	$16.09
Ophthalmology: Pediatric	3	1	*	1	1	*
Ophthalmology: Retina	11	2	*	3	3	*
Orthopedic (Non-surgical)	0	*	*	12	7	$16.96
Orthopedic Surgery: General	119	28	$23.19	108	32	$22.38
Ortho Surg: Foot & Ankle	13	11	$18.22	4	3	*
Ortho Surg: Hand	24	17	$22.87	8	6	*
Ortho Surg: Hip & Joint	22	11	$22.10	7	4	*
Ortho Surg: Oncology	0	*	*	0	*	*
Ortho Surg: Pediatric	4	3	*	1	1	*
Ortho Surg: Spine	13	11	$27.49	10	7	$29.93
Ortho Surg: Trauma	5	3	*	1	1	*
Ortho Surg: Sports Med	43	16	$24.42	13	7	$23.33
Otorhinolaryngology	5	2	*	84	36	$23.15
Otorhinolaryngology: Pediatric	0	*	*	1	1	*
Pathology: Anatomic & Clinical	0	*	*	20	7	$23.15
Pathology: Anatomic	0	*	*	5	2	*
Pathology: Clinical	5	1	*	8	2	*

*Please note that the Total RVU information provided by the Anesthesiology practices are ASA units. Anesthesiology practices are not represented in Physician Work RVU tables.

Table 57: Physician Compensation per Total RVU (CMS RBRVS Method) by Group Type (continued)

	Single-specialty			Multispecialty		
	Physicians	Medical Practices	Median	Physicians	Medical Practices	Median
Pediatrics: General	90	15	$18.80	411	69	$19.05
Ped: Adolescent Medicine	0	*	*	1	1	*
Ped: Allergy/Immunology	2	1	*	1	1	*
Ped: Cardiology	5	1	*	11	4	$31.92
Ped: Child Development	*	*	*	5	1	*
Ped: Critical Care/Intensivist	8	1	*	5	2	*
Ped: Emergency Medicine	0	*	*	0	*	*
Ped: Endocrinology	1	1	*	2	2	*
Ped: Gastroenterology	4	1	*	5	3	*
Ped: Genetics	*	*	*	5	3	*
Ped: Hematology/Oncology	2	1	*	8	5	*
Ped: Hospitalist	0	*	*	6	3	*
Ped: Infectious Disease	0	*	*	2	1	*
Ped: Neonatal Medicine	16	2	*	11	3	$35.01
Ped: Nephrology	0	*	*	4	2	*
Ped: Neurology	4	2	*	6	3	*
Ped: Pulmonology	6	2	*	2	2	*
Ped: Rheumatology	0	*	*	1	1	*
Ped: Sports Medicine	*	*	*	0	*	*
Physiatry (Phys Med & Rehab)	11	6	$16.30	33	17	$27.84
Podiatry: General	0	*	*	41	22	$16.97
Podiatry: Surg-Foot & Ankle	2	1	*	15	7	$19.03
Podiatry: Surg-Forefoot Only	1	1	*	2	1	*
Psychiatry: General	0	*	*	63	20	$31.29
Psychiatry: Child & Adolescent	0	*	*	7	5	*
Psychiatry: Geriatric	*	*	*	5	2	*
Pulmonary Medicine	6	3	*	76	30	$22.38
Pulmonary Med: Critical Care	1	1	*	25	11	$21.41
Radiation Oncology	12	2	*	8	4	*
Radiology: Diagnostic-Inv	47	7	$27.46	22	7	$33.05
Radiology: Diagnostic-Noninv	38	7	$33.53	42	10	$24.55
Radiology: Nuclear Medicine	13	4	$24.80	4	3	*
Rheumatology	15	4	$24.60	48	31	$22.01
Sleep Medicine	0	*	*	2	2	*
Surgery: General	45	10	$22.71	189	54	$21.19
Surg: Cardiovascular	12	4	$27.85	31	12	$34.77
Surg: Cardiovascular-Pediatric	2	2	*	0	*	*
Surg: Colon and Rectal	1	1	*	4	3	*
Surg: Neurological	28	6	$28.12	34	12	$28.62
Surg: Oncology	0	*	*	1	1	*
Surg: Oral	3	1	*	0	*	*
Surg: Pediatric	0	*	*	7	3	*
Surg: Plastic & Reconstruction	7	3	*	22	13	$23.52
Surg: Plastic & Recon-Hand	0	*	*	0	*	*
Surg: Plastic & Recon-Pediatric	1	1	*	0	*	*
Surg: Thoracic (primary)	16	1	*	1	1	*
Surg: Transplant	4	1	*	1	1	*
Surg: Trauma	0	*	*	8	2	*
Surg: Trauma-Burn	6	2	*	0	*	*
Surg: Vascular (primary)	4	2	*	24	10	$26.71
Urgent Care	3	1	*	124	35	$19.88
Urology	15	3	$39.99	68	32	$22.07
Urology: Pediatric	1	1	*	11	2	*

Table 58: Physician Work RVUs (CMS RBRVS Method)

	Physicians	Medical Practices	Mean	Std. Dev.	25th %tile	Median	75th %tile	90th %tile
Allergy/Immunology	67	42	4,235	2,034	2,953	3,631	4,868	7,544
Cardiology: Electrophysiology	34	23	8,824	2,727	6,962	8,724	11,222	12,608
Cardiology: Invasive	177	53	7,874	2,762	5,674	7,625	9,789	11,689
Cardiology: Inv-Intervntnl	238	58	8,978	2,612	7,199	8,859	10,748	12,645
Cardiology: Noninvasive	181	57	6,475	2,323	4,786	6,085	7,957	9,764
Critical Care: Intensivist	16	8	4,196	1,335	3,061	4,287	5,320	6,259
Dentistry	3	1	*	*	*	*	*	*
Dermatology	137	63	6,948	2,514	5,153	6,658	8,483	10,458
Dermatology: MOHS Surgery	7	7	*	*	*	*	*	*
Emergency Medicine	159	20	4,987	1,816	3,780	4,670	5,884	7,812
Endocrinology/Metabolism	95	56	4,257	1,366	3,354	3,976	4,840	6,059
Family Practice (w/ OB)	699	90	4,244	1,173	3,331	4,139	4,985	5,865
Family Practice (w/o OB)	1,859	155	4,044	1,169	3,266	3,923	4,671	5,693
Family Practice: Sports Med	10	6	5,229	1,779	3,693	5,264	6,827	7,447
Gastroenterology	233	78	7,815	2,366	6,385	7,671	9,121	10,904
Gastroenterology: Hepatology	21	4	9,189	2,469	7,088	8,808	11,254	12,604
Geriatrics	25	10	3,608	1,126	2,720	3,518	4,592	5,306
Hematology/Oncology	147	49	4,477	2,105	3,169	3,895	5,060	7,020
Hem/Onc: Oncology (only)	33	13	4,218	1,597	3,248	3,934	5,146	6,756
Infectious Disease	60	35	5,121	2,961	3,221	3,924	5,554	9,974
Internal Medicine: General	1,687	151	4,009	1,169	3,230	3,856	4,636	5,574
Internal Med: Hospitalist	166	36	3,677	1,408	2,861	3,273	4,254	5,606
Internal Med: Pediatric	33	14	4,157	1,685	2,978	3,678	5,410	7,174
Nephrology	88	36	6,732	2,924	4,511	5,935	8,093	11,647
Neurology	209	69	4,682	1,771	3,535	4,296	5,697	6,820
OBGYN: General	531	92	6,384	2,056	4,969	6,230	7,515	9,033
OBGYN: Gynecology (only)	76	28	4,892	1,638	3,706	4,711	5,954	6,993
OBGYN: Gyn Oncology	10	6	5,478	1,772	4,256	5,193	6,579	8,814
OBGYN: Maternal & Fetal Med	33	10	6,929	2,457	5,045	7,513	8,416	10,117
OBGYN: Repro Endocrinology	8	5	*	*	*	*	*	*
Occupational Medicine	30	19	3,244	1,213	2,246	2,971	3,960	4,973
Ophthalmology	162	55	7,393	2,612	5,488	7,377	9,130	10,763
Ophthalmology: Pediatric	7	5	*	*	*	*	*	*
Ophthalmology: Retina	10	6	11,887	1,823	10,729	12,145	12,849	14,775
Orthopedic (Non-surgical)	18	11	6,780	2,606	4,138	6,427	9,058	10,348
Orthopedic Surgery: General	272	72	7,294	2,460	5,494	7,132	8,841	10,526
Ortho Surg: Foot & Ankle	13	11	8,004	2,556	6,172	7,101	9,831	12,442
Ortho Surg: Hand	28	22	7,617	2,572	5,759	7,149	8,868	11,512
Ortho Surg: Hip & Joint	31	16	7,810	2,139	6,471	7,482	9,420	11,026
Ortho Surg: Oncology	0	*	*	*	*	*	*	*
Ortho Surg: Pediatric	10	7	7,760	2,274	6,413	7,895	9,588	10,542
Ortho Surg: Spine	25	18	9,125	2,079	7,832	8,491	10,175	12,726
Ortho Surg: Trauma	9	4	*	*	*	*	*	*
Ortho Surg: Sports Med	64	28	6,950	2,828	5,005	6,782	8,213	10,928
Otorhinolaryngology	147	61	6,592	2,434	4,934	6,273	8,018	9,753
Otorhinolaryngology: Pediatric	0	*	*	*	*	*	*	*
Pathology: Anatomic & Clinical	49	14	5,297	2,232	3,824	4,803	6,938	8,624
Pathology: Anatomic	15	5	4,935	1,817	3,697	4,605	6,485	8,229
Pathology: Clinical	34	6	4,514	1,050	3,912	4,293	4,791	6,195

Table 58: Physician Work RVUs (CMS RBRVS Method) (continued)

	Physicians	Medical Practices	Mean	Std. Dev.	25th %tile	Median	75th %tile	90th %tile
Pediatrics: General	677	106	4,267	1,240	3,458	4,152	5,034	5,910
Ped: Adolescent Medicine	59	6	4,105	1,001	3,493	4,041	4,630	5,456
Ped: Allergy/Immunology	6	6	*	*	*	*	*	*
Ped: Cardiology	23	10	4,413	1,430	3,126	4,083	5,624	6,441
Ped: Child Development	9	5	*	*	*	*	*	*
Ped: Critical Care/Intensivist	14	7	3,893	1,138	3,142	3,906	4,543	5,669
Ped: Emergency Medicine	0	*	*	*	*	*	*	*
Ped: Endocrinology	8	8	*	*	*	*	*	*
Ped: Gastroenterology	6	4	*	*	*	*	*	*
Ped: Genetics	3	2	*	*	*	*	*	*
Ped: Hematology/Oncology	11	8	2,843	490	2,509	2,731	3,184	3,596
Ped: Hospitalist	4	3	*	*	*	*	*	*
Ped: Infectious Disease	3	2	*	*	*	*	*	*
Ped: Neonatal Medicine	33	12	6,302	3,055	4,035	5,989	8,586	10,700
Ped: Nephrology	3	3	*	*	*	*	*	*
Ped: Neurology	18	10	4,487	1,915	3,390	4,019	5,601	7,829
Ped: Pulmonology	6	5	*	*	*	*	*	*
Ped: Rheumatology	0	*	*	*	*	*	*	*
Ped: Sports Medicine	0	*	*	*	*	*	*	*
Physiatry (Phys Med & Rehab)	67	32	4,463	1,712	2,982	4,363	5,512	7,250
Podiatry: General	66	35	4,488	1,738	3,433	4,096	5,232	6,576
Podiatry: Surg-Foot & Ankle	19	11	5,074	980	4,227	4,884	5,817	6,954
Podiatry: Surg-Forefoot Only	4	3	*	*	*	*	*	*
Psychiatry: General	141	38	3,662	1,433	2,698	3,453	4,328	5,420
Psychiatry: Child & Adolescent	16	10	4,111	1,409	3,297	3,774	4,468	6,819
Psychiatry: Geriatric	7	4	*	*	*	*	*	*
Pulmonary Medicine	132	53	5,950	2,154	4,364	5,664	7,155	9,162
Pulmonary Med: Critical Care	49	16	5,655	1,682	4,601	5,370	7,275	7,886
Radiation Oncology	40	17	9,145	2,445	7,675	8,373	10,637	13,800
Radiology: Diagnostic-Inv	159	25	9,701	2,610	7,934	9,594	11,528	13,298
Radiology: Diagnostic-Noninv	177	32	7,949	3,037	5,266	8,144	10,028	11,859
Radiology: Nuclear Medicine	14	10	6,359	2,377	4,396	5,592	7,706	10,637
Rheumatology	104	59	4,352	1,629	3,379	4,097	4,952	5,940
Sleep Medicine	2	2	*	*	*	*	*	*
Surgery: General	374	94	7,022	2,255	5,525	6,809	8,297	9,834
Surg: Cardiovascular	70	27	8,753	2,902	6,584	8,903	11,146	12,788
Surg: Cardiovascular-Pediatric	1	1	*	*	*	*	*	*
Surg: Colon and Rectal	9	5	*	*	*	*	*	*
Surg: Neurological	67	25	8,337	2,336	6,190	8,455	10,201	11,530
Surg: Oncology	1	1	*	*	*	*	*	*
Surg: Oral	1	1	*	*	*	*	*	*
Surg: Pediatric	7	5	*	*	*	*	*	*
Surg: Plastic & Reconstruction	44	27	6,040	2,227	4,536	5,947	7,636	9,731
Surg: Plastic & Recon-Hand	3	2	*	*	*	*	*	*
Surg: Plastic & Recon-Pediatric	0	*	*	*	*	*	*	*
Surg: Thoracic (primary)	22	5	10,591	3,280	8,061	11,296	13,249	14,693
Surg: Transplant	7	5	*	*	*	*	*	*
Surg: Trauma	11	4	6,693	2,389	6,346	7,088	7,492	10,817
Surg: Trauma-Burn	2	2	*	*	*	*	*	*
Surg: Vascular (primary)	36	16	7,172	2,405	5,252	7,201	9,047	10,799
Urgent Care	195	50	4,364	1,459	3,166	4,360	5,484	6,349
Urology	151	56	6,741	2,219	5,447	6,593	7,983	9,613
Urology: Pediatric	10	2	*	*	*	*	*	*

MEDICAL GROUP MANAGEMENT ASSOCIATION™

Table 59: Physician Work RVUs (CMS RBRVS Method) by Group Type

	Single-specialty			Multispecialty		
	Physicians	Medical Practices	Median	Physicians	Medical Practices	Median
Allergy/Immunology	2	1	*	65	41	3,650
Cardiology: Electrophysiology	17	12	10,932	17	11	7,356
Cardiology: Invasive	89	21	7,623	88	32	7,626
Cardiology: Inv-Intervntnl	139	28	8,984	99	30	8,618
Cardiology: Noninvasive	76	22	6,031	105	35	6,103
Critical Care: Intensivist	0	*	*	16	8	4,287
Dentistry	0	*	*	3	1	*
Dermatology	4	1	*	133	62	6,629
Dermatology: MOHS Surgery	0	*	*	7	7	*
Emergency Medicine	33	3	5,336	126	17	4,452
Endocrinology/Metabolism	2	2	*	93	54	3,989
Family Practice (w/ OB)	82	18	3,391	617	72	4,223
Family Practice (w/o OB)	143	29	4,090	1,716	126	3,917
Family Practice: Sports Med	5	2	*	5	4	*
Gastroenterology	37	7	8,037	196	71	7,635
Gastroenterology: Hepatology	18	3	9,144	3	1	*
Geriatrics	0	*	*	25	10	3,518
Hematology/Oncology	38	6	4,447	109	43	3,869
Hem/Onc: Oncology (only)	11	2	*	22	11	3,957
Infectious Disease	12	5	7,689	48	30	3,820
Internal Medicine: General	68	17	3,745	1,619	134	3,865
Internal Med: Hospitalist	0	*	*	166	36	3,273
Internal Med: Pediatric	0	*	*	33	14	3,678
Nephrology	14	3	9,017	74	33	5,572
Neurology	53	9	4,973	156	60	4,219
OBGYN: General	57	6	5,827	474	86	6,251
OBGYN: Gynecology (only)	3	2	*	73	26	4,702
OBGYN: Gyn Oncology	0	*	*	10	6	5,193
OBGYN: Maternal & Fetal Med	3	1	*	30	9	7,579
OBGYN: Repro Endocrinology	1	1	*	7	4	*
Occupational Medicine	0	*	*	30	19	2,971
Ophthalmology	23	3	9,122	139	52	7,257
Ophthalmology: Pediatric	3	1	*	4	4	*
Ophthalmology: Retina	5	2	*	5	4	*
Orthopedic (Non-surgical)	0	*	*	18	11	6,427
Orthopedic Surgery: General	83	17	7,388	189	55	6,892
Ortho Surg: Foot & Ankle	8	7	*	5	4	*
Ortho Surg: Hand	14	11	6,714	14	11	7,536
Ortho Surg: Hip & Joint	18	9	7,447	13	7	7,727
Ortho Surg: Oncology	0	*	*	0	*	*
Ortho Surg: Pediatric	6	3	*	4	4	*
Ortho Surg: Spine	13	9	8,285	12	9	8,984
Ortho Surg: Trauma	4	2	*	5	2	*
Ortho Surg: Sports Med	34	13	7,385	30	15	5,763
Otorhinolaryngology	1	1	*	146	60	6,258
Otorhinolaryngology: Pediatric	0	*	*	0	*	*
Pathology: Anatomic & Clinical	6	1	*	43	13	5,680
Pathology: Anatomic	5	1	*	10	4	4,673
Pathology: Clinical	2	1	*	32	5	4,260

Table 59: Physician Work RVUs (CMS RBRVS Method) by Group Type (continued)

	Single-specialty			Multispecialty		
	Physicians	Medical Practices	Median	Physicians	Medical Practices	Median
Pediatrics: General	42	8	4,008	635	98	4,160
Ped: Adolescent Medicine	0	*	*	59	6	4,041
Ped: Allergy/Immunology	0	*	*	6	6	*
Ped: Cardiology	7	2	*	16	8	3,711
Ped: Child Development	*	*	*	9	5	*
Ped: Critical Care/Intensivist	0	*	*	14	7	3,906
Ped: Emergency Medicine	0	*	*	0	*	*
Ped: Endocrinology	1	1	*	7	7	*
Ped: Gastroenterology	0	*	*	6	4	*
Ped: Genetics	*	*	*	3	2	*
Ped: Hematology/Oncology	3	1	*	8	7	*
Ped: Hospitalist	0	*	*	4	3	*
Ped: Infectious Disease	0	*	*	3	2	*
Ped: Neonatal Medicine	0	*	*	33	12	5,989
Ped: Nephrology	0	*	*	3	3	*
Ped: Neurology	3	1	*	15	9	3,921
Ped: Pulmonology	0	*	*	6	5	*
Ped: Rheumatology	0	*	*	0	*	*
Ped: Sports Medicine	*	*	*	0	*	*
Physiatry (Phys Med & Rehab)	8	4	*	59	28	4,471
Podiatry: General	0	*	*	66	35	4,096
Podiatry: Surg-Foot & Ankle	0	*	*	19	11	4,884
Podiatry: Surg-Forefoot Only	1	1	*	3	2	*
Psychiatry: General	0	*	*	141	38	3,453
Psychiatry: Child & Adolescent	0	*	*	16	10	3,774
Psychiatry: Geriatric	*	*	*	7	4	*
Pulmonary Medicine	6	3	*	126	50	5,805
Pulmonary Med: Critical Care	20	4	5,126	29	12	5,389
Radiation Oncology	14	4	9,567	26	13	8,202
Radiology: Diagnostic-Inv	77	8	10,967	82	17	8,660
Radiology: Diagnostic-Noninv	60	8	8,913	117	24	7,722
Radiology: Nuclear Medicine	4	3	*	10	7	5,592
Rheumatology	6	2	*	98	57	4,068
Sleep Medicine	0	*	*	2	2	*
Surgery: General	52	8	8,058	322	86	6,562
Surg: Cardiovascular	21	6	11,770	49	21	6,975
Surg: Cardiovascular-Pediatric	1	1	*	0	*	*
Surg: Colon and Rectal	0	*	*	9	5	*
Surg: Neurological	19	3	10,092	48	22	7,393
Surg: Oncology	0	*	*	1	1	*
Surg: Oral	0	*	*	1	1	*
Surg: Pediatric	1	1	*	6	4	*
Surg: Plastic & Reconstruction	3	2	*	41	25	6,002
Surg: Plastic & Recon-Hand	0	*	*	3	2	*
Surg: Plastic & Recon-Pediatric	0	*	*	0	*	*
Surg: Thoracic (primary)	18	2	*	4	3	*
Surg: Transplant	0	*	*	7	5	*
Surg: Trauma	3	1	*	8	3	*
Surg: Trauma-Burn	1	1	*	1	1	*
Surg: Vascular (primary)	3	1	*	33	15	7,311
Urgent Care	3	1	*	192	49	4,427
Urology	24	4	7,775	127	52	6,468
Urology: Pediatric	1	1	*	9	1	*

     MEDICAL GROUP MANAGEMENT ASSOCIATION™

Table 60: Physician Work RVUs (CMS RBRVS Method) by Hospital Ownership

	Hospital Owned			Non-hospital Owned		
	Physicians	Medical Practices	Median	Physicians	Medical Practices	Median
Allergy/Immunology	16	12	3,301	51	30	3,864
Cardiology: Electrophysiology	4	3	*	30	20	8,319
Cardiology: Invasive	29	8	7,626	148	45	7,600
Cardiology: Inv-Intervntnl	48	10	9,121	190	48	8,802
Cardiology: Noninvasive	36	11	6,512	138	45	6,083
Critical Care: Intensivist	10	4	4,062	6	4	*
Dentistry	0	*	*	3	1	*
Dermatology	39	20	6,004	96	42	7,217
Dermatology: MOHS Surgery	2	2	*	5	5	*
Emergency Medicine	68	8	4,452	91	12	4,911
Endocrinology/Metabolism	46	23	3,957	49	33	3,989
Family Practice (w/ OB)	281	40	3,924	418	50	4,216
Family Practice (w/o OB)	1,080	69	3,836	779	86	4,061
Family Practice: Sports Med	5	4	*	5	2	*
Gastroenterology	61	22	7,084	169	55	7,849
Gastroenterology: Hepatology	*	*	*	21	4	8,808
Geriatrics	9	4	*	16	6	3,977
Hematology/Oncology	36	13	3,341	109	35	4,351
Hem/Onc: Oncology (only)	6	3	*	27	10	3,867
Infectious Disease	17	11	3,555	43	24	4,430
Internal Medicine: General	706	62	3,809	933	88	3,990
Internal Med: Hospitalist	117	19	3,230	49	17	3,654
Internal Med: Pediatric	19	9	3,617	14	5	3,891
Nephrology	32	11	5,174	56	25	6,618
Neurology	47	20	4,190	160	48	4,390
OBGYN: General	193	38	5,808	317	53	6,621
OBGYN: Gynecology (only)	55	12	5,156	21	16	4,098
OBGYN: Gyn Oncology	5	3	*	5	3	*
OBGYN: Maternal & Fetal Med	22	6	7,923	11	4	5,343
OBGYN: Repro Endocrinology	4	2	*	2	2	*
Occupational Medicine	11	5	2,801	19	14	3,475
Ophthalmology	37	15	7,047	120	39	7,658
Ophthalmology: Pediatric	1	1	*	6	4	*
Ophthalmology: Retina	1	1	*	9	5	*
Orthopedic (Non-surgical)	7	5	*	11	6	8,968
Orthopedic Surgery: General	50	18	6,973	218	53	7,220
Ortho Surg: Foot & Ankle	*	*	*	13	11	7,101
Ortho Surg: Hand	3	3	*	25	19	6,886
Ortho Surg: Hip & Joint	3	1	*	28	15	7,412
Ortho Surg: Oncology	*	*	*	0	*	*
Ortho Surg: Pediatric	4	2	*	6	5	*
Ortho Surg: Spine	3	3	*	22	15	8,454
Ortho Surg: Trauma	4	1	*	3	2	*
Ortho Surg: Sports Med	9	6	*	51	21	6,706
Otorhinolaryngology	44	17	6,393	101	43	6,202
Otorhinolaryngology: Pediatric	*	*	*	0	*	*
Pathology: Anatomic & Clinical	18	4	3,946	31	10	5,910
Pathology: Anatomic	3	1	*	12	4	4,605
Pathology: Clinical	8	3	*	26	3	4,325

Table 60: Physician Work RVUs (CMS RBRVS Method) by Hospital Ownership (continued)

	Hospital Owned			Non-hospital Owned		
	Physicians	Medical Practices	Median	Physicians	Medical Practices	Median
Pediatrics: General	311	45	4,152	351	60	4,250
Ped: Adolescent Medicine	8	3	*	51	3	4,041
Ped: Allergy/Immunology	2	2	*	4	4	*
Ped: Cardiology	4	1	*	19	9	4,683
Ped: Child Development	3	3	*	6	2	*
Ped: Critical Care/Intensivist	2	1	*	12	6	3,906
Ped: Emergency Medicine	0	*	*	*	*	*
Ped: Endocrinology	5	5	*	3	3	*
Ped: Gastroenterology	5	3	*	1	1	*
Ped: Genetics	1	1	*	2	1	*
Ped: Hematology/Oncology	6	3	*	5	5	*
Ped: Hospitalist	2	1	*	2	2	*
Ped: Infectious Disease	2	1	*	1	1	*
Ped: Neonatal Medicine	22	7	6,288	11	5	4,616
Ped: Nephrology	2	2	*	1	1	*
Ped: Neurology	10	6	4,123	8	4	*
Ped: Pulmonology	4	3	*	2	2	*
Ped: Rheumatology	*	*	*	0	*	*
Ped: Sports Medicine	*	*	*	0	*	*
Physiatry (Phys Med & Rehab)	28	11	4,111	39	21	4,363
Podiatry: General	31	14	3,830	33	20	4,418
Podiatry: Surg-Foot & Ankle	6	4	*	13	7	4,836
Podiatry: Surg-Forefoot Only	0	*	*	4	3	*
Psychiatry: General	55	20	3,453	76	17	3,451
Psychiatry: Child & Adolescent	8	5	*	8	5	*
Psychiatry: Geriatric	2	2	*	5	2	*
Pulmonary Medicine	35	17	5,392	97	36	5,788
Pulmonary Med: Critical Care	9	4	*	40	12	5,699
Radiation Oncology	12	6	8,014	28	11	9,084
Radiology: Diagnostic-Inv	29	7	7,726	130	18	10,207
Radiology: Diagnostic-Noninv	39	7	6,091	138	25	8,527
Radiology: Nuclear Medicine	7	3	*	7	7	*
Rheumatology	39	21	4,072	64	37	4,158
Sleep Medicine	1	1	*	1	1	*
Surgery: General	109	32	6,127	260	61	7,208
Surg: Cardiovascular	18	8	6,741	52	19	9,738
Surg: Cardiovascular-Pediatric	0	*	*	1	1	*
Surg: Colon and Rectal	0	*	*	9	5	*
Surg: Neurological	19	10	8,653	48	15	8,243
Surg: Oncology	*	*	*	1	1	*
Surg: Oral	0	*	*	1	1	*
Surg: Pediatric	5	3	*	2	2	*
Surg: Plastic & Reconstruction	13	7	5,879	31	20	6,002
Surg: Plastic & Recon-Hand	1	1	*	2	1	*
Surg: Plastic & Recon-Pediatric	*	*	*	0	*	*
Surg: Thoracic (primary)	1	1	*	21	4	11,412
Surg: Transplant	4	3	*	3	2	*
Surg: Trauma	9	3	*	2	1	*
Surg: Trauma-Burn	1	1	*	1	1	*
Surg: Vascular (primary)	13	8	7,317	23	8	6,646
Urgent Care	70	18	4,258	125	32	4,472
Urology	31	15	6,534	118	40	6,675
Urology: Pediatric	9	1	*	1	1	*

Table 61: Physician Work RVUs (CMS RBRVS Method) by Percent of Capitation Revenue

	No capitation		10% or less		11% to 50%		51% or more	
	Physicians	Median	Physicians	Median	Physicians	Median	Physicians	Median
Allergy/Immunology	27	4,310	18	3,911	15	3,343	7	*
Cardiology: Electrophysiology	17	9,508	11	8,045	5	*	1	*
Cardiology: Invasive	109	7,868	46	7,357	18	6,718	4	*
Cardiology: Inv-Intervntnl	166	8,805	56	8,838	12	9,358	3	*
Cardiology: Noninvasive	90	6,042	41	7,019	37	5,385	13	5,749
Critical Care: Intensivist	1	*	5	*	7	*	3	*
Dentistry	0	*	3	*	0	*	0	*
Dermatology	58	6,328	36	6,801	34	6,806	9	*
Dermatology: MOHS Surgery	4	*	3	*	0	*	0	*
Emergency Medicine	45	4,927	54	5,484	60	4,074	0	*
Endocrinology/Metabolism	37	3,807	26	4,146	26	3,667	5	*
Family Practice (w/ OB)	258	4,216	230	4,333	206	3,658	4	*
Family Practice (w/o OB)	800	3,915	444	3,968	497	3,842	105	4,449
Family Practice: Sports Med	4	*	4	*	2	*	*	*
Gastroenterology	123	7,977	47	7,209	50	6,887	13	8,140
Gastroenterology: Hepatology	21	8,808	0	*	0	*	0	*
Geriatrics	1	*	9	*	15	4,070	0	*
Hematology/Oncology	62	4,190	41	3,720	30	3,673	5	*
Hem/Onc: Oncology (only)	21	4,198	0	*	8	*	4	*
Infectious Disease	24	3,727	19	4,886	15	3,977	2	*
Internal Medicine: General	667	3,746	419	4,041	447	3,947	140	3,660
Internal Med: Hospitalist	82	3,196	60	3,412	10	3,516	14	*
Internal Med: Pediatric	15	3,606	14	4,278	4	*	0	*
Nephrology	39	6,812	27	5,518	20	5,004	1	*
Neurology	98	4,832	46	4,036	52	4,290	13	3,941
OBGYN: General	221	6,281	114	6,498	145	6,090	51	5,336
OBGYN: Gynecology (only)	56	5,220	7	*	8	*	5	*
OBGYN: Gyn Oncology	1	*	6	*	3	*	*	*
OBGYN: Maternal & Fetal Med	21	7,016	4	*	8	*	*	*
OBGYN: Repro Endocrinology	3	*	1	*	2	*	2	*
Occupational Medicine	18	2,942	2	*	7	*	3	*
Ophthalmology	74	7,287	35	8,135	33	7,047	20	7,300
Ophthalmology: Pediatric	4	*	1	*	2	*	0	*
Ophthalmology: Retina	5	*	2	*	3	*	0	*
Orthopedic (Non-surgical)	7	*	4	*	1	*	6	*
Orthopedic Surgery: General	150	7,297	55	6,590	55	7,028	12	7,091
Ortho Surg: Foot & Ankle	8	*	2	*	3	*	*	*
Ortho Surg: Hand	18	6,714	3	*	6	*	1	*
Ortho Surg: Hip & Joint	24	7,526	4	*	2	*	1	*
Ortho Surg: Oncology	0	*	*	*	*	*	*	*
Ortho Surg: Pediatric	5	*	3	*	2	*	0	*
Ortho Surg: Spine	18	8,109	1	*	5	*	1	*
Ortho Surg: Trauma	4	*	*	*	5	*	*	*
Ortho Surg: Sports Med	49	7,227	6	*	5	*	3	*
Otorhinolaryngology	60	6,470	34	6,543	41	6,124	12	5,468
Otorhinolaryngology: Pediatric	0	*	*	*	*	*	*	*
Pathology: Anatomic & Clinical	12	4,605	23	5,850	11	6,112	3	*
Pathology: Anatomic	12	4,471	0	*	3	*	*	*
Pathology: Clinical	4	*	4	*	26	4,260	*	*

Table 61: Physician Work RVUs (CMS RBRVS Method) by Percent of Capitation Revenue (continued)

	No capitation		10% or less		11% to 50%		51% or more	
	Physicians	Median	Physicians	Median	Physicians	Median	Physicians	Median
Pediatrics: General	273	4,208	129	3,896	217	4,439	57	4,033
Ped: Adolescent Medicine	13	*	31	4,041	15	*	*	*
Ped: Allergy/Immunology	1	*	1	*	4	*	*	*
Ped: Cardiology	7	*	9	*	7	*	0	*
Ped: Child Development	1	*	2	*	6	*	*	*
Ped: Critical Care/Intensivist	1	*	6	*	7	*	*	*
Ped: Emergency Medicine	0	*	*	*	*	*	*	*
Ped: Endocrinology	3	*	2	*	3	*	*	*
Ped: Gastroenterology	1	*	1	*	4	*	*	*
Ped: Genetics	2	*	1	*	*	*	*	*
Ped: Hematology/Oncology	4	*	5	*	2	*	0	*
Ped: Hospitalist	0	*	2	*	2	*	0	*
Ped: Infectious Disease	*	*	3	*	*	*	*	*
Ped: Neonatal Medicine	9	*	13	8,362	11	5,028	0	*
Ped: Nephrology	0	*	1	*	2	*	*	*
Ped: Neurology	8	*	4	*	6	*	*	*
Ped: Pulmonology	1	*	1	*	4	*	*	*
Ped: Rheumatology	*	*	0	*	0	*	*	*
Ped: Sports Medicine	0	*	*	*	*	*	*	*
Physiatry (Phys Med & Rehab)	35	3,808	15	5,002	15	3,884	2	*
Podiatry: General	28	3,973	15	4,168	14	4,044	9	*
Podiatry: Surg-Foot & Ankle	5	*	6	*	5	*	3	*
Podiatry: Surg-Forefoot Only	1	*	3	*	*	*	0	*
Psychiatry: General	38	3,718	37	3,453	52	3,060	14	3,516
Psychiatry: Child & Adolescent	5	*	6	*	4	*	1	*
Psychiatry: Geriatric	4	*	1	*	1	*	*	*
Pulmonary Medicine	54	5,912	37	6,433	35	4,539	6	*
Pulmonary Med: Critical Care	38	5,627	3	*	8	*	0	*
Radiation Oncology	21	8,359	7	*	11	8,756	1	*
Radiology: Diagnostic-Inv	79	9,697	17	8,454	57	10,833	6	*
Radiology: Diagnostic-Noninv	90	8,521	36	8,451	51	6,445	0	*
Radiology: Nuclear Medicine	5	*	4	*	3	*	1	*
Rheumatology	44	4,013	33	4,716	19	3,924	7	*
Sleep Medicine	2	*	0	*	0	*	*	*
Surgery: General	190	7,151	84	7,160	78	6,242	21	6,866
Surg: Cardiovascular	29	9,721	15	9,004	24	8,041	2	*
Surg: Cardiovascular-Pediatric	0	*	1	*	0	*	*	*
Surg: Colon and Rectal	0	*	4	*	4	*	0	*
Surg: Neurological	41	8,653	14	6,798	12	7,034	0	*
Surg: Oncology	1	*	*	*	0	*	*	*
Surg: Oral	1	*	0	*	0	*	0	*
Surg: Pediatric	0	*	2	*	5	*	*	*
Surg: Plastic & Reconstruction	13	6,053	14	6,206	16	5,595	1	*
Surg: Plastic & Recon-Hand	1	*	*	*	2	*	*	*
Surg: Plastic & Recon-Pediatric	0	*	0	*	*	*	*	*
Surg: Thoracic (primary)	21	11,412	1	*	0	*	0	*
Surg: Transplant	1	*	3	*	3	*	*	*
Surg: Trauma	3	*	3	*	5	*	*	*
Surg: Trauma-Burn	0	*	1	*	1	*	*	*
Surg: Vascular (primary)	14	6,944	7	*	15	6,646	0	*
Urgent Care	83	4,817	53	3,578	41	4,085	16	5,328
Urology	77	6,728	38	6,589	27	6,593	9	*
Urology: Pediatric	1	*	0	*	9	*	*	*

Table 62: Physician Compensation per Physician Work RVU (CMS RBRVS Method)

	Physicians	Medical Practices	Mean	Std. Dev.	25th %tile	Median	75th %tile	90th %tile
Allergy/Immunology	65	41	$67.81	$27.55	$45.72	$67.91	$88.93	$108.27
Cardiology: Electrophysiology	34	23	$40.26	$10.85	$31.41	$37.32	$47.38	$53.91
Cardiology: Invasive	176	53	$51.92	$20.70	$38.27	$48.11	$60.20	$73.90
Cardiology: Inv-Intervntnl	236	57	$50.13	$18.43	$38.67	$47.51	$57.27	$70.52
Cardiology: Noninvasive	180	57	$50.84	$18.51	$38.93	$48.68	$58.82	$69.86
Critical Care: Intensivist	16	8	$53.12	$21.39	$37.36	$47.59	$61.55	$95.87
Dentistry	3	1	*	*	*	*	*	*
Dermatology	134	62	$42.39	$14.68	$33.93	$39.45	$47.78	$55.84
Dermatology: MOHS Surgery	6	6	*	*	*	*	*	*
Emergency Medicine	159	20	$48.73	$20.44	$35.96	$43.34	$54.09	$79.41
Endocrinology/Metabolism	95	56	$45.77	$14.75	$37.35	$42.88	$52.46	$64.10
Family Practice (w/ OB)	699	90	$40.60	$8.73	$34.87	$39.77	$44.81	$51.16
Family Practice (w/o OB)	1,847	154	$39.69	$9.77	$34.20	$38.51	$43.41	$50.13
Family Practice: Sports Med	10	6	$46.89	$13.32	$37.18	$41.87	$53.84	$75.33
Gastroenterology	228	76	$45.98	$15.31	$35.45	$42.67	$52.12	$67.27
Gastroenterology: Hepatology	21	4	$39.85	$8.18	$34.03	$39.07	$47.13	$49.12
Geriatrics	25	10	$42.35	$10.64	$34.10	$41.38	$50.54	$57.32
Hematology/Oncology	136	48	$84.56	$39.08	$55.75	$76.06	$100.43	$143.97
Hem/Onc: Oncology (only)	33	13	$89.48	$37.74	$59.66	$83.25	$110.99	$142.74
Infectious Disease	60	35	$44.84	$18.36	$32.63	$43.55	$57.97	$68.88
Internal Medicine: General	1,680	150	$42.29	$13.05	$34.81	$40.06	$46.27	$56.06
Internal Med: Hospitalist	166	36	$51.13	$16.95	$42.08	$49.71	$56.77	$68.81
Internal Med: Pediatric	33	14	$42.18	$13.38	$33.60	$39.34	$45.06	$68.09
Nephrology	87	35	$39.16	$13.34	$31.48	$39.57	$43.44	$52.93
Neurology	207	68	$47.91	$18.96	$35.66	$43.97	$55.73	$72.60
OBGYN: General	529	91	$42.50	$15.25	$33.96	$40.17	$46.64	$54.45
OBGYN: Gynecology (only)	76	28	$45.84	$15.39	$40.17	$42.40	$47.01	$62.83
OBGYN: Gyn Oncology	10	6	$65.51	$23.64	$51.06	$61.05	$68.08	$121.83
OBGYN: Maternal & Fetal Med	32	10	$62.35	$27.67	$42.90	$57.26	$80.60	$94.44
OBGYN: Repro Endocrinology	8	5	*	*	*	*	*	*
Occupational Medicine	30	19	$55.96	$22.76	$36.62	$50.27	$67.33	$101.72
Ophthalmology	159	54	$40.03	$16.79	$31.50	$36.20	$46.13	$56.84
Ophthalmology: Pediatric	7	5	*	*	*	*	*	*
Ophthalmology: Retina	10	6	$41.76	$11.22	$31.35	$44.23	$52.67	$55.85
Orthopedic (Non-surgical)	18	11	$43.16	$10.30	$35.56	$37.96	$51.15	$63.01
Orthopedic Surgery: General	267	71	$53.73	$23.27	$42.67	$49.85	$58.73	$68.04
Ortho Surg: Foot & Ankle	13	11	$55.36	$23.31	$36.73	$49.32	$64.51	$102.10
Ortho Surg: Hand	28	22	$61.49	$28.08	$41.06	$56.30	$76.05	$102.07
Ortho Surg: Hip & Joint	31	16	$50.75	$22.27	$38.90	$46.73	$57.03	$64.92
Ortho Surg: Oncology	0	*	*	*	*	*	*	*
Ortho Surg: Pediatric	10	7	$49.01	$26.30	$32.73	$37.71	$66.50	$105.06
Ortho Surg: Spine	22	17	$50.04	$17.02	$33.79	$52.31	$65.23	$70.51
Ortho Surg: Trauma	9	4	*	*	*	*	*	*
Ortho Surg: Sports Med	62	28	$53.34	$20.08	$37.88	$49.07	$66.96	$84.04
Otorhinolaryngology	146	60	$49.94	$20.37	$39.64	$45.87	$55.15	$67.91
Otorhinolaryngology: Pediatric	0	*	*	*	*	*	*	*
Pathology: Anatomic & Clinical	49	14	$61.93	$33.31	$37.60	$48.19	$75.48	$131.14
Pathology: Anatomic	15	5	$58.95	$32.06	$37.47	$47.40	$74.76	$107.60
Pathology: Clinical	34	6	$38.81	$14.20	$28.92	$35.28	$42.65	$67.21

Table 62: Physician Compensation per Physician Work RVU (CMS RBRVS Method) (continued)

	Physicians	Medical Practices	Mean	Std. Dev.	25th %tile	Median	75th %tile	90th %tile
Pediatrics: General	673	105	$38.94	$11.13	$31.77	$37.33	$43.71	$50.96
Ped: Adolescent Medicine	59	6	$36.47	$8.62	$31.98	$35.57	$38.44	$42.65
Ped: Allergy/Immunology	6	6	*	*	*	*	*	*
Ped: Cardiology	23	10	$56.13	$21.27	$38.62	$54.85	$71.38	$87.80
Ped: Child Development	9	5	*	*	*	*	*	*
Ped: Critical Care/Intensivist	14	7	$50.32	$16.58	$37.19	$46.97	$59.23	$82.40
Ped: Emergency Medicine	0	*	*	*	*	*	*	*
Ped: Endocrinology	8	8	*	*	*	*	*	*
Ped: Gastroenterology	6	4	*	*	*	*	*	*
Ped: Genetics	3	2	*	*	*	*	*	*
Ped: Hematology/Oncology	11	8	$59.50	$10.23	$53.47	$58.93	$68.18	$76.10
Ped: Hospitalist	4	3	*	*	*	*	*	*
Ped: Infectious Disease	3	2	*	*	*	*	*	*
Ped: Neonatal Medicine	33	12	$46.32	$17.89	$33.42	$45.71	$59.35	$73.52
Ped: Nephrology	3	3	*	*	*	*	*	*
Ped: Neurology	18	10	$48.68	$19.01	$38.98	$41.71	$50.27	$89.37
Ped: Pulmonology	6	5	*	*	*	*	*	*
Ped: Rheumatology	0	*	*	*	*	*	*	*
Ped: Sports Medicine	0	*	*	*	*	*	*	*
Physiatry (Phys Med & Rehab)	67	32	$52.52	$16.92	$38.53	$49.88	$67.13	$76.13
Podiatry: General	65	34	$38.55	$9.65	$31.50	$36.49	$44.80	$54.06
Podiatry: Surg-Foot & Ankle	19	11	$36.85	$13.25	$23.86	$36.31	$41.77	$61.26
Podiatry: Surg-Forefoot Only	4	3	*	*	*	*	*	*
Psychiatry: General	140	38	$49.34	$17.91	$38.84	$45.06	$54.09	$70.54
Psychiatry: Child & Adolescent	15	10	$51.60	$13.84	$40.30	$48.67	$61.94	$77.30
Psychiatry: Geriatric	7	4	*	*	*	*	*	*
Pulmonary Medicine	130	52	$42.18	$16.73	$31.95	$38.31	$46.48	$66.38
Pulmonary Med: Critical Care	49	16	$48.08	$30.49	$33.48	$37.22	$51.79	$63.11
Radiation Oncology	40	17	$47.05	$22.46	$34.00	$41.12	$50.99	$81.42
Radiology: Diagnostic-Inv	157	24	$43.86	$14.12	$33.63	$42.83	$52.50	$67.13
Radiology: Diagnostic-Noninv	177	32	$54.13	$24.09	$40.74	$50.50	$62.07	$79.01
Radiology: Nuclear Medicine	14	10	$47.61	$16.31	$38.10	$44.50	$55.95	$78.12
Rheumatology	103	58	$48.42	$19.68	$35.96	$44.44	$54.32	$69.29
Sleep Medicine	2	2	*	*	*	*	*	*
Surgery: General	369	93	$42.94	$12.25	$34.65	$41.65	$48.46	$57.79
Surg: Cardiovascular	70	27	$57.12	$25.36	$41.80	$52.55	$64.85	$89.12
Surg: Cardiovascular-Pediatric	1	1	*	*	*	*	*	*
Surg: Colon and Rectal	9	5	*	*	*	*	*	*
Surg: Neurological	67	25	$57.76	$19.45	$45.97	$53.03	$65.51	$88.37
Surg: Oncology	1	1	*	*	*	*	*	*
Surg: Oral	0	*	*	*	*	*	*	*
Surg: Pediatric	6	4	*	*	*	*	*	*
Surg: Plastic & Reconstruction	44	27	$52.66	$21.81	$35.77	$50.01	$66.06	$88.27
Surg: Plastic & Recon-Hand	3	2	*	*	*	*	*	*
Surg: Plastic & Recon-Pediatric	0	*	*	*	*	*	*	*
Surg: Thoracic (primary)	22	5	$48.12	$18.20	$30.54	$51.46	$60.18	$71.02
Surg: Transplant	7	5	*	*	*	*	*	*
Surg: Trauma	11	4	$59.17	$33.89	$34.33	$50.97	$71.66	$132.57
Surg: Trauma-Burn	2	2	*	*	*	*	*	*
Surg: Vascular (primary)	36	16	$47.49	$14.85	$36.60	$43.71	$52.65	$70.87
Urgent Care	195	50	$41.43	$12.58	$32.88	$38.38	$46.78	$57.13
Urology	148	55	$50.51	$20.37	$39.66	$47.33	$55.45	$71.06
Urology: Pediatric	10	2	*	*	*	*	*	*

MEDICAL GROUP MANAGEMENT ASSOCIATION™

Table 63: Physician Compensation per Physician Work RVU (CMS RBRVS Method) by Group Type

	Single-specialty			Multispecialty		
	Physicians	Medical Practices	Median	Physicians	Medical Practices	Median
Allergy/Immunology	2	1	*	63	40	$67.67
Cardiology: Electrophysiology	17	12	$38.93	17	11	$37.30
Cardiology: Invasive	88	21	$48.55	88	32	$47.85
Cardiology: Inv-Intervntnl	139	28	$44.99	97	29	$50.86
Cardiology: Noninvasive	76	22	$49.70	104	35	$47.63
Critical Care: Intensivist	0	*	*	16	8	$47.59
Dentistry	0	*	*	3	1	*
Dermatology	4	1	*	130	61	$39.45
Dermatology: MOHS Surgery	0	*	*	6	6	*
Emergency Medicine	33	3	$37.50	126	17	$44.10
Endocrinology/Metabolism	2	2	*	93	54	$42.55
Family Practice (w/ OB)	82	18	$39.29	617	72	$39.95
Family Practice (w/o OB)	143	29	$35.78	1,704	125	$38.69
Family Practice: Sports Med	5	2	*	5	4	*
Gastroenterology	37	7	$48.02	191	69	$42.38
Gastroenterology: Hepatology	18	3	$39.01	3	1	*
Geriatrics	0	*	*	25	10	$41.38
Hematology/Oncology	28	6	$99.77	108	42	$72.86
Hem/Onc: Oncology (only)	11	2	*	22	11	$68.53
Infectious Disease	12	5	$25.99	48	30	$44.16
Internal Medicine: General	68	17	$45.05	1,612	133	$40.00
Internal Med: Hospitalist	0	*	*	166	36	$49.71
Internal Med: Pediatric	0	*	*	33	14	$39.34
Nephrology	14	3	$27.41	73	32	$39.96
Neurology	53	9	$48.27	154	59	$41.63
OBGYN: General	57	6	$37.50	472	85	$40.28
OBGYN: Gynecology (only)	3	2	*	73	26	$42.21
OBGYN: Gyn Oncology	0	*	*	10	6	$61.05
OBGYN: Maternal & Fetal Med	3	1	*	29	9	$54.92
OBGYN: Repro Endocrinology	1	1	*	7	4	*
Occupational Medicine	0	*	*	30	19	$50.27
Ophthalmology	23	3	$40.58	136	51	$35.68
Ophthalmology: Pediatric	3	1	*	4	4	*
Ophthalmology: Retina	5	2	*	5	4	*
Orthopedic (Non-surgical)	0	*	*	18	11	$37.96
Orthopedic Surgery: General	82	17	$49.14	185	54	$50.40
Ortho Surg: Foot & Ankle	8	7	*	5	4	*
Ortho Surg: Hand	14	11	$56.30	14	11	$56.20
Ortho Surg: Hip & Joint	18	9	$44.04	13	7	$52.77
Ortho Surg: Oncology	0	*	*	0	*	*
Ortho Surg: Pediatric	6	3	*	4	4	*
Ortho Surg: Spine	11	8	$53.03	11	9	$51.59
Ortho Surg: Trauma	4	2	*	5	2	*
Ortho Surg: Sports Med	32	13	$56.20	30	15	$43.93
Otorhinolaryngology	1	1	*	145	59	$45.88
Otorhinolaryngology: Pediatric	0	*	*	0	*	*
Pathology: Anatomic & Clinical	6	1	*	43	13	$47.64
Pathology: Anatomic	5	1	*	10	4	$39.17
Pathology: Clinical	2	1	*	32	5	$35.68

Table 63: Physician Compensation per Physician Work RVU (CMS RBRVS Method) by Group Type (continued)

	Single-specialty			Multispecialty		
	Physicians	Medical Practices	Median	Physicians	Medical Practices	Median
Pediatrics: General	42	8	$37.76	631	97	$37.31
Ped: Adolescent Medicine	0	*	*	59	6	$35.57
Ped: Allergy/Immunology	0	*	*	6	6	*
Ped: Cardiology	7	2	*	16	8	$56.33
Ped: Child Development	*	*	*	9	5	*
Ped: Critical Care/Intensivist	0	*	*	14	7	$46.97
Ped: Emergency Medicine	0	*	*	0	*	*
Ped: Endocrinology	1	1	*	7	7	*
Ped: Gastroenterology	0	*	*	6	4	*
Ped: Genetics	*	*	*	3	2	*
Ped: Hematology/Oncology	3	1	*	8	7	*
Ped: Hospitalist	0	*	*	4	3	*
Ped: Infectious Disease	0	*	*	3	2	*
Ped: Neonatal Medicine	0	*	*	33	12	$45.71
Ped: Nephrology	0	*	*	3	3	*
Ped: Neurology	3	1	*	15	9	$40.69
Ped: Pulmonology	0	*	*	6	5	*
Ped: Rheumatology	0	*	*	0	*	*
Ped: Sports Medicine	*	*	*	0	*	*
Physiatry (Phys Med & Rehab)	8	4	*	59	28	$48.44
Podiatry: General	0	*	*	65	34	$36.49
Podiatry: Surg-Foot & Ankle	0	*	*	19	11	$36.31
Podiatry: Surg-Forefoot Only	1	1	*	3	2	*
Psychiatry: General	0	*	*	140	38	$45.06
Psychiatry: Child & Adolescent	0	*	*	15	10	$48.67
Psychiatry: Geriatric	*	*	*	7	4	*
Pulmonary Medicine	6	3	*	124	49	$37.60
Pulmonary Med: Critical Care	20	4	$35.01	29	12	$45.97
Radiation Oncology	14	4	$38.94	26	13	$41.12
Radiology: Diagnostic-Inv	77	8	$35.40	80	16	$47.77
Radiology: Diagnostic-Noninv	60	8	$49.10	117	24	$52.23
Radiology: Nuclear Medicine	4	3	*	10	7	$44.50
Rheumatology	6	2	*	97	56	$45.41
Sleep Medicine	0	*	*	2	2	*
Surgery: General	52	8	$38.11	317	85	$42.24
Surg: Cardiovascular	21	6	$41.27	49	21	$59.04
Surg: Cardiovascular-Pediatric	1	1	*	0	*	*
Surg: Colon and Rectal	0	*	*	9	5	*
Surg: Neurological	19	3	$54.52	48	22	$52.49
Surg: Oncology	0	*	*	1	1	*
Surg: Oral	0	*	*	0	*	*
Surg: Pediatric	0	*	*	6	4	*
Surg: Plastic & Reconstruction	3	2	*	41	25	$47.55
Surg: Plastic & Recon-Hand	0	*	*	3	2	*
Surg: Plastic & Recon-Pediatric	0	*	*	0	*	*
Surg: Thoracic (primary)	18	2	*	4	3	*
Surg: Transplant	0	*	*	7	5	*
Surg: Trauma	3	1	*	8	3	*
Surg: Trauma-Burn	1	1	*	1	1	*
Surg: Vascular (primary)	3	1	*	33	15	$42.13
Urgent Care	3	1	*	192	49	$38.38
Urology	23	4	$52.83	125	51	$45.79
Urology: Pediatric	1	1	*	9	1	*

THIS PAGE INTENTIONALLY LEFT BLANK

PHYSICIAN TIME WORKED

Table 64: Physician Weeks Worked per Year

	Physicians	Medical Practices	Mean	Std. Dev.	25th %tile	Median	75th %tile	90th %tile
Allergy/Immunology	135	68	46.89	2.46	46.00	48.00	48.00	49.00
Anesthesiology	1,322	88	44.31	2.70	42.80	44.00	46.00	48.00
Anesth: Pain Management	81	30	44.77	2.89	44.00	45.00	46.50	48.00
Anesth: Pediatric	34	5	44.91	2.78	43.00	43.00	47.00	50.00
Cardiology: Electrophysiology	130	73	45.25	2.70	44.00	46.00	47.00	48.90
Cardiology: Invasive	482	125	45.43	2.32	44.00	46.00	47.00	48.00
Cardiology: Inv-Intervntnl	607	139	45.48	2.37	44.00	46.00	47.00	48.00
Cardiology: Noninvasive	442	132	45.89	2.29	44.00	46.00	48.00	49.00
Critical Care: Intensivist	15	8	46.74	1.28	46.00	46.00	48.00	48.52
Dentistry	21	6	45.73	1.96	45.00	45.00	47.50	48.34
Dermatology	205	104	46.36	2.55	45.00	46.00	48.00	49.00
Dermatology: MOHS Surgery	19	17	46.78	1.77	46.00	47.00	48.00	48.10
Emergency Medicine	269	26	45.20	2.30	44.00	45.60	47.00	48.00
Endocrinology/Metabolism	142	83	46.57	2.12	46.00	47.00	48.00	48.00
Family Practice (w/ OB)	943	184	46.53	2.16	46.00	47.00	48.00	49.00
Family Practice (w/o OB)	3,335	441	46.58	2.06	46.00	47.00	48.00	49.00
Family Practice: Sports Med	25	19	46.22	2.94	45.80	46.00	48.00	49.40
Gastroenterology	506	153	46.38	2.24	45.00	47.00	48.00	49.00
Gastroenterology: Hepatology	70	15	46.56	1.35	46.00	47.00	47.25	48.00
Geriatrics	36	20	46.24	2.35	44.47	46.05	48.00	48.60
Hematology/Oncology	284	98	46.25	2.17	45.65	46.00	48.00	48.00
Hem/Onc: Oncology (only)	72	28	46.64	1.40	46.00	46.00	47.00	48.00
Infectious Disease	102	51	46.48	2.09	46.00	46.00	48.00	49.00
Internal Medicine: General	2,888	370	46.70	1.97	46.00	47.00	48.00	49.00
Internal Med: Hospitalist	257	55	46.85	1.84	46.00	46.00	48.00	49.00
Internal Med: Pediatric	78	31	47.54	1.97	46.00	48.00	48.25	50.00
Nephrology	176	65	45.91	2.07	45.00	46.00	47.00	48.00
Neurology	373	116	46.63	2.10	45.00	47.00	48.00	49.00
OBGYN: General	1,035	230	46.49	2.13	46.00	46.60	48.00	48.80
OBGYN: Gynecology (only)	164	62	46.01	2.17	45.00	46.00	48.00	48.00
OBGYN: Gyn Oncology	13	8	47.38	1.39	46.00	48.00	48.50	49.00
OBGYN: Maternal & Fetal Med	38	11	46.34	1.44	46.00	46.00	47.25	48.00
OBGYN: Repro Endocrinology	27	10	46.70	2.18	44.00	48.00	48.00	50.00
Occupational Medicine	90	38	46.22	1.65	46.00	46.00	47.80	48.00
Ophthalmology	373	114	46.19	2.58	45.00	46.00	48.00	49.00
Ophthalmology: Pediatric	19	14	46.32	2.31	45.00	46.00	48.00	49.00
Ophthalmology: Retina	65	24	46.50	1.90	46.00	47.00	48.00	49.00
Orthopedic (Non-surgical)	41	23	46.82	2.18	46.00	47.00	48.00	49.80
Orthopedic Surgery: General	642	181	46.34	2.54	45.00	47.00	48.00	49.00
Ortho Surg: Foot & Ankle	50	43	46.01	2.52	45.00	46.00	48.00	49.00
Ortho Surg: Hand	119	71	46.02	2.82	45.00	46.00	48.00	49.00
Ortho Surg: Hip & Joint	109	57	45.50	3.06	44.00	46.00	48.00	49.00
Ortho Surg: Oncology	3	3	*	*	*	*	*	*
Ortho Surg: Pediatric	38	24	46.88	1.97	46.00	47.45	48.00	49.10
Ortho Surg: Spine	114	71	46.26	2.56	45.00	46.50	48.00	49.00
Ortho Surg: Trauma	23	15	46.48	2.59	44.00	46.00	49.00	50.00
Ortho Surg: Sports Med	188	88	46.21	2.59	45.00	46.25	48.00	49.00
Otorhinolaryngology	310	103	47.09	2.09	46.00	48.00	48.00	49.00
Otorhinolaryngology: Pediatric	14	3	45.36	1.50	43.75	46.00	46.00	47.00
Pathology: Anatomic & Clinical	150	30	45.26	2.50	43.63	46.00	47.00	48.00
Pathology: Anatomic	57	11	45.58	2.56	44.00	45.00	48.00	48.00
Pathology: Clinical	51	13	46.37	2.10	45.00	47.00	48.00	48.00

Table 64: Physician Weeks Worked per Year (continued)

	Physicians	Medical Practices	Mean	Std. Dev.	25th %tile	Median	75th %tile	90th %tile
Pediatrics: General	1,576	271	46.83	1.97	46.00	47.00	48.00	49.00
Ped: Adolescent Medicine	45	10	46.76	1.42	46.00	47.00	48.00	48.00
Ped: Allergy/Immunology	7	5	*	*	*	*	*	*
Ped: Cardiology	37	16	46.43	2.77	45.00	47.00	48.00	48.40
Ped: Child Development	9	5	*	*	*	*	*	*
Ped: Critical Care/Intensivist	55	14	46.02	1.76	44.00	46.00	48.00	48.00
Ped: Emergency Medicine	8	2	*	*	*	*	*	*
Ped: Endocrinology	16	10	47.00	1.51	46.00	48.00	48.00	48.00
Ped: Gastroenterology	15	7	47.33	1.45	47.00	48.00	48.00	48.00
Ped: Genetics	10	4	47.80	1.48	46.00	48.00	48.50	50.00
Ped: Hematology/Oncology	37	15	46.90	1.66	46.00	48.00	48.00	48.00
Ped: Hospitalist	20	9	47.60	1.31	47.00	48.00	48.00	49.80
Ped: Infectious Disease	5	3	*	*	*	*	*	*
Ped: Neonatal Medicine	49	11	46.24	1.39	45.00	46.00	47.50	48.00
Ped: Nephrology	7	4	*	*	*	*	*	*
Ped: Neurology	19	11	46.32	2.11	46.00	47.00	48.00	48.00
Ped: Pulmonology	15	8	45.87	1.81	44.00	46.00	48.00	48.00
Ped: Rheumatology	4	3	*	*	*	*	*	*
Ped: Sports Medicine	1	1	*	*	*	*	*	*
Physiatry (Phys Med & Rehab)	117	60	46.56	2.20	46.00	47.00	48.00	48.00
Podiatry: General	77	43	46.07	1.92	45.00	46.00	48.00	48.00
Podiatry: Surg-Foot & Ankle	39	19	46.71	2.11	45.10	48.00	48.00	49.00
Podiatry: Surg-Forefoot Only	13	4	46.96	1.36	46.00	48.00	48.00	48.30
Psychiatry: General	190	47	45.83	2.00	44.26	46.00	47.00	48.00
Psychiatry: Child & Adolescent	21	12	46.49	1.90	44.60	47.00	48.00	49.60
Psychiatry: Geriatric	11	6	46.00	3.77	44.00	47.00	49.00	49.00
Pulmonary Medicine	209	98	46.57	2.09	45.25	47.00	48.00	49.00
Pulmonary Med: Critical Care	134	39	46.57	2.55	46.00	47.00	48.00	50.00
Radiation Oncology	81	25	43.93	3.60	42.00	45.00	46.00	48.00
Radiology: Diagnostic-Inv	285	44	41.84	3.67	39.00	40.00	45.00	48.00
Radiology: Diagnostic-Noninv	405	68	43.37	2.93	41.00	44.00	45.00	46.76
Radiology: Nuclear Medicine	37	20	45.16	2.39	44.00	45.00	48.00	48.00
Rheumatology	189	102	46.51	2.15	46.00	47.00	48.00	48.00
Sleep Medicine	14	6	46.21	2.01	46.00	46.50	47.25	48.50
Surgery: General	672	199	46.36	2.16	45.00	46.60	48.00	48.20
Surg: Cardiovascular	118	35	45.07	2.81	43.00	45.00	48.00	48.00
Surg: Cardiovascular-Pediatric	5	5	*	*	*	*	*	*
Surg: Colon and Rectal	28	15	45.89	2.48	45.00	46.50	48.00	48.00
Surg: Neurological	157	50	45.88	3.00	45.00	46.80	48.00	49.00
Surg: Oncology	3	3	*	*	*	*	*	*
Surg: Oral	17	7	47.01	1.32	45.50	48.00	48.00	48.00
Surg: Pediatric	14	7	46.43	1.55	45.00	46.00	48.00	48.00
Surg: Plastic & Reconstruction	59	35	46.98	1.59	45.60	47.00	48.00	49.00
Surg: Plastic & Recon-Hand	15	5	45.93	2.15	46.00	46.00	48.00	48.40
Surg: Plastic & Recon-Pediatric	4	2	*	*	*	*	*	*
Surg: Thoracic (primary)	37	13	47.23	1.21	46.30	47.00	48.00	49.00
Surg: Transplant	12	5	47.67	.78	48.00	48.00	48.00	48.00
Surg: Trauma	20	6	46.79	1.59	46.00	48.00	48.00	48.00
Surg: Trauma-Burn	12	5	46.23	2.58	44.50	47.90	48.00	48.00
Surg: Vascular (primary)	97	43	46.01	2.10	44.00	46.00	48.00	48.16
Urgent Care	277	73	46.91	2.18	46.00	47.00	48.00	49.00
Urology	338	103	46.46	2.05	45.00	46.00	48.00	49.00
Urology: Pediatric	13	4	47.85	.55	48.00	48.00	48.00	48.00

Table 65: Physician Weeks Worked per Year by Years in Specialty

	1 to 2 years		3 to 7 years		8 to 17 years		18 years or more	
	Physicians	Median	Physicians	Median	Physicians	Median	Physicians	Median
Allergy/Immunology	6	*	20	48.00	55	48.00	56	48.00
Anesthesiology	109	43.00	209	44.00	499	44.00	260	44.00
Anesth: Pain Management	6	*	15	46.00	39	44.00	12	44.50
Anesth: Pediatric	2	*	7	*	14	43.00	6	*
Cardiology: Electrophysiology	5	*	32	45.00	57	46.00	23	45.00
Cardiology: Invasive	21	46.60	123	46.00	170	46.00	142	46.00
Cardiology: Inv-Intervntnl	21	46.00	101	46.00	250	46.00	211	46.00
Cardiology: Noninvasive	12	45.49	70	45.00	109	46.00	193	46.00
Critical Care: Intensivist	0	*	3	*	6	*	2	*
Dentistry	0	*	1	*	9	*	11	45.00
Dermatology	11	46.00	40	48.00	80	46.15	74	47.00
Dermatology: MOHS Surgery	2	*	6	*	5	*	6	*
Emergency Medicine	39	46.00	78	47.00	110	45.00	68	45.60
Endocrinology/Metabolism	7	*	24	48.00	56	47.00	44	47.00
Family Practice (w/ OB)	97	47.00	299	48.00	343	47.00	247	47.00
Family Practice (w/o OB)	234	47.00	709	47.00	1,080	47.00	1,067	47.00
Family Practice: Sports Med	3	*	4	*	11	48.00	5	*
Gastroenterology	26	48.00	81	47.00	190	47.00	175	46.00
Gastroenterology: Hepatology	3	*	8	*	29	47.00	35	46.00
Geriatrics	3	*	2	*	22	47.50	11	48.00
Hematology/Oncology	10	46.00	52	46.00	96	46.35	104	46.00
Hem/Onc: Oncology (only)	0	*	10	47.00	28	46.00	31	47.00
Infectious Disease	10	48.00	23	47.00	37	47.00	28	46.00
Internal Medicine: General	203	47.00	682	47.00	933	47.00	873	47.00
Internal Med: Hospitalist	46	47.00	94	47.00	85	48.00	35	46.00
Internal Med: Pediatric	16	47.00	35	48.00	17	48.00	5	*
Nephrology	11	47.00	33	46.00	56	46.00	61	46.00
Neurology	23	46.00	82	47.00	141	47.00	105	47.00
OBGYN: General	66	48.00	266	47.00	401	47.00	263	47.00
OBGYN: Gynecology (only)	3	*	11	48.00	42	46.00	102	46.00
OBGYN: Gyn Oncology	2	*	1	*	4	*	4	*
OBGYN: Maternal & Fetal Med	3	*	7	*	16	46.00	14	46.00
OBGYN: Repro Endocrinology	2	*	4	*	10	46.00	4	*
Occupational Medicine	3	*	21	46.37	36	46.00	36	46.15
Ophthalmology	14	45.50	87	47.10	149	46.00	120	46.75
Ophthalmology: Pediatric	*	*	7	*	10	47.50	4	*
Ophthalmology: Retina	2	*	14	46.00	32	47.00	18	46.50
Orthopedic (Non-surgical)	2	*	11	47.00	12	47.00	16	47.50
Orthopedic Surgery: General	32	48.00	109	48.00	216	47.00	287	47.00
Ortho Surg: Foot & Ankle	8	*	17	46.00	23	46.00	5	*
Ortho Surg: Hand	4	*	38	47.00	46	46.00	35	47.00
Ortho Surg: Hip & Joint	3	*	14	46.50	48	46.00	43	46.00
Ortho Surg: Oncology	1	*	*	*	1	*	1	*
Ortho Surg: Pediatric	2	*	14	47.80	15	48.00	7	*
Ortho Surg: Spine	8	*	23	46.00	53	47.00	33	48.00
Ortho Surg: Trauma	1	*	11	48.00	6	*	5	*
Ortho Surg: Sports Med	18	48.00	49	47.00	97	47.00	37	46.00
Otorhinolaryngology	19	48.00	64	48.00	99	48.00	140	48.00
Otorhinolaryngology: Pediatric	1	*	2	*	7	*	6	*
Pathology: Anatomic & Clinical	7	*	26	46.00	52	46.00	67	45.40
Pathology: Anatomic	*	*	10	45.00	18	45.00	26	45.50
Pathology: Clinical	2	*	8	*	18	47.00	23	46.00

Table 65: Physician Weeks Worked per Year by Years in Specialty (continued)

	1 to 2 years		3 to 7 years		8 to 17 years		18 years or more	
	Physicians	Median	Physicians	Median	Physicians	Median	Physicians	Median
Pediatrics: General	96	47.00	360	48.00	512	48.00	525	47.40
Ped: Adolescent Medicine	3	*	12	46.50	14	47.00	11	48.00
Ped: Allergy/Immunology	*	*	1	*	3	*	3	*
Ped: Cardiology	2	*	11	48.00	10	46.00	11	46.00
Ped: Child Development	0	*	2	*	1	*	1	*
Ped: Critical Care/Intensivist	3	*	11	47.00	38	46.00	4	*
Ped: Emergency Medicine	*	*	1	*	5	*	2	*
Ped: Endocrinology	3	*	5	*	3	*	4	*
Ped: Gastroenterology	1	*	7	*	3	*	3	*
Ped: Genetics	1	*	4	*	2	*	3	*
Ped: Hematology/Oncology	0	*	11	48.00	14	48.00	10	46.00
Ped: Hospitalist	3	*	8	*	5	*	5	*
Ped: Infectious Disease	1	*	0	*	3	*	1	*
Ped: Neonatal Medicine	0	*	11	48.00	23	45.00	14	46.50
Ped: Nephrology	*	*	1	*	4	*	1	*
Ped: Neurology	3	*	7	*	6	*	3	*
Ped: Pulmonology	1	*	6	*	6	*	2	*
Ped: Rheumatology	*	*	2	*	2	*	*	*
Ped: Sports Medicine	*	*	*	*	1	*	*	*
Physiatry (Phys Med & Rehab)	11	47.00	30	47.00	51	47.00	19	47.00
Podiatry: General	9	*	19	48.00	28	46.00	19	46.00
Podiatry: Surg-Foot & Ankle	0	*	15	48.00	20	46.50	8	*
Podiatry: Surg-Forefoot Only	1	*	1	*	7	*	4	*
Psychiatry: General	16	46.55	39	45.80	66	45.55	52	45.00
Psychiatry: Child & Adolescent	2	*	5	*	8	*	4	*
Psychiatry: Geriatric	*	*	1	*	5	*	6	*
Pulmonary Medicine	5	*	26	46.00	85	46.80	69	48.00
Pulmonary Med: Critical Care	7	*	25	47.00	58	47.00	37	47.00
Radiation Oncology	3	*	19	45.00	34	45.00	19	44.00
Radiology: Diagnostic-Inv	16	40.00	56	39.00	114	40.00	82	42.00
Radiology: Diagnostic-Noninv	16	44.00	74	43.00	150	44.00	131	44.00
Radiology: Nuclear Medicine	2	*	3	*	11	44.00	19	45.90
Rheumatology	6	*	28	46.95	57	47.00	80	48.00
Sleep Medicine	2	*	3	*	3	*	5	*
Surgery: General	43	47.00	131	46.80	231	47.00	227	47.00
Surg: Cardiovascular	4	*	30	44.00	58	45.00	28	46.00
Surg: Cardiovascular-Pediatric	1	*	1	*	3	*	*	*
Surg: Colon and Rectal	1	*	5	*	11	48.00	10	45.00
Surg: Neurological	10	47.30	39	46.30	57	47.00	44	46.50
Surg: Oncology	*	*	1	*	2	*	*	*
Surg: Oral	1	*	3	*	6	*	6	*
Surg: Pediatric	3	*	5	*	3	*	7	*
Surg: Plastic & Reconstruction	3	*	18	48.00	15	48.00	21	47.00
Surg: Plastic & Recon-Hand	*	*	2	*	8	*	5	*
Surg: Plastic & Recon-Pediatric	*	*	2	*	2	*	*	*
Surg: Thoracic (primary)	1	*	9	*	15	47.00	10	47.00
Surg: Transplant	2	*	1	*	6	*	3	*
Surg: Trauma	2	*	5	*	10	47.00	3	*
Surg: Trauma-Burn	2	*	1	*	2	*	7	*
Surg: Vascular (primary)	6	*	21	47.00	36	45.50	25	46.00
Urgent Care	17	48.00	70	48.00	109	47.00	81	47.00
Urology	18	47.50	61	46.00	123	46.00	130	47.00
Urology: Pediatric	*	*	2	*	2	*	*	*

MEDICAL GROUP MANAGEMENT ASSOCIATION™

Table 66: Physician Hours Worked per Week

	Physicians	Medical Practices	Mean	Std. Dev.	25th %tile	Median	75th %tile	90th %tile
Allergy/Immunology	127	67	39.54	5.39	36.00	40.00	40.00	45.00
Anesthesiology	1,344	91	47.80	8.83	40.00	50.00	55.00	60.00
Anesth: Pain Management	85	31	42.84	7.58	40.00	40.00	45.00	51.40
Anesth: Pediatric	35	5	42.25	7.51	40.00	42.39	46.86	50.00
Cardiology: Electrophysiology	126	74	50.43	9.53	40.00	50.00	60.00	60.00
Cardiology: Invasive	479	125	47.90	9.77	40.00	48.00	55.00	60.00
Cardiology: Inv-Intervntnl	609	134	49.94	9.94	40.00	50.00	60.00	60.00
Cardiology: Noninvasive	432	136	46.95	10.42	40.00	45.00	55.00	60.00
Critical Care: Intensivist	21	10	38.76	5.31	40.00	40.00	40.00	40.00
Dentistry	39	8	40.10	5.00	36.00	40.00	40.00	45.00
Dermatology	207	104	38.32	6.48	36.00	40.00	40.00	45.00
Dermatology: MOHS Surgery	18	16	37.83	8.73	35.75	40.00	40.00	41.50
Emergency Medicine	326	33	38.20	7.13	35.11	36.00	40.00	41.68
Endocrinology/Metabolism	137	81	40.74	7.09	36.00	40.00	40.00	50.00
Family Practice (w/ OB)	971	189	41.72	8.10	40.00	40.00	45.00	53.00
Family Practice (w/o OB)	3,530	450	39.67	5.61	36.00	40.00	40.00	48.00
Family Practice: Sports Med	24	21	41.06	8.58	36.23	40.00	43.50	53.00
Gastroenterology	515	149	45.63	9.78	40.00	40.00	50.00	60.00
Gastroenterology: Hepatology	63	15	49.35	12.26	40.00	50.00	60.00	60.00
Geriatrics	44	21	39.55	6.40	36.00	40.00	40.00	40.00
Hematology/Oncology	298	101	44.23	10.33	40.00	40.00	50.00	60.00
Hem/Onc: Oncology (only)	72	28	47.40	9.81	40.00	40.50	50.00	67.00
Infectious Disease	102	52	44.92	11.04	40.00	40.00	50.00	62.80
Internal Medicine: General	3,037	376	40.35	6.45	36.00	40.00	40.00	50.00
Internal Med: Hospitalist	265	57	40.66	6.81	36.00	40.00	40.00	50.00
Internal Med: Pediatric	86	31	39.30	4.93	36.00	40.00	40.00	44.00
Nephrology	179	65	47.18	11.38	40.00	45.00	60.00	60.00
Neurology	386	108	42.79	8.97	40.00	40.00	50.00	55.00
OBGYN: General	1,099	230	42.60	8.99	40.00	40.00	45.00	55.00
OBGYN: Gynecology (only)	161	60	37.85	6.58	36.00	36.92	40.00	41.60
OBGYN: Gyn Oncology	11	8	43.36	9.03	40.00	40.00	55.00	59.00
OBGYN: Maternal & Fetal Med	44	14	41.55	7.76	39.25	40.00	40.00	52.50
OBGYN: Repro Endocrinology	29	11	41.45	4.86	40.00	40.00	40.00	55.00
Occupational Medicine	86	38	39.79	7.01	36.00	40.00	40.03	50.00
Ophthalmology	385	117	39.09	5.53	36.00	40.00	40.00	44.00
Ophthalmology: Pediatric	24	17	39.92	4.23	38.50	40.00	40.00	47.00
Ophthalmology: Retina	67	26	41.88	9.16	40.00	40.00	46.00	50.00
Orthopedic (Non-surgical)	44	25	39.09	6.68	36.00	40.00	40.00	50.00
Orthopedic Surgery: General	625	184	45.06	9.74	40.00	40.00	50.00	60.00
Ortho Surg: Foot & Ankle	52	45	46.56	8.93	40.00	44.50	50.00	60.00
Ortho Surg: Hand	124	73	46.56	9.02	40.00	45.00	54.75	60.00
Ortho Surg: Hip & Joint	109	58	45.39	10.58	40.00	40.00	50.00	60.00
Ortho Surg: Oncology	3	3	*	*	*	*	*	*
Ortho Surg: Pediatric	33	24	48.06	11.86	40.00	40.00	60.00	70.00
Ortho Surg: Spine	119	71	47.02	11.09	40.00	44.00	55.00	60.00
Ortho Surg: Trauma	30	18	49.70	11.97	40.00	50.00	60.00	60.00
Ortho Surg: Sports Med	205	97	47.78	9.00	40.00	48.00	55.00	60.00
Otorhinolaryngology	313	103	41.70	7.87	40.00	40.00	45.00	50.00
Otorhinolaryngology: Pediatric	16	3	48.56	11.29	50.00	55.00	55.00	55.00
Pathology: Anatomic & Clinical	157	30	41.06	6.77	40.00	40.00	40.00	50.00
Pathology: Anatomic	60	11	40.57	5.50	40.00	40.00	43.75	45.00
Pathology: Clinical	69	14	42.32	7.91	40.00	40.00	40.00	55.00

Table 66: Physician Hours Worked per Week (continued)

	Physicians	Medical Practices	Mean	Std. Dev.	25th %tile	Median	75th %tile	90th %tile
Pediatrics: General	1,576	271	46.83	1.97	46.00	47.00	48.00	49.00
Ped: Adolescent Medicine	45	10	46.76	1.42	46.00	47.00	48.00	48.00
Ped: Allergy/Immunology	7	5	*	*	*	*	*	*
Ped: Cardiology	37	16	46.43	2.77	45.00	47.00	48.00	48.40
Ped: Child Development	9	5	*	*	*	*	*	*
Ped: Critical Care/Intensivist	55	14	46.02	1.76	44.00	46.00	48.00	48.00
Ped: Emergency Medicine	8	2	*	*	*	*	*	*
Ped: Endocrinology	16	10	47.00	1.51	46.00	48.00	48.00	48.00
Ped: Gastroenterology	15	7	47.33	1.45	47.00	48.00	48.00	48.00
Ped: Genetics	10	4	47.80	1.48	46.00	48.00	48.50	50.00
Ped: Hematology/Oncology	37	15	46.90	1.66	46.00	48.00	48.00	48.00
Ped: Hospitalist	20	9	47.60	1.31	47.00	48.00	48.00	49.80
Ped: Infectious Disease	5	3	*	*	*	*	*	*
Ped: Neonatal Medicine	49	11	46.24	1.39	45.00	46.00	47.50	48.00
Ped: Nephrology	7	4	*	*	*	*	*	*
Ped: Neurology	19	11	46.32	2.11	46.00	47.00	48.00	48.00
Ped: Pulmonology	15	8	45.87	1.81	44.00	46.00	48.00	48.00
Ped: Rheumatology	4	3	*	*	*	*	*	*
Ped: Sports Medicine	1	1	*	*	*	*	*	*
Physiatry (Phys Med & Rehab)	117	60	46.56	2.20	46.00	47.00	48.00	48.00
Podiatry: General	77	43	46.07	1.92	45.00	46.00	48.00	48.00
Podiatry: Surg-Foot & Ankle	39	19	46.71	2.11	45.10	48.00	48.00	49.00
Podiatry: Surg-Forefoot Only	13	4	46.96	1.36	46.00	48.00	48.00	48.30
Psychiatry: General	190	47	45.83	2.00	44.26	46.00	47.00	48.00
Psychiatry: Child & Adolescent	21	12	46.49	1.90	44.60	47.00	48.00	49.60
Psychiatry: Geriatric	11	6	46.00	3.77	44.00	47.00	49.00	49.00
Pulmonary Medicine	209	98	46.57	2.09	45.25	47.00	48.00	49.00
Pulmonary Med: Critical Care	134	39	46.57	2.55	46.00	47.00	48.00	50.00
Radiation Oncology	81	25	43.93	3.60	42.00	45.00	46.00	48.00
Radiology: Diagnostic-Inv	285	44	41.84	3.67	39.00	40.00	45.00	48.00
Radiology: Diagnostic-Noninv	405	68	43.37	2.93	41.00	44.00	45.00	46.76
Radiology: Nuclear Medicine	37	20	45.16	2.39	44.00	45.00	48.00	48.00
Rheumatology	189	102	46.51	2.15	46.00	47.00	48.00	48.00
Sleep Medicine	14	6	46.21	2.01	46.00	46.50	47.25	48.50
Surgery: General	672	199	46.36	2.16	45.00	46.60	48.00	48.20
Surg: Cardiovascular	118	35	45.07	2.81	43.00	45.00	48.00	48.00
Surg: Cardiovascular-Pediatric	5	5	*	*	*	*	*	*
Surg: Colon and Rectal	28	15	45.89	2.48	45.00	46.50	48.00	48.00
Surg: Neurological	157	50	45.88	3.00	45.00	46.80	48.00	49.00
Surg: Oncology	3	3	*	*	*	*	*	*
Surg: Oral	17	7	47.01	1.32	45.50	48.00	48.00	48.00
Surg: Pediatric	14	7	46.43	1.55	45.00	46.00	48.00	48.00
Surg: Plastic & Reconstruction	59	35	46.98	1.59	45.60	47.00	48.00	49.00
Surg: Plastic & Recon-Hand	15	5	45.93	2.15	46.00	46.00	48.00	48.40
Surg: Plastic & Recon-Pediatric	4	2	*	*	*	*	*	*
Surg: Thoracic (primary)	37	13	47.23	1.21	46.30	47.00	48.00	49.00
Surg: Transplant	12	5	47.67	.78	48.00	48.00	48.00	48.00
Surg: Trauma	20	6	46.79	1.59	46.00	48.00	48.00	48.00
Surg: Trauma-Burn	12	5	46.23	2.58	44.50	47.90	48.00	48.00
Surg: Vascular (primary)	97	43	46.01	2.10	44.00	46.00	48.00	48.16
Urgent Care	277	73	46.91	2.18	46.00	47.00	48.00	49.00
Urology	338	103	46.46	2.05	45.00	46.00	48.00	49.00
Urology: Pediatric	13	4	47.85	.55	48.00	48.00	48.00	48.00

Table 67: Physician Hours Worked per Week by Years in Specialty

	1 to 2 years		3 to 7 years		8 to 17 years		18 years or more	
	Physicians	Median	Physicians	Median	Physicians	Median	Physicians	Median
Allergy/Immunology	6	*	18	40.00	47	40.00	50	40.00
Anesthesiology	104	55.00	208	50.00	487	50.00	272	46.00
Anesth: Pain Management	7	*	18	40.00	37	44.00	13	43.00
Anesth: Pediatric	2	*	7	*	15	40.00	6	*
Cardiology: Electrophysiology	3	*	33	50.00	54	50.00	18	50.00
Cardiology: Invasive	19	50.00	121	50.00	153	45.00	136	45.00
Cardiology: Inv-Intervntnl	21	50.00	98	50.00	233	50.00	197	50.00
Cardiology: Noninvasive	8	*	49	50.00	105	50.00	192	40.00
Critical Care: Intensivist	0	*	3	*	9	*	5	*
Dentistry	1	*	1	*	6	*	12	42.50
Dermatology	10	40.00	34	40.00	74	40.00	74	40.00
Dermatology: MOHS Surgery	1	*	5	*	6	*	6	*
Emergency Medicine	38	35.31	84	36.49	114	36.00	70	36.44
Endocrinology/Metabolism	8	*	23	40.00	45	40.00	41	40.00
Family Practice (w/ OB)	87	40.00	286	40.00	312	40.00	221	40.00
Family Practice (w/o OB)	234	40.00	687	40.00	1,059	40.00	1,056	40.00
Family Practice: Sports Med	3	*	3	*	10	40.00	5	*
Gastroenterology	27	40.00	81	40.00	194	40.00	162	40.00
Gastroenterology: Hepatology	3	*	7	*	24	50.00	29	50.00
Geriatrics	3	*	2	*	20	40.00	11	40.00
Hematology/Oncology	10	42.50	53	40.00	99	40.00	99	40.00
Hem/Onc: Oncology (only)	0	*	10	50.00	28	45.00	30	45.25
Infectious Disease	9	*	23	40.00	36	50.00	28	40.00
Internal Medicine: General	195	40.00	643	40.00	891	40.00	839	40.00
Internal Med: Hospitalist	45	40.00	86	40.00	82	40.00	33	36.00
Internal Med: Pediatric	16	40.00	33	40.00	19	40.00	5	*
Nephrology	12	50.00	32	46.75	57	45.00	62	45.00
Neurology	22	40.00	73	40.00	145	40.00	106	40.00
OBGYN: General	64	40.00	261	40.00	389	40.00	254	40.00
OBGYN: Gynecology (only)	3	*	11	40.00	42	40.00	96	36.00
OBGYN: Gyn Oncology	2	*	1	*	4	*	4	*
OBGYN: Maternal & Fetal Med	3	*	9	*	17	40.00	14	38.00
OBGYN: Repro Endocrinology	2	*	4	*	11	40.00	5	*
Occupational Medicine	1	*	16	40.00	35	40.00	33	40.00
Ophthalmology	13	36.00	82	40.00	145	40.00	120	40.00
Ophthalmology: Pediatric	*	*	7	*	11	40.00	4	*
Ophthalmology: Retina	2	*	14	40.00	33	44.00	17	40.00
Orthopedic (Non-surgical)	2	*	11	40.00	12	40.00	16	36.00
Orthopedic Surgery: General	31	45.00	98	40.00	204	40.00	265	40.00
Ortho Surg: Foot & Ankle	8	*	15	44.00	23	44.00	5	*
Ortho Surg: Hand	4	*	37	50.00	44	45.00	37	40.00
Ortho Surg: Hip & Joint	3	*	14	40.00	47	40.00	41	40.00
Ortho Surg: Oncology	1	*	*	*	1	*	1	*
Ortho Surg: Pediatric	2	*	10	47.50	14	40.00	6	*
Ortho Surg: Spine	9	*	24	47.50	53	40.00	30	40.00
Ortho Surg: Trauma	1	*	13	50.00	9	*	6	*
Ortho Surg: Sports Med	17	50.00	49	50.00	97	47.00	37	45.00
Otorhinolaryngology	17	40.00	54	40.00	95	40.00	130	40.00
Otorhinolaryngology: Pediatric	1	*	2	*	7	*	6	*
Pathology: Anatomic & Clinical	7	*	27	40.00	56	40.00	61	40.00
Pathology: Anatomic	*	*	10	40.00	19	40.00	28	40.00
Pathology: Clinical	3	*	9	*	24	40.00	29	40.00

Table 67: Physician Hours Worked per Week by Years in Specialty (continued)

	1 to 2 years		3 to 7 years		8 to 17 years		18 years or more	
	Physicians	Median	Physicians	Median	Physicians	Median	Physicians	Median
Pediatrics: General	91	40.00	343	40.00	492	40.00	514	40.00
Ped: Adolescent Medicine	2	*	9	*	8	*	9	*
Ped: Allergy/Immunology	*	*	1	*	3	*	3	*
Ped: Cardiology	2	*	12	40.00	8	*	9	*
Ped: Child Development	1	*	4	*	1	*	1	*
Ped: Critical Care/Intensivist	3	*	12	43.00	39	40.00	5	*
Ped: Emergency Medicine	*	*	1	*	5	*	2	*
Ped: Endocrinology	3	*	5	*	3	*	5	*
Ped: Gastroenterology	1	*	9	*	6	*	5	*
Ped: Genetics	1	*	4	*	2	*	3	*
Ped: Hematology/Oncology	0	*	11	40.00	14	40.00	9	*
Ped: Hospitalist	3	*	8	*	4	*	5	*
Ped: Infectious Disease	1	*	0	*	3	*	1	*
Ped: Neonatal Medicine	0	*	11	40.00	27	50.00	15	40.00
Ped: Nephrology	*	*	1	*	4	*	2	*
Ped: Neurology	3	*	7	*	9	*	3	*
Ped: Pulmonology	1	*	6	*	8	*	2	*
Ped: Rheumatology	*	*	2	*	2	*	*	*
Ped: Sports Medicine	*	*	*	*	1	*	*	*
Physiatry (Phys Med & Rehab)	12	40.00	28	40.00	45	40.00	19	40.00
Podiatry: General	8	*	20	40.00	30	40.00	19	36.00
Podiatry: Surg-Foot & Ankle	0	*	13	40.00	15	40.00	8	*
Podiatry: Surg-Forefoot Only	1	*	1	*	7	*	4	*
Psychiatry: General	18	40.00	39	40.00	76	40.00	53	40.00
Psychiatry: Child & Adolescent	1	*	4	*	6	*	4	*
Psychiatry: Geriatric	*	*	1	*	5	*	7	*
Pulmonary Medicine	3	*	24	40.00	75	40.00	69	40.00
Pulmonary Med: Critical Care	7	*	25	50.00	56	50.00	36	50.00
Radiation Oncology	3	*	21	44.00	35	40.00	20	40.00
Radiology: Diagnostic-Inv	19	45.00	58	44.00	123	44.00	85	40.00
Radiology: Diagnostic-Noninv	18	40.00	74	40.00	150	40.00	145	40.00
Radiology: Nuclear Medicine	2	*	4	*	11	50.00	19	40.00
Rheumatology	6	*	22	40.00	53	40.00	79	40.00
Sleep Medicine	2	*	3	*	3	*	5	*
Surgery: General	35	40.00	127	40.00	213	40.00	228	40.00
Surg: Cardiovascular	5	*	30	50.00	61	48.00	34	40.00
Surg: Cardiovascular-Pediatric	1	*	1	*	3	*	*	*
Surg: Colon and Rectal	1	*	4	*	11	50.00	10	40.00
Surg: Neurological	7	*	36	42.50	58	50.00	43	40.00
Surg: Oncology	*	*	1	*	2	*	*	*
Surg: Oral	1	*	2	*	7	*	9	*
Surg: Pediatric	3	*	6	*	4	*	7	*
Surg: Plastic & Reconstruction	2	*	16	40.00	17	40.00	18	40.00
Surg: Plastic & Recon-Hand	*	*	2	*	8	*	5	*
Surg: Plastic & Recon-Pediatric	*	*	2	*	2	*	*	*
Surg: Thoracic (primary)	1	*	9	*	14	40.00	10	40.00
Surg: Transplant	2	*	1	*	7	*	3	*
Surg: Trauma	2	*	5	*	10	40.00	3	*
Surg: Trauma-Burn	2	*	1	*	2	*	7	*
Surg: Vascular (primary)	5	*	23	48.00	37	40.00	23	50.00
Urgent Care	11	40.00	56	40.00	89	40.00	79	40.00
Urology	15	40.00	54	40.00	115	45.00	122	40.00
Urology: Pediatric	*	*	2	*	2	*	*	*

THIS PAGE INTENTIONALLY LEFT BLANK

SPECIALTY SUMMARY TABLES

SPECIALTY SUMMARY TABLES

MEDICAL GROUP MANAGEMENT ASSOCIATION™

ALLERGY

Table 68A: Compensation

	Physicians	Medical Practices	Mean	Std. Dev.	25th %tile	Median	75th %tile	90th %tile
Overall	185	94	$300,319	$212,916	$182,988	$235,316	$341,037	$499,421
1 to 2 Years in Specialty	8	7	*	*	*	*	*	*
Group Type								
Single-specialty	48	11	$435,260	$326,927	$231,699	$340,160	$567,866	$678,834
Multispecialty	137	83	$253,040	$125,370	$180,281	$214,693	$303,573	$403,443
Geographic Section								
Eastern	26	10	$334,962	$176,263	$197,712	$305,845	$390,028	$650,993
Midwest	52	36	$261,373	$111,801	$183,135	$239,487	$328,167	$417,891
Southern	58	24	$347,808	$237,958	$186,152	$305,208	$372,428	$636,704
Western	49	24	$267,055	$266,319	$173,836	$197,263	$242,383	$372,228
Capitation								
No capitation	78	43	$342,218	$285,070	$178,457	$268,830	$387,750	$578,170
10% or less	49	23	$317,281	$165,631	$188,528	$300,306	$352,087	$643,411
11% to 50%	30	17	$244,969	$89,909	$167,220	$227,656	$319,596	$403,246
51% or more	18	10	$224,200	$62,901	$191,728	$208,919	$271,640	$309,841

Table 68B: Gross Charges (TC/NPP Excluded)

	Physicians	Medical Practices	Mean	Std. Dev.	25th %tile	Median	75th %tile	90th %tile
Overall	75	52	$755,485	$387,550	$468,718	$692,340	$910,459	$1,288,175
1 to 2 Years in Specialty	3	3	*	*	*	*	*	*
Group Type								
Single-specialty	8	4	*	*	*	*	*	*
Multispecialty	67	48	$717,729	$378,837	$460,758	$621,905	$877,580	$1,206,543
Geographic Section								
Eastern	8	6	*	*	*	*	*	*
Midwest	29	23	$670,513	$233,178	$462,742	$618,005	$831,713	$1,036,735
Southern	17	11	$909,249	$604,748	$453,755	$715,877	$1,290,218	$2,101,925
Western	21	12	$715,158	$324,872	$510,453	$633,505	$874,681	$1,258,632
Capitation								
No capitation	36	23	$794,988	$468,728	$457,069	$630,709	$951,909	$1,371,218
10% or less	20	15	$759,085	$225,437	$632,183	$781,469	$883,593	$1,104,481
11% to 50%	13	10	$757,045	$400,921	$425,489	$621,905	$997,471	$1,537,738
51% or more	6	4	*	*	*	*	*	*

Table 68C: Compensation to Gross Charges Ratio (TC/NPP Excluded)

	Physicians	Medical Practices	Mean	Std. Dev.	25th %tile	Median	75th %tile	90th %tile
Overall	71	50	.358	.104	.288	.358	.417	.491
1 to 2 Years in Specialty	3	3	*	*	*	*	*	*
Group Type								
Single-specialty	8	4	*	*	*	*	*	*
Multispecialty	63	46	.367	.104	.295	.363	.434	.523
Geographic Section								
Eastern	8	6	*	*	*	*	*	*
Midwest	29	23	.376	.120	.305	.363	.446	.574
Southern	13	9	.380	.086	.342	.389	.430	.513
Western	21	12	.329	.094	.254	.313	.416	.442
Capitation								
No capitation	32	21	.332	.090	.246	.345	.393	.455
10% or less	20	15	.369	.086	.299	.362	.430	.491
11% to 50%	13	10	.342	.109	.240	.359	.416	.523
51% or more	6	4	*	*	*	*	*	*

ANESTHESIOLOGY

Table 69A: Compensation

	Physicians	Medical Practices	Mean	Std. Dev.	25th %tile	Median	75th %tile	90th %tile
Overall	1,702	118	$330,299	$114,693	$250,769	$305,676	$394,371	$485,910
1 to 2 Years in Specialty	155	35	$265,039	$74,276	$216,849	$249,823	$321,842	$367,969
Group Type								
Single-specialty	1,227	68	$342,915	$122,644	$258,798	$330,823	$417,750	$521,127
Multispecialty	475	50	$297,708	$82,614	$244,631	$277,647	$330,745	$417,964
Geographic Section								
Eastern	264	19	$282,105	$71,516	$243,175	$270,000	$330,823	$383,334
Midwest	450	39	$376,120	$108,555	$293,027	$380,758	$454,485	$545,000
Southern	511	38	$362,746	$137,467	$272,696	$346,000	$438,120	$539,819
Western	477	22	$278,984	$76,008	$228,910	$261,514	$315,000	$369,937
Capitation								
No capitation	1,232	89	$344,771	$123,010	$260,207	$330,823	$418,620	$524,506
10% or less	136	13	$341,021	$89,627	$268,520	$336,543	$411,960	$465,722
11% to 50%	162	12	$270,624	$72,108	$228,238	$261,550	$292,750	$346,057
51% or more	30	3	$284,593	$62,620	$242,775	$265,596	$306,060	$368,780

Table 69B: Gross Charges (TC/NPP Excluded)

	Physicians	Medical Practices	Mean	Std. Dev.	25th %tile	Median	75th %tile	90th %tile
Overall	350	42	$832,548	$400,004	$601,119	$769,094	$951,775	$1,133,038
1 to 2 Years in Specialty	21	10	$731,796	$318,568	$560,587	$685,046	$828,914	$1,158,896
Group Type								
Single-specialty	157	12	$853,868	$437,949	$602,482	$780,719	$956,283	$1,157,173
Multispecialty	193	30	$815,205	$366,507	$595,545	$753,665	$946,690	$1,132,437
Geographic Section								
Eastern	34	4	$755,423	$283,406	$616,425	$743,526	$944,197	$1,015,729
Midwest	158	21	$868,711	$347,676	$667,600	$810,532	$961,104	$1,136,708
Southern	74	9	$957,841	$615,936	$552,307	$804,216	$1,097,225	$2,060,767
Western	84	8	$685,367	$194,126	$523,264	$624,941	$825,987	$976,781
Capitation								
No capitation	249	27	$826,521	$384,858	$600,808	$750,956	$936,114	$1,133,238
10% or less	46	8	$654,525	$264,910	$466,149	$616,946	$820,332	$917,047
11% to 50%	48	6	$1,040,158	$508,951	$733,982	$903,386	$1,050,117	$2,421,911
51% or more	7	1	*	*	*	*	*	*

Table 69C: Compensation to Gross Charges Ratio (TC/NPP Excluded)

	Physicians	Medical Practices	Mean	Std. Dev.	25th %tile	Median	75th %tile	90th %tile
Overall	335	40	.433	.140	.320	.424	.532	.623
1 to 2 Years in Specialty	17	8	.368	.089	.297	.385	.440	.467
Group Type	335	40	.433	.140	.320	.424	.532	.623
Single-specialty	149	12	.444	.155	.318	.440	.579	.656
Multispecialty	186	28	.425	.126	.321	.417	.510	.596
Geographic Section	335	40	.433	.140	.320	.424	.532	.623
Eastern	31	3	.378	.126	.276	.342	.423	.579
Midwest	153	21	.439	.138	.308	.449	.536	.609
Southern	67	8	.413	.136	.327	.418	.506	.595
Western	84	8	.459	.145	.353	.419	.588	.688
Capitation	335	40	.433	.140	.320	.424	.532	.623
No capitation	240	27	.455	.138	.350	.458	.563	.636
10% or less	40	6	.454	.126	.360	.414	.565	.613
11% to 50%	48	6	.304	.077	.258	.280	.353	.444
51% or more	7	1	*	*	*	*	*	*

CARDIOLOGY: INVASIVE

Table 70A: Compensation

	Physicians	Medical Practices	Mean	Std. Dev.	25th %tile	Median	75th %tile	90th %tile
Overall	601	151	$393,408	$172,447	$286,216	$360,988	$437,260	$608,337
1 to 2 Years in Specialty	29	21	$246,373	$69,765	$197,103	$238,586	$297,794	$350,000
Group Type								
Single-specialty	276	69	$386,387	$164,619	$285,975	$372,212	$430,596	$581,419
Multispecialty	325	82	$399,371	$178,862	$286,703	$350,000	$446,060	$696,924
Geographic Section								
Eastern	96	28	$350,058	$111,226	$260,250	$353,849	$400,699	$516,423
Midwest	177	39	$416,319	$169,200	$311,450	$383,000	$490,031	$629,602
Southern	188	50	$435,934	$217,055	$296,452	$378,270	$478,840	$812,861
Western	140	34	$337,060	$112,553	$274,608	$315,885	$382,721	$452,931
Capitation								
No capitation	386	100	$419,721	$192,758	$291,144	$381,108	$479,959	$667,344
10% or less	128	32	$359,075	$126,785	$289,153	$338,762	$399,665	$495,326
11% to 50%	31	14	$353,325	$125,984	$270,337	$330,430	$406,009	$534,818
51% or more	18	4	$316,270	$81,053	$274,000	$296,952	$338,800	$487,743

Table 70B: Gross Charges (TC/NPP Excluded)

	Physicians	Medical Practices	Mean	Std. Dev.	25th %tile	Median	75th %tile	90th %tile
Overall	106	41	$1,520,015	$736,571	$963,416	$1,438,519	$1,977,603	$2,459,859
1 to 2 Years in Specialty	0	0	*	*	*	*	*	*
Group Type	106	41	$1,520,015	$736,571	$963,416	$1,438,519	$1,977,603	$2,459,859
Single-specialty	31	11	$1,137,785	$496,551	$742,200	$1,028,511	$1,489,114	$1,976,704
Multispecialty	75	30	$1,678,003	$763,778	$1,118,453	$1,502,760	$2,022,512	$2,762,356
Geographic Section	106	41	$1,520,015	$736,571	$963,416	$1,438,519	$1,977,603	$2,459,859
Eastern	13	7	$1,521,300	$554,962	$1,094,104	$1,500,680	$1,980,758	$2,418,427
Midwest	41	17	$1,463,265	$839,134	$787,626	$1,279,480	$1,917,807	$2,762,206
Southern	38	13	$1,609,144	$763,073	$946,800	$1,589,394	$2,033,497	$2,658,090
Western	14	4	$1,443,097	$483,865	$1,108,750	$1,426,153	$1,619,888	$2,298,063
Capitation	106	41	$1,520,015	$736,571	$963,416	$1,438,519	$1,977,603	$2,459,859
No capitation	54	22	$1,455,419	$679,162	$936,729	$1,421,660	$1,741,686	$2,250,867
10% or less	45	16	$1,507,668	$739,161	$890,589	$1,329,419	$2,022,512	$2,473,569
11% to 50%	3	2	*	*	*	*	*	*
51% or more	4	1	*	*	*	*	*	*

Table 70C: Compensation to Gross Charges Ratio (TC/NPP Excluded)

	Physicians	Medical Practices	Mean	Std. Dev.	25th %tile	Median	75th %tile	90th %tile
Overall	98	40	0.301	0.109	0.214	0.279	0.364	0.429
1 to 2 Years in Specialty	0	0	*	*	*	*	*	*
Group Type	98	40	0.301	0.109	0.214	0.279	0.364	0.429
Single-specialty	30	11	0.327	0.123	0.25	0.285	0.405	0.47
Multispecialty	68	29	0.29	0.1	0.207	0.276	0.35	0.418
Geographic Section	98	40	0.301	0.109	0.214	0.279	0.364	0.429
Eastern	11	7	0.292	0.112	0.181	0.274	0.401	0.488
Midwest	37	16	0.332	0.11	0.261	0.3	0.412	0.467
Southern	37	13	0.292	0.114	0.211	0.246	0.35	0.425
Western	13	4	0.251	0.058	0.203	0.251	0.291	0.351
Capitation	98	40	0.301	0.109	0.214	0.279	0.364	0.429
No capitation	52	22	0.284	0.078	0.216	0.272	0.314	0.413
10% or less	42	16	0.333	0.133	0.238	0.308	0.384	0.51
11% to 50%	1	1	*	*	*	*	*	*
51% or more	3	1	*	*	*	*	*	*

CARDIOLOGY: INVASIVE/INTERVENTIONAL

Table 71A: Compensation

	Physicians	Medical Practices	Mean	Std. Dev.	25th %tile	Median	75th %tile	90th %tile
Overall	720	157	$478,112	$215,985	$351,011	$422,123	$568,144	$749,273
1 to 2 Years in Specialty	26	24	$285,874	$110,905	$216,892	$259,500	$328,554	$437,914
Group Type								
Single-specialty	461	89	$465,722	$200,271	$354,161	$420,683	$529,900	$727,209
Multispecialty	259	68	$500,165	$240,272	$344,090	$443,490	$603,804	$772,031
Geographic Section								
Eastern	95	28	$399,486	$142,511	$290,860	$385,000	$500,000	$597,222
Midwest	228	47	$485,423	$228,372	$354,356	$426,210	$568,144	$731,446
Southern	275	53	$523,590	$235,988	$370,948	$447,984	$635,584	$800,000
Western	122	29	$423,163	$157,392	$331,855	$368,949	$480,745	$659,709
Capitation								
No capitation	510	109	$495,477	$215,640	$359,237	$434,333	$594,919	$769,222
10% or less	159	32	$449,236	$233,555	$339,612	$372,196	$508,910	$620,487
11% to 50%	27	11	$413,724	$128,462	$339,000	$365,000	$526,528	$603,790
51% or more	8	3	*	*	*	*	*	*

Table 71B: Gross Charges (TC/NPP Excluded)

	Physicians	Medical Practices	Mean	Std. Dev.	25th %tile	Median	75th %tile	90th %tile
Overall	135	44	$1,766,340	$733,792	$1,318,414	$1,627,381	$2,022,512	$3,077,450
1 to 2 Years in Specialty	5	5	*	*	*	*	*	*
Group Type								
Single-specialty	64	16	$1,675,104	$695,954	$1,308,755	$1,604,131	$1,920,173	$2,287,285
Multispecialty	71	28	$1,848,580	$761,814	$1,333,351	$1,653,642	$2,157,954	$3,143,034
Geographic Section								
Eastern	21	9	$1,816,526	$740,446	$1,350,437	$1,649,403	$1,987,000	$3,365,017
Midwest	49	15	$1,689,312	$796,453	$1,191,838	$1,558,809	$2,071,472	$3,108,473
Southern	51	15	$1,854,802	$715,722	$1,370,741	$1,733,228	$2,021,053	$3,239,227
Western	14	5	$1,638,402	$565,291	$1,311,500	$1,504,000	$2,083,418	$2,517,881
Capitation								
No capitation	78	26	$1,687,249	$717,688	$1,298,758	$1,582,773	$1,945,793	$2,465,692
10% or less	46	13	$1,727,421	$565,952	$1,347,825	$1,621,115	$2,022,512	$2,476,137
11% to 50%	7	3	*	*	*	*	*	*
51% or more	3	1	*	*	*	*	*	*

Table 71C: Compensation to Gross Charges Ratio (TC/NPP Excluded)

	Physicians	Medical Practices	Mean	Std. Dev.	25th %tile	Median	75th %tile	90th %tile
Overall	124	42	.309	.120	.221	.279	.372	.471
1 to 2 Years in Specialty	5	5	*	*	*	*	*	*
Group Type								
Single-specialty	60	16	.314	.124	.221	.277	.395	.467
Multispecialty	64	26	.305	.116	.217	.282	.361	.489
Geographic Section								
Eastern	18	8	.248	.076	.181	.236	.297	.376
Midwest	46	15	.352	.137	.239	.304	.456	.540
Southern	47	14	.305	.114	.220	.288	.357	.440
Western	13	5	.255	.045	.215	.259	.297	.314
Capitation								
No capitation	72	25	.319	.113	.244	.297	.381	.466
10% or less	44	13	.291	.118	.207	.239	.350	.468
11% to 50%	4	2	*	*	*	*	*	*
51% or more	3	1	*	*	*	*	*	*

MEDICAL GROUP MANAGEMENT ASSOCIATION™

CARDIOLOGY: NONINVASIVE

Table 72A: Compensation

	Physicians	Medical Practices	Mean	Std. Dev.	25th %tile	Median	75th %tile	90th %tile
Overall	582	166	$336,094	$144,407	$241,128	$307,618	$391,404	$518,613
1 to 2 Years in Specialty	16	12	$245,326	$73,294	$204,492	$227,414	$259,838	$387,451
Group Type								
Single-specialty	305	76	$356,755	$130,228	$252,656	$355,610	$419,850	$536,141
Multispecialty	277	90	$313,345	$155,650	$230,173	$284,709	$359,347	$498,036
Geographic Section								
Eastern	227	41	$332,748	$136,908	$231,606	$296,800	$390,000	$510,494
Midwest	144	44	$338,510	$170,466	$259,067	$308,451	$399,133	$501,836
Southern	135	51	$367,509	$146,163	$257,750	$350,114	$457,056	$583,913
Western	76	30	$285,706	$84,228	$229,405	$278,831	$338,449	$391,130
Capitation								
No capitation	336	94	$348,891	$135,019	$252,370	$344,329	$401,836	$564,887
10% or less	126	40	$342,325	$140,799	$235,058	$327,571	$459,051	$508,400
11% to 50%	75	24	$293,628	$203,418	$198,972	$275,000	$321,832	$430,397
51% or more	21	7	$315,889	$83,616	$259,112	$296,321	$368,465	$454,377

Table 72B: Gross Charges (TC/NPP Excluded)

	Physicians	Medical Practices	Mean	Std. Dev.	25th %tile	Median	75th %tile	90th %tile
Overall	107	45	$1,301,793	$735,311	$712,437	$1,177,541	$1,616,884	$2,202,524
1 to 2 Years in Specialty	2	2	*	*	*	*	*	*
Group Type								
Single-specialty	26	10	$1,042,261	$402,149	$660,266	$1,045,657	$1,330,367	$1,566,472
Multispecialty	81	35	$1,385,100	$798,090	$731,686	$1,274,158	$1,707,798	$2,509,509
Geographic Section								
Eastern	28	7	$1,304,133	$771,622	$656,275	$1,103,519	$1,671,825	$2,576,150
Midwest	31	15	$1,601,734	$911,763	$901,539	$1,338,606	$2,004,384	$3,110,070
Southern	30	14	$1,193,891	$538,259	$869,831	$1,243,833	$1,480,193	$1,683,562
Western	18	9	$961,427	$396,423	$649,486	$882,303	$1,241,205	$1,651,073
Capitation								
No capitation	48	19	$1,187,099	$674,994	$663,403	$1,031,622	$1,531,813	$2,019,313
10% or less	28	15	$1,089,076	$499,425	$631,504	$1,153,382	$1,469,330	$1,789,547
11% to 50%	25	8	$1,819,429	$907,101	$1,136,909	$1,611,661	$2,399,278	$3,431,379
51% or more	6	3	*	*	*	*	*	*

Table 72C: Compensation to Gross Charges Ratio (TC/NPP Excluded)

	Physicians	Medical Practices	Mean	Std. Dev.	25th %tile	Median	75th %tile	90th %tile
Overall	89	44	.347	.141	.247	.302	.414	.515
1 to 2 Years in Specialty	1	1	*	*	*	*	*	*
Group Type								
Single-specialty	25	10	.383	.162	.245	.331	.481	.644
Multispecialty	64	34	.333	.131	.247	.294	.398	.490
Geographic Section								
Eastern	20	7	.338	.168	.200	.273	.440	.616
Midwest	24	15	.322	.148	.240	.275	.396	.490
Southern	28	14	.365	.146	.251	.307	.455	.636
Western	17	8	.363	.079	.326	.379	.403	.459
Capitation								
No capitation	46	19	.344	.125	.258	.302	.407	.522
10% or less	23	14	.414	.174	.290	.399	.467	.718
11% to 50%	14	8	.257	.096	.187	.244	.252	.471
51% or more	6	3	*	*	*	*	*	*

DERMATOLOGY

Table 73A: Compensation

	Physicians	Medical Practices	Mean	Std. Dev.	25th %tile	Median	75th %tile	90th %tile
Overall	313	140	$304,158	$154,148	$205,795	$262,782	$367,894	$477,400
1 to 2 Years in Specialty	16	13	$208,813	$82,355	$140,979	$202,476	$283,848	$341,316
Group Type								
Single-specialty	25	10	$452,604	$244,671	$284,247	$392,934	$554,943	$843,582
Multispecialty	288	130	$291,272	$136,891	$203,327	$256,846	$353,497	$457,348
Geographic Section								
Eastern	48	24	$261,819	$111,556	$175,000	$226,037	$321,683	$438,970
Midwest	103	52	$311,753	$160,482	$203,500	$273,665	$389,289	$527,432
Southern	50	25	$340,123	$179,165	$214,241	$275,839	$387,775	$687,313
Western	112	39	$299,264	$149,157	$216,543	$262,791	$351,643	$456,984
Capitation								
No capitation	124	67	$358,481	$185,647	$216,336	$329,894	$443,910	$649,550
10% or less	63	34	$277,581	$145,881	$192,700	$243,990	$318,145	$436,463
11% to 50%	64	24	$260,515	$114,283	$176,550	$239,299	$321,254	$406,969
51% or more	37	14	$276,971	$104,497	$219,013	$244,695	$326,007	$400,168

Table 73B: Gross Charges (TC/NPP Excluded)

	Physicians	Medical Practices	Mean	Std. Dev.	25th %tile	Median	75th %tile	90th %tile
Overall	143	74	$968,470	$390,432	$697,902	$910,607	$1,235,982	$1,433,257
1 to 2 Years in Specialty	8	8	*	*	*	*	*	*
Group Type								
Single-specialty	8	5	*	*	*	*	*	*
Multispecialty	135	69	$960,295	$377,298	$697,902	$924,862	$1,231,861	$1,419,529
Geographic Section								
Eastern	20	9	$1,047,784	$316,807	$823,549	$1,069,499	$1,238,504	$1,504,177
Midwest	66	34	$985,403	$384,983	$733,309	$957,562	$1,250,578	$1,502,469
Southern	21	14	$1,076,474	$390,154	$794,843	$927,932	$1,381,831	$1,828,624
Western	36	17	$830,360	$413,509	$525,940	$733,665	$1,126,290	$1,313,972
Capitation								
No capitation	69	38	$896,110	$375,916	$657,547	$831,042	$1,097,162	$1,393,500
10% or less	41	21	$998,481	$424,522	$684,640	$977,590	$1,297,060	$1,505,561
11% to 50%	27	11	$1,040,259	$302,778	$781,996	$988,506	$1,299,180	$1,459,193
51% or more	6	4	*	*	*	*	*	*

Table 73C: Compensation to Gross Charges Ratio (TC/NPP Excluded)

	Physicians	Medical Practices	Mean	Std. Dev.	25th %tile	Median	75th %tile	90th %tile
Overall	135	71	.317	.096	.249	.297	.365	.433
1 to 2 Years in Specialty	5	5	*	*	*	*	*	*
Group Type								
Single-specialty	6	4	*	*	*	*	*	*
Multispecialty	129	67	.312	.090	.248	.297	.351	.416
Geographic Section								
Eastern	19	8	.309	.121	.230	.274	.322	.547
Midwest	64	34	.313	.079	.261	.315	.366	.414
Southern	17	12	.319	.059	.277	.317	.356	.403
Western	35	17	.330	.122	.241	.288	.391	.528
Capitation								
No capitation	65	36	.349	.090	.283	.347	.401	.469
10% or less	39	20	.315	.101	.251	.298	.334	.412
11% to 50%	25	11	.237	.048	.201	.226	.281	.299
51% or more	6	4	*	*	*	*	*	*

EMERGENCY MEDICINE

Table 74A: Compensation

	Physicians	Medical Practices	Mean	Std. Dev.	25th %tile	Median	75th %tile	90th %tile
Overall	556	49	$224,400	$60,151	$187,351	$211,709	$247,280	$289,470
1 to 2 Years in Specialty	76	19	$190,237	$35,774	$175,694	$184,376	$198,663	$232,389
Group Type								
Single-specialty	136	10	$254,344	$85,733	$187,690	$240,575	$305,308	$373,984
Multispecialty	420	39	$214,704	$45,157	$187,351	$208,795	$233,903	$269,747
Geographic Section								
Eastern	157	13	$201,548	$39,381	$179,030	$194,230	$219,035	$251,627
Midwest	141	18	$234,572	$55,973	$201,808	$223,162	$261,511	$289,954
Southern	59	7	$281,186	$74,163	$232,826	$270,820	$348,715	$378,567
Western	199	11	$218,385	$60,072	$186,472	$210,385	$231,631	$273,226
Capitation								
No capitation	221	24	$243,756	$81,396	$186,407	$228,753	$280,640	$366,957
10% or less	84	11	$219,335	$34,587	$194,062	$216,706	$243,412	$270,167
11% to 50%	112	11	$205,213	$42,344	$174,624	$196,319	$217,664	$269,477
51% or more	18	2	$215,051	$32,460	$191,150	$197,546	$237,438	$273,818

Table 74B: Gross Charges (TC/NPP Excluded)

	Physicians	Medical Practices	Mean	Std. Dev.	25th %tile	Median	75th %tile	90th %tile
Overall	182	18	$638,688	$248,863	$450,732	$612,001	$814,959	$979,533
1 to 2 Years in Specialty	13	7	$705,454	$247,904	$507,255	$619,601	$942,955	$1,102,543
Group Type								
Single-specialty	68	5	$790,990	$244,509	$607,900	$793,065	$949,646	$1,092,688
Multispecialty	114	13	$547,842	$203,641	$410,123	$538,102	$667,406	$846,045
Geographic Section								
Eastern	51	5	$490,051	$240,340	$346,105	$412,737	$582,208	$924,531
Midwest	58	7	$590,882	$158,761	$505,470	$588,767	$698,491	$815,492
Southern	25	1	$851,215	$96,660	$766,613	$851,024	$937,938	$976,233
Western	48	5	$743,691	$282,202	$527,561	$683,902	$976,780	$1,135,208
Capitation								
No capitation	83	7	$766,373	$232,962	$604,000	$758,371	$910,562	$1,072,466
10% or less	41	6	$545,864	$200,322	$428,439	$577,378	$693,332	$807,592
11% to 50%	58	5	$521,583	$215,722	$382,966	$479,234	$631,602	$916,585

Table 74C: Compensation to Gross Charges Ratio (TC/NPP Excluded)

	Physicians	Medical Practices	Mean	Std. Dev.	25th %tile	Median	75th %tile	90th %tile
Overall	175	18	.399	.137	.310	.387	.473	.542
1 to 2 Years in Specialty	13	7	.296	.073	.247	.277	.349	.427
Group Type								
Single-specialty	68	5	.362	.093	.283	.345	.430	.503
Multispecialty	107	13	.422	.155	.321	.400	.498	.586
Geographic Section								
Eastern	46	5	.439	.185	.345	.420	.509	.733
Midwest	56	7	.420	.128	.328	.407	.499	.584
Southern	25	1	.381	.108	.282	.411	.466	.518
Western	48	5	.345	.080	.280	.324	.393	.483
Capitation								
No capitation	83	7	.364	.110	.287	.335	.422	.494
10% or less	39	6	.448	.161	.348	.404	.516	.617
11% to 50%	53	5	.418	.143	.336	.438	.497	.581

ENDOCRINOLOGY/METABOLISM

Table 75A: Compensation

	Physicians	Medical Practices	Mean	Std. Dev.	25th %tile	Median	75th %tile	90th %tile
Overall	207	114	$187,529	$80,820	$141,417	$170,000	$213,878	$273,685
1 to 2 Years in Specialty	9	9	*	*	*	*	*	*
Group Type								
Single-specialty	12	9	$228,931	$185,866	$152,815	$173,508	$221,651	$645,596
Multispecialty	195	105	$184,982	$69,747	$141,414	$168,239	$213,878	$272,132
Geographic Section								
Eastern	42	25	$153,174	$29,835	$137,084	$150,034	$177,732	$194,935
Midwest	59	36	$200,791	$75,657	$144,080	$175,828	$237,434	$297,678
Southern	50	26	$216,234	$122,076	$146,516	$182,706	$256,456	$287,310
Western	56	27	$173,695	$49,544	$138,536	$162,758	$198,052	$245,461
Capitation								
No capitation	81	52	$196,231	$97,514	$141,094	$172,813	$228,423	$287,031
10% or less	59	34	$186,849	$83,567	$140,145	$162,136	$213,878	$262,189
11% to 50%	42	20	$173,430	$56,708	$136,622	$149,994	$213,734	$250,998
51% or more	10	6	$177,859	$44,795	$149,312	$172,016	$187,553	$281,806

Table 75B: Gross Charges (TC/NPP Excluded)

	Physicians	Medical Practices	Mean	Std. Dev.	25th %tile	Median	75th %tile	90th %tile
Overall	93	57	$535,439	$342,352	$368,910	$452,417	$579,287	$881,686
1 to 2 Years in Specialty	1	1	*	*	*	*	*	*
Group Type								
Single-specialty	1	1	*	*	*	*	*	*
Multispecialty	92	56	$537,811	$343,459	$370,452	$454,747	$580,596	$887,369
Geographic Section								
Eastern	17	12	$556,136	$512,426	$352,784	$452,417	$578,096	$994,781
Midwest	35	23	$539,395	$274,941	$371,431	$444,604	$613,076	$1,025,566
Southern	24	12	$560,705	$378,558	$340,055	$468,196	$618,780	$947,272
Western	17	10	$470,928	$197,083	$337,138	$403,158	$554,710	$755,572
Capitation								
No capitation	43	27	$579,257	$358,699	$359,718	$488,298	$626,098	$1,121,555
10% or less	29	17	$544,045	$396,926	$378,685	$461,942	$579,287	$782,564
11% to 50%	17	10	$389,351	$94,287	$347,344	$397,300	$440,722	$536,860
51% or more	3	2	*	*	*	*	*	*

Table 75C: Compensation to Gross Charges Ratio (TC/NPP Excluded)

	Physicians	Medical Practices	Mean	Std. Dev.	25th %tile	Median	75th %tile	90th %tile
Overall	89	55	.402	.134	.311	.393	.485	.588
1 to 2 Years in Specialty	1	1	*	*	*	*	*	*
Group Type								
Single-specialty	1	1	*	*	*	*	*	*
Multispecialty	88	54	.401	.134	.311	.388	.484	.588
Geographic Section								
Eastern	15	11	.398	.160	.315	.342	.449	.700
Midwest	34	23	.399	.122	.324	.404	.482	.549
Southern	23	11	.437	.145	.311	.440	.501	.639
Western	17	10	.366	.115	.267	.326	.481	.553
Capitation								
No capitation	40	25	.365	.119	.249	.349	.468	.531
10% or less	28	17	.437	.124	.342	.426	.492	.607
11% to 50%	17	10	.430	.162	.303	.393	.521	.746
51% or more	3	2	*	*	*	*	*	*

FAMILY PRACTICE (WITH OB)

Table 76A: Compensation

	Physicians	Medical Practices	Mean	Std. Dev.	25th %tile	Median	75th %tile	90th %tile
Overall	1,301	219	$167,228	$49,458	$131,429	$156,829	$193,368	$236,076
1 to 2 Years in Specialty	107	61	$137,704	$30,528	$115,141	$136,320	$155,305	$173,299
Group Type								
Single-specialty	282	69	$159,936	$53,297	$124,754	$151,787	$182,688	$227,920
Multispecialty	1,019	150	$169,246	$48,175	$134,795	$158,711	$197,155	$238,239
Geographic Section								
Eastern	105	24	$149,766	$42,911	$121,503	$135,784	$166,735	$228,799
Midwest	743	112	$172,521	$49,281	$137,359	$162,450	$202,010	$242,723
Southern	187	25	$170,487	$52,639	$132,830	$154,999	$198,060	$243,765
Western	266	58	$157,046	$47,130	$126,849	$148,717	$181,563	$213,639
Capitation								
No capitation	546	119	$169,632	$48,761	$133,827	$160,119	$200,544	$242,631
10% or less	344	47	$172,873	$53,076	$134,874	$161,712	$201,540	$247,427
11% to 50%	341	47	$163,208	$48,536	$128,190	$154,962	$188,229	$227,430
51% or more	54	2	$144,080	$25,142	$124,534	$139,690	$154,735	$174,007

Table 76B: Gross Charges (TC/NPP Excluded)

	Physicians	Medical Practices	Mean	Std. Dev.	25th %tile	Median	75th %tile	90th %tile
Overall	625	91	$471,771	$148,217	$373,947	$442,429	$549,518	$666,733
1 to 2 Years in Specialty	58	27	$436,211	$115,139	$358,855	$412,793	$506,548	$600,016
Group Type								
Single-specialty	89	24	$433,173	$165,701	$317,328	$378,508	$511,894	$691,815
Multispecialty	536	67	$478,180	$144,284	$382,834	$452,174	$550,906	$664,909
Geographic Section								
Eastern	49	13	$410,088	$108,397	$337,705	$393,399	$466,757	$579,022
Midwest	423	52	$475,112	$153,859	$374,348	$438,782	$549,597	$671,766
Southern	41	5	$506,652	$138,136	$409,767	$490,467	$588,229	$682,782
Western	112	21	$473,370	$139,171	$376,181	$446,608	$575,051	$675,511
Capitation								
No capitation	268	48	$485,274	$168,136	$374,638	$446,748	$561,973	$696,539
10% or less	184	21	$459,523	$121,999	$377,390	$449,088	$525,028	$615,983
11% to 50%	168	20	$465,350	$140,770	$372,704	$433,144	$558,478	$666,440
51% or more	4	1	*	*	*	*	*	*

Table 76C: Compensation to Gross Charges Ratio (TC/NPP Excluded)

	Physicians	Medical Practices	Mean	Std. Dev.	25th %tile	Median	75th %tile	90th %tile
Overall	621	91	.371	.092	.306	.369	.426	.482
1 to 2 Years in Specialty	58	27	.341	.095	.269	.339	.397	.461
Group Type								
Single-specialty	85	24	.387	.126	.264	.416	.480	.542
Multispecialty	536	67	.369	.086	.310	.367	.413	.467
Geographic Section								
Eastern	49	13	.371	.109	.295	.364	.441	.514
Midwest	419	52	.384	.087	.331	.380	.431	.484
Southern	41	5	.334	.092	.259	.337	.384	.423
Western	112	21	.336	.094	.266	.304	.396	.459
Capitation								
No capitation	268	48	.369	.092	.296	.367	.421	.493
10% or less	184	21	.387	.077	.352	.382	.426	.469
11% to 50%	164	20	.355	.106	.289	.335	.429	.498
51% or more	4	1	*	*	*	*	*	*

FAMILY PRACTICE (WITHOUT OB)

Table 77A: Compensation

	Physicians	Medical Practices	Mean	Std. Dev.	25th %tile	Median	75th %tile	90th %tile
Overall	4,321	517	$163,151	$57,997	$125,907	$150,267	$185,844	$234,961
1 to 2 Years in Specialty	290	128	$132,989	$33,759	$114,945	$129,069	$141,916	$167,051
Group Type								
Single-specialty	714	192	$171,227	$72,791	$125,285	$154,068	$199,069	$260,087
Multispecialty	3,607	325	$161,553	$54,466	$125,971	$150,000	$184,663	$228,742
Geographic Section								
Eastern	758	104	$156,676	$56,944	$120,953	$142,018	$176,972	$228,716
Midwest	1,660	193	$157,892	$50,395	$123,877	$148,281	$180,294	$223,411
Southern	938	126	$186,206	$76,870	$134,342	$167,314	$219,236	$281,258
Western	965	94	$154,876	$41,794	$126,531	$149,397	$177,432	$206,322
Capitation								
No capitation	1,982	270	$170,037	$64,476	$128,997	$154,516	$195,703	$246,002
10% or less	990	116	$155,734	$54,313	$120,478	$144,076	$180,494	$224,988
11% to 50%	934	92	$157,888	$51,875	$123,914	$145,945	$180,360	$230,661
51% or more	242	17	$162,269	$39,262	$132,282	$160,966	$181,147	$207,378

Table 77B: Gross Charges (TC/NPP Excluded)

	Physicians	Medical Practices	Mean	Std. Dev.	25th %tile	Median	75th %tile	90th %tile
Overall	1,745	186	$470,099	$193,994	$342,647	$431,376	$550,066	$717,076
1 to 2 Years in Specialty	67	43	$360,647	$111,643	$262,964	$347,761	$452,480	$513,532
Group Type								
Single-specialty	180	43	$438,425	$141,381	$334,284	$412,776	$517,444	$630,715
Multispecialty	1,565	143	$473,742	$198,868	$344,980	$434,075	$552,844	$733,360
Geographic Section								
Eastern	349	42	$397,954	$134,276	$304,292	$371,300	$464,227	$581,752
Midwest	859	82	$499,518	$220,951	$348,157	$447,475	$597,613	$813,465
Southern	214	27	$468,162	$206,036	$349,460	$434,376	$551,292	$688,984
Western	323	35	$471,097	$135,003	$376,824	$465,809	$547,769	$627,667
Capitation								
No capitation	905	98	$513,484	$224,135	$353,752	$463,456	$622,436	$820,251
10% or less	411	50	$422,599	$150,310	$333,991	$404,089	$498,959	$602,895
11% to 50%	358	28	$421,695	$128,805	$323,454	$409,132	$504,009	$593,771
51% or more	56	7	$439,918	$155,987	$350,617	$427,893	$518,848	$610,747

Table 77C: Compensation to Gross Charges Ratio (TC/NPP Excluded)

	Physicians	Medical Practices	Mean	Std. Dev.	25th %tile	Median	75th %tile	90th %tile
Overall	1,709	185	.369	.115	.290	.370	.430	.504
1 to 2 Years in Specialty	67	43	.397	.125	.296	.380	.462	.590
Group Type								
Single-specialty	178	43	.366	.095	.298	.373	.414	.480
Multispecialty	1,531	142	.369	.117	.290	.368	.431	.505
Geographic Section								
Eastern	347	42	.393	.117	.317	.382	.451	.547
Midwest	843	82	.359	.117	.276	.367	.426	.498
Southern	198	26	.389	.115	.306	.391	.445	.506
Western	321	35	.355	.104	.279	.348	.405	.474
Capitation								
No capitation	873	97	.351	.124	.249	.358	.416	.503
10% or less	410	50	.389	.101	.321	.386	.440	.501
11% to 50%	356	28	.380	.104	.316	.358	.433	.511
51% or more	55	7	.403	.095	.350	.372	.458	.534

MEDICAL GROUP MANAGEMENT ASSOCIATION™

GASTROENTEROLOGY

Table 78A: Compensation

	Physicians	Medical Practices	Mean	Std. Dev.	25th %tile	Median	75th %tile	90th %tile
Overall	720	201	$358,576	$164,116	$250,036	$321,023	$432,604	$559,629
1 to 2 Years in Specialty	44	29	$291,945	$173,445	$190,744	$232,846	$297,144	$533,075
Group Type								
Single-specialty	235	31	$366,721	$148,782	$275,809	$337,688	$452,129	$549,692
Multispecialty	485	170	$354,629	$171,061	$245,569	$309,572	$424,560	$561,311
Geographic Section								
Eastern	143	40	$339,782	$146,016	$230,000	$302,467	$428,900	$554,200
Midwest	233	69	$392,984	$191,646	$276,982	$339,397	$473,708	$593,737
Southern	153	46	$378,302	$179,585	$231,468	$352,659	$471,422	$611,734
Western	191	46	$314,872	$106,731	$243,857	$291,963	$369,369	$477,158
Capitation								
No capitation	436	113	$388,231	$184,465	$266,312	$348,255	$489,916	$596,293
10% or less	105	47	$339,782	$121,131	$258,233	$315,788	$409,500	$488,516
11% to 50%	97	26	$309,240	$104,458	$231,738	$296,951	$372,540	$473,815
51% or more	33	13	$318,043	$125,542	$253,057	$284,000	$329,456	$543,487

Table 78B: Gross Charges (TC/NPP Excluded)

	Physicians	Medical Practices	Mean	Std. Dev.	25th %tile	Median	75th %tile	90th %tile
Overall	331	102	$1,478,564	$544,511	$1,130,255	$1,433,899	$1,732,198	$2,213,022
1 to 2 Years in Specialty	18	15	$1,314,294	$374,743	$1,103,926	$1,203,231	$1,545,028	$1,752,687
Group Type								
Single-specialty	122	16	$1,400,250	$466,161	$1,158,023	$1,404,389	$1,668,830	$2,035,387
Multispecialty	209	86	$1,524,279	$581,622	$1,106,408	$1,444,512	$1,806,240	$2,431,136
Geographic Section								
Eastern	48	17	$1,341,593	$628,621	$955,343	$1,474,525	$1,734,543	$2,145,450
Midwest	132	42	$1,594,586	$581,278	$1,216,177	$1,480,029	$1,799,807	$2,457,517
Southern	91	25	$1,511,843	$451,004	$1,231,504	$1,433,899	$1,799,279	$2,144,120
Western	60	18	$1,282,421	$443,671	$981,199	$1,229,912	$1,622,228	$1,855,029
Capitation								
No capitation	221	57	$1,427,535	$529,680	$1,102,009	$1,390,000	$1,699,512	$2,111,686
10% or less	57	27	$1,551,038	$560,457	$1,093,037	$1,544,577	$1,844,390	$2,333,382
11% to 50%	44	12	$1,628,719	$562,118	$1,291,637	$1,534,150	$1,791,392	$2,449,920
51% or more	8	5	*	*	*	*	*	*

Table 78C: Compensation to Gross Charges Ratio (TC/NPP Excluded)

	Physicians	Medical Practices	Mean	Std. Dev.	25th %tile	Median	75th %tile	90th %tile
Overall	289	98	.272	.085	.216	.258	.305	.375
1 to 2 Years in Specialty	13	12	.223	.052	.168	.222	.262	.304
Group Type								
Single-specialty	100	16	.297	.106	.234	.283	.328	.409
Multispecialty	189	82	.259	.069	.208	.242	.294	.362
Geographic Section								
Eastern	36	16	.258	.143	.180	.208	.295	.398
Midwest	120	41	.273	.076	.221	.254	.312	.378
Southern	77	24	.277	.081	.225	.259	.294	.393
Western	56	17	.273	.058	.229	.277	.315	.346
Capitation								
No capitation	196	55	.282	.090	.228	.270	.314	.382
10% or less	53	26	.259	.072	.207	.242	.299	.374
11% to 50%	32	12	.225	.059	.181	.215	.239	.346
51% or more	7	4	*	*	*	*	*	*

HEMATOLOGY/ONCOLOGY

Table 79A: Compensation

	Physicians	Medical Practices	Mean	Std. Dev.	25th %tile	Median	75th %tile	90th %tile
Overall	399	124	$394,361	$256,944	$218,052	$299,319	$472,384	$817,611
1 to 2 Years in Specialty	24	14	$238,660	$109,444	$177,651	$192,310	$244,634	$457,420
Group Type								
Single-specialty	130	29	$535,391	$297,280	$301,416	$462,386	$802,878	$980,278
Multispecialty	269	95	$326,206	$202,967	$208,917	$246,299	$380,577	$564,220
Geographic Section								
Eastern	73	24	$335,495	$205,568	$198,750	$250,000	$379,400	$795,365
Midwest	139	48	$496,728	$323,526	$240,590	$379,872	$774,446	$984,820
Southern	87	28	$370,392	$198,250	$204,204	$327,723	$469,963	$714,967
Western	100	24	$315,897	$175,057	$209,492	$243,174	$374,145	$541,638
Capitation								
No capitation	206	72	$495,554	$291,846	$264,877	$400,321	$743,925	$928,945
10% or less	78	29	$346,302	$206,261	$211,257	$267,495	$430,490	$700,286
11% to 50%	52	14	$249,522	$86,951	$188,397	$234,472	$293,559	$380,043
51% or more	14	6	$234,576	$79,029	$172,230	$221,737	$300,318	$348,179

Table 79B: Gross Charges (TC/NPP Excluded)

	Physicians	Medical Practices	Mean	Std. Dev.	25th %tile	Median	75th %tile	90th %tile
Overall	171	59	$701,389	$430,746	$427,039	$612,245	$849,100	$1,191,675
1 to 2 Years in Specialty	6	5	*	*	*	*	*	*
Group Type								
Single-specialty	57	9	$777,804	$414,072	$532,037	$685,000	$946,490	$1,350,000
Multispecialty	114	50	$663,181	$435,599	$374,296	$568,557	$786,039	$1,156,323
Geographic Section								
Eastern	20	7	$489,865	$454,260	$290,492	$347,182	$593,722	$659,183
Midwest	74	26	$658,047	$357,979	$439,307	$633,345	$780,572	$1,052,708
Southern	50	16	$864,259	$539,163	$530,756	$718,491	$1,083,729	$1,656,000
Western	27	10	$675,249	$251,447	$523,495	$588,203	$849,100	$1,103,996
Capitation								
No capitation	86	31	$826,873	$523,568	$483,880	$687,165	$1,040,925	$1,540,272
10% or less	45	18	$604,159	$256,547	$453,208	$575,282	$698,777	$933,933
11% to 50%	28	6	$478,809	$249,229	$290,492	$364,185	$621,337	$815,664
51% or more	3	2	*	*	*	*	*	*

Table 79C: Compensation to Gross Charges Ratio (TC/NPP Excluded)

	Physicians	Medical Practices	Mean	Std. Dev.	25th %tile	Median	75th %tile	90th %tile
Overall	132	51	.523	.193	.387	.472	.648	.831
1 to 2 Years in Specialty	5	4	*	*	*	*	*	*
Group Type								
Single-specialty	35	8	.514	.214	.361	.433	.753	.861
Multispecialty	97	43	.526	.187	.398	.482	.647	.825
Geographic Section								
Eastern	18	5	.648	.186	.481	.633	.813	.922
Midwest	46	21	.476	.164	.375	.444	.577	.667
Southern	44	15	.503	.205	.359	.429	.591	.863
Western	24	10	.554	.195	.405	.510	.714	.909
Capitation								
No capitation	57	26	.527	.220	.373	.471	.704	.897
10% or less	36	15	.482	.129	.407	.449	.526	.608
11% to 50%	27	6	.569	.216	.359	.551	.788	.876
51% or more	3	2	*	*	*	*	*	*

INFECTIOUS DISEASE

Table 80A: Compensation

	Physicians	Medical Practices	Mean	Std. Dev.	25th %tile	Median	75th %tile	90th %tile
Overall	146	70	$224,149	$161,429	$140,000	$180,286	$222,954	$409,353
1 to 2 Years in Specialty	11	9	$150,385	$32,437	$131,500	$140,000	$160,000	$214,590
Group Type								
Single-specialty	41	12	$288,871	$233,713	$164,180	$214,544	$324,641	$531,991
Multispecialty	105	58	$198,877	$114,141	$139,201	$173,939	$215,014	$272,970
Geographic Section								
Eastern	35	14	$249,039	$247,023	$130,000	$171,591	$235,200	$498,548
Midwest	39	24	$220,833	$119,376	$141,537	$181,095	$243,250	$420,117
Southern	27	15	$266,813	$190,489	$152,778	$190,602	$329,849	$475,127
Western	45	17	$182,066	$39,314	$146,914	$178,539	$213,079	$232,073
Capitation								
No capitation	70	36	$269,542	$216,783	$140,622	$201,376	$308,193	$464,281
10% or less	25	15	$186,795	$49,558	$140,500	$184,780	$227,815	$264,088
11% to 50%	29	15	$179,838	$81,650	$134,047	$157,400	$200,405	$237,795
51% or more	7	3	*	*	*	*	*	*

Table 80B: Gross Charges (TC/NPP Excluded)

	Physicians	Medical Practices	Mean	Std. Dev.	25th %tile	Median	75th %tile	90th %tile
Overall	77	39	$557,042	$276,458	$343,041	$515,902	$743,323	$1,014,818
1 to 2 Years in Specialty	6	4	*	*	*	*	*	*
Group Type								
Single-specialty	34	9	$687,817	$282,952	$481,962	$627,104	$860,979	$1,173,705
Multispecialty	43	30	$453,638	$224,952	$294,230	$404,419	$538,834	$813,659
Geographic Section								
Eastern	21	9	$490,593	$252,202	$294,244	$488,272	$619,701	$837,929
Midwest	25	16	$508,419	$230,689	$340,419	$494,991	$617,383	$896,724
Southern	16	8	$749,119	$374,149	$487,284	$748,657	$1,107,508	$1,200,661
Western	15	6	$526,225	$169,684	$404,419	$511,981	$621,235	$796,110
Capitation								
No capitation	42	20	$617,276	$309,517	$373,959	$529,724	$846,255	$1,154,399
10% or less	19	11	$462,223	$201,254	$321,712	$463,032	$606,429	$765,512
11% to 50%	14	7	$527,010	$232,339	$342,618	$499,960	$702,085	$938,747
51% or more	2	1	*	*	*	*	*	*

Table 80C: Compensation to Gross Charges Ratio (TC/NPP Excluded)

	Physicians	Medical Practices	Mean	Std. Dev.	25th %tile	Median	75th %tile	90th %tile
Overall	75	37	.426	.178	.297	.372	.520	.734
1 to 2 Years in Specialty	5	3	*	*	*	*	*	*
Group Type								
Single-specialty	34	9	.387	.164	.268	.346	.445	.670
Multispecialty	41	28	.459	.183	.322	.395	.581	.753
Geographic Section								
Eastern	20	8	.424	.145	.339	.393	.470	.735
Midwest	25	16	.480	.220	.313	.395	.715	.790
Southern	15	7	.379	.162	.261	.346	.520	.655
Western	15	6	.387	.139	.292	.341	.444	.665
Capitation								
No capitation	41	19	.419	.171	.300	.370	.505	.729
10% or less	18	10	.416	.140	.319	.375	.489	.684
11% to 50%	14	7	.449	.233	.265	.369	.717	.816
51% or more	2	1	*	*	*	*	*	*

INTERNAL MEDICINE: GENERAL

Table 81A: Compensation

	Physicians	Medical Practices	Mean	Std. Dev.	25th %tile	Median	75th %tile	90th %tile
Overall	4,357	438	$165,861	$57,421	$130,229	$154,756	$186,241	$232,886
1 to 2 Years in Specialty	410	121	$134,856	$30,532	$120,289	$129,029	$140,132	$161,118
Group Type								
Single-specialty	295	68	$174,429	$70,531	$129,335	$160,000	$205,447	$256,456
Multispecialty	4,062	370	$165,239	$56,310	$130,318	$154,469	$185,200	$230,825
Geographic Section								
Eastern	864	96	$159,333	$58,474	$123,992	$147,377	$181,269	$222,542
Midwest	1,313	160	$164,597	$56,535	$129,974	$153,856	$184,969	$234,919
Southern	796	92	$180,101	$69,942	$134,954	$163,199	$210,168	$270,260
Western	1,384	90	$162,947	$47,474	$132,050	$154,619	$180,814	$211,303
Capitation								
No capitation	1,608	221	$174,117	$70,242	$130,013	$157,935	$199,931	$257,521
10% or less	885	105	$162,503	$54,065	$127,992	$151,972	$185,710	$234,223
11% to 50%	883	81	$158,259	$49,886	$126,860	$150,140	$179,000	$218,657
51% or more	387	19	$167,533	$46,717	$134,557	$158,789	$184,740	$238,022

Table 81B: Gross Charges (TC/NPP Excluded)

	Physicians	Medical Practices	Mean	Std. Dev.	25th %tile	Median	75th %tile	90th %tile
Overall	1,535	181	$460,411	$192,357	$338,669	$426,044	$539,407	$678,261
1 to 2 Years in Specialty	84	54	$356,724	$128,083	$271,456	$381,625	$434,744	$519,257
Group Type								
Single-specialty	56	20	$514,976	$256,736	$324,521	$461,764	$662,645	$862,023
Multispecialty	1,479	161	$458,345	$189,297	$339,325	$425,866	$536,207	$672,156
Geographic Section								
Eastern	322	36	$449,073	$229,512	$333,210	$420,931	$520,033	$662,686
Midwest	645	77	$460,018	$196,654	$331,592	$410,707	$540,940	$723,275
Southern	236	31	$446,747	$165,175	$336,134	$426,254	$519,974	$670,491
Western	332	37	$481,883	$158,312	$377,161	$459,286	$568,958	$675,010
Capitation								
No capitation	659	90	$474,619	$225,154	$335,840	$425,321	$569,684	$738,075
10% or less	432	49	$453,332	$166,746	$344,498	$431,365	$526,160	$677,940
11% to 50%	355	31	$440,936	$161,326	$335,656	$421,734	$519,575	$623,533
51% or more	69	6	$485,833	$156,391	$375,426	$438,402	$590,765	$702,897

Table 81C: Compensation to Gross Charges Ratio (TC/NPP Excluded)

	Physicians	Medical Practices	Mean	Std. Dev.	25th %tile	Median	75th %tile	90th %tile
Overall	1,511	180	.380	.116	.302	.370	.442	.514
1 to 2 Years in Specialty	80	50	.399	.148	.293	.347	.462	.636
Group Type								
Single-specialty	53	20	.372	.136	.269	.344	.463	.583
Multispecialty	1,458	160	.380	.115	.304	.370	.442	.513
Geographic Section								
Eastern	315	36	.376	.134	.291	.346	.420	.536
Midwest	638	77	.389	.115	.319	.385	.445	.516
Southern	227	30	.399	.101	.319	.394	.463	.529
Western	331	37	.354	.103	.280	.332	.426	.486
Capitation								
No capitation	642	89	.369	.111	.290	.371	.440	.498
10% or less	427	49	.385	.105	.307	.381	.442	.516
11% to 50%	353	31	.384	.131	.303	.347	.431	.536
51% or more	69	6	.426	.119	.338	.425	.482	.561

INTERNAL MEDICINE: HOSPITALIST

Table 82A: Compensation

	Physicians	Medical Practices	Mean	Std. Dev.	25th %tile	Median	75th %tile	90th %tile
Overall	350	79	$180,456	$61,303	$147,521	$161,955	$196,036	$248,434
1 to 2 Years in Specialty	59	31	$152,052	$25,485	$139,908	$149,999	$161,629	$183,333
Group Type								
Single-specialty	6	2	*	*	*	*	*	*
Multispecialty	344	77	$180,803	$61,760	$147,270	$162,581	$196,426	$249,172
Geographic Section								
Eastern	47	18	$163,581	$47,850	$130,000	$151,052	$187,970	$241,644
Midwest	134	25	$174,946	$40,310	$149,999	$165,000	$189,837	$238,400
Southern	96	17	$204,593	$91,401	$151,335	$169,007	$223,039	$334,663
Western	73	19	$169,695	$39,906	$143,171	$157,140	$184,822	$231,586
Capitation								
No capitation	169	30	$189,296	$74,126	$149,253	$165,000	$210,848	$262,712
10% or less	77	23	$172,219	$45,564	$147,714	$160,690	$177,871	$253,984
11% to 50%	46	14	$162,924	$46,271	$130,779	$150,160	$178,307	$226,286
51% or more	47	9	$176,656	$39,777	$146,685	$168,112	$193,107	$231,248

Table 82B: Gross Charges (TC/NPP Excluded)

	Physicians	Medical Practices	Mean	Std. Dev.	25th %tile	Median	75th %tile	90th %tile
Overall	154	37	$374,521	$148,930	$264,142	$345,936	$452,784	$604,887
1 to 2 Years in Specialty	24	14	$357,181	$140,343	$261,659	$314,182	$476,147	$610,371
Group Type								
Multispecialty	154	37	$374,521	$148,930	$264,142	$345,936	$452,784	$604,887
Geographic Section								
Eastern	20	7	$446,013	$177,983	$293,510	$425,582	$606,136	$700,310
Midwest	87	18	$371,185	$126,199	$278,667	$346,201	$446,646	$554,505
Southern	20	5	$432,268	$201,151	$313,803	$355,811	$528,777	$856,457
Western	27	7	$289,541	$105,317	$205,855	$264,822	$360,631	$473,715
Capitation								
No capitation	95	18	$388,771	$158,481	$290,884	$351,638	$475,060	$619,852
10% or less	45	12	$354,524	$131,756	$260,017	$320,494	$396,232	$546,551
11% to 50%	10	5	$375,232	$108,360	$283,516	$402,933	$471,783	$511,324
51% or more	4	2	*	*	*	*	*	*

Table 82C: Compensation to Gross Charges Ratio (TC/NPP Excluded)

	Physicians	Medical Practices	Mean	Std. Dev.	25th %tile	Median	75th %tile	90th %tile
Overall	151	37	.505	.154	.395	.484	.603	.728
1 to 2 Years in Specialty	24	14	.490	.152	.364	.505	.598	.711
Group Type								
Multispecialty	151	37	.505	.154	.395	.484	.603	.728
Geographic Section								
Eastern	20	7	.426	.146	.321	.382	.497	.663
Midwest	86	18	.503	.136	.425	.477	.591	.676
Southern	20	5	.490	.197	.289	.499	.721	.735
Western	25	7	.587	.152	.473	.564	.714	.809
Capitation								
No capitation	94	18	.482	.155	.387	.449	.554	.720
10% or less	45	12	.558	.134	.482	.573	.658	.735
11% to 50%	10	5	.433	.117	.332	.428	.497	.660
51% or more	2	2	*	*	*	*	*	*

NEPHROLOGY

Table 83A: Compensation

	Physicians	Medical Practices	Mean	Std. Dev.	25th %tile	Median	75th %tile	90th %tile
Overall	268	86	$261,919	$136,797	$185,990	$227,385	$302,463	$400,000
1 to 2 Years in Specialty	24	13	$177,977	$45,948	$149,898	$175,943	$202,691	$219,872
Group Type								
Single-specialty	68	11	$267,744	$111,997	$186,716	$242,700	$368,375	$400,000
Multispecialty	200	75	$259,938	$144,462	$184,960	$217,657	$299,873	$376,954
Geographic Section								
Eastern	63	18	$245,969	$102,033	$163,637	$226,362	$279,540	$412,825
Midwest	67	31	$253,841	$93,190	$185,000	$216,745	$314,079	$371,985
Southern	71	20	$326,009	$211,543	$186,716	$267,500	$400,000	$444,986
Western	67	17	$217,077	$54,852	$184,946	$213,633	$251,946	$286,237
Capitation								
No capitation	138	44	$290,064	$173,561	$186,716	$242,700	$351,442	$444,403
10% or less	41	18	$242,413	$78,366	$182,984	$216,250	$301,652	$364,393
11% to 50%	51	17	$224,233	$76,147	$178,092	$200,932	$262,745	$368,375
51% or more	8	4	*	*	*	*	*	*

Table 83B: Gross Charges (TC/NPP Excluded)

	Physicians	Medical Practices	Mean	Std. Dev.	25th %tile	Median	75th %tile	90th %tile
Overall	134	47	$754,814	$292,372	$535,890	$732,353	$944,198	$1,083,826
1 to 2 Years in Specialty	8	7	*	*	*	*	*	*
Group Type								
Single-specialty	45	6	$872,560	$242,273	$748,356	$844,672	$985,932	$1,191,249
Multispecialty	89	41	$695,280	$298,614	$468,043	$631,881	$886,913	$1,063,936
Geographic Section								
Eastern	44	10	$822,838	$244,927	$657,853	$788,774	$928,461	$1,159,892
Midwest	39	19	$715,338	$374,411	$435,010	$664,312	$916,100	$1,236,970
Southern	37	13	$745,667	$266,987	$510,304	$787,137	$975,651	$1,026,609
Western	14	5	$675,169	$203,818	$559,352	$614,056	$789,671	$1,064,169
Capitation								
No capitation	83	24	$747,768	$261,826	$534,515	$761,577	$893,731	$988,594
10% or less	22	12	$663,813	$295,413	$432,564	$607,664	$950,257	$1,143,649
11% to 50%	27	9	$838,434	$363,951	$568,026	$769,890	$1,160,881	$1,317,931
51% or more	1	1	*	*	*	*	*	*

Table 83C: Compensation to Gross Charges Ratio (TC/NPP Excluded)

	Physicians	Medical Practices	Mean	Std. Dev.	25th %tile	Median	75th %tile	90th %tile
Overall	131	46	.359	.163	.259	.322	.406	.613
1 to 2 Years in Specialty	8	7	*	*	*	*	*	*
Group Type								
Single-specialty	44	6	.278	.088	.198	.274	.344	.384
Multispecialty	87	40	.400	.177	.290	.343	.453	.683
Geographic Section								
Eastern	43	10	.285	.076	.202	.296	.345	.363
Midwest	38	19	.424	.176	.300	.355	.466	.701
Southern	36	12	.402	.208	.231	.346	.527	.699
Western	14	5	.300	.058	.255	.295	.342	.392
Capitation								
No capitation	82	23	.363	.181	.241	.317	.423	.679
10% or less	22	12	.398	.171	.289	.374	.469	.643
11% to 50%	25	9	.318	.065	.282	.320	.345	.393
51% or more	1	1	*	*	*	*	*	*

NEUROLOGY

Table 84A: Compensation

	Physicians	Medical Practices	Mean	Std. Dev.	25th %tile	Median	75th %tile	90th %tile
Overall	522	150	$213,082	$97,235	$156,843	$185,666	$236,655	$317,607
1 to 2 Years in Specialty	30	22	$163,443	$43,384	$134,966	$154,843	$195,239	$238,732
Group Type								
Single-specialty	135	21	$224,932	$108,573	$150,357	$191,459	$259,466	$384,337
Multispecialty	387	129	$208,948	$92,752	$157,014	$184,576	$228,786	$297,874
Geographic Section								
Eastern	137	24	$196,753	$64,824	$160,041	$185,200	$219,303	$282,848
Midwest	189	58	$235,244	$116,907	$158,909	$201,071	$259,393	$397,418
Southern	88	35	$210,811	$107,175	$147,118	$184,892	$248,417	$306,287
Western	108	33	$196,860	$76,575	$156,905	$178,937	$205,931	$309,123
Capitation								
No capitation	254	85	$226,456	$107,478	$159,818	$198,593	$256,669	$358,171
10% or less	102	35	$200,391	$82,273	$151,430	$176,880	$230,145	$297,132
11% to 50%	107	17	$208,883	$103,047	$154,718	$177,692	$225,265	$287,297
51% or more	32	12	$192,536	$46,508	$168,125	$178,570	$201,334	$285,003

Table 84B: Gross Charges (TC/NPP Excluded)

	Physicians	Medical Practices	Mean	Std. Dev.	25th %tile	Median	75th %tile	90th %tile
Overall	224	75	$709,576	$398,689	$489,938	$624,120	$820,499	$1,076,906
1 to 2 Years in Specialty	10	9	$593,780	$213,806	$474,782	$595,574	$748,221	$905,259
Group Type								
Single-specialty	60	9	$682,841	$321,921	$473,510	$648,053	$859,675	$1,205,861
Multispecialty	164	66	$719,357	$423,784	$495,043	$598,657	$801,921	$1,029,159
Geographic Section								
Eastern	38	11	$632,738	$211,759	$490,593	$572,156	$884,740	$929,411
Midwest	126	39	$734,329	$469,288	$481,651	$649,697	$824,328	$1,233,153
Southern	28	13	$770,660	$343,589	$545,164	$671,812	$922,766	$1,469,087
Western	32	12	$649,909	$286,867	$508,853	$546,578	$746,881	$1,035,635
Capitation								
No capitation	115	41	$726,956	$317,833	$504,926	$646,591	$826,330	$1,111,809
10% or less	61	21	$595,679	$301,802	$383,851	$551,773	$767,784	$915,694
11% to 50%	38	9	$888,235	$654,624	$525,710	$652,817	$939,682	$1,856,180
51% or more	10	4	$525,571	$160,600	$433,912	$482,767	$532,925	$919,634

Table 84C: Compensation to Gross Charges Ratio (TC/NPP Excluded)

	Physicians	Medical Practices	Mean	Std. Dev.	25th %tile	Median	75th %tile	90th %tile
Overall	222	74	.346	.133	.260	.319	.392	.555
1 to 2 Years in Specialty	10	9	.308	.129	.211	.280	.335	.610
Group Type								
Single-specialty	60	9	.392	.198	.235	.318	.466	.715
Multispecialty	162	65	.329	.093	.264	.320	.383	.454
Geographic Section								
Eastern	38	11	.312	.100	.242	.291	.349	.476
Midwest	126	39	.359	.152	.257	.324	.401	.587
Southern	26	12	.323	.107	.234	.309	.388	.470
Western	32	12	.355	.091	.292	.344	.406	.466
Capitation								
No capitation	113	40	.337	.108	.264	.320	.388	.468
10% or less	61	21	.395	.182	.264	.347	.453	.709
11% to 50%	38	9	.279	.064	.233	.279	.312	.379
51% or more	10	4	.413	.096	.356	.391	.457	.586

OBSTETRICS/GYNECOLOGY

Table 85A: Compensation

	Physicians	Medical Practices	Mean	Std. Dev.	25th %tile	Median	75th %tile	90th %tile
Overall	1,638	284	$257,933	$107,545	$192,370	$233,061	$293,390	$385,521
1 to 2 Years in Specialty	116	57	$186,950	$41,305	$164,017	$181,709	$203,219	$230,796
Group Type								
Single-specialty	451	88	$269,023	$140,182	$185,880	$238,953	$310,253	$419,767
Multispecialty	1,187	196	$253,720	$91,889	$195,505	$232,132	$288,080	$372,687
Geographic Section								
Eastern	282	50	$225,012	$120,589	$170,484	$204,736	$246,703	$324,252
Midwest	543	108	$277,035	$103,632	$210,308	$258,904	$324,765	$411,481
Southern	298	58	$289,022	$126,653	$208,532	$255,778	$329,896	$466,139
Western	515	68	$237,832	$79,669	$187,223	$221,800	$267,348	$326,743
Capitation								
No capitation	777	177	$272,872	$116,275	$195,519	$247,649	$317,342	$416,613
10% or less	240	48	$251,751	$93,760	$185,455	$230,471	$304,841	$388,872
11% to 50%	285	40	$254,822	$129,457	$187,422	$233,385	$292,090	$385,729
51% or more	140	16	$241,980	$78,886	$198,683	$220,471	$271,212	$316,679

Table 85B: Gross Charges (TC/NPP Excluded)

	Physicians	Medical Practices	Mean	Std. Dev.	25th %tile	Median	75th %tile	90th %tile
Overall	538	115	$923,820	$405,281	$679,740	$874,092	$1,079,366	$1,361,118
1 to 2 Years in Specialty	27	22	$802,572	$299,315	$610,784	$762,113	$902,450	$1,195,503
Group Type								
Single-specialty	110	23	$1,045,818	$629,983	$682,464	$945,543	$1,197,962	$1,759,594
Multispecialty	428	92	$892,465	$316,916	$679,078	$871,501	$1,044,241	$1,287,463
Geographic Section								
Eastern	107	18	$829,694	$275,304	$650,559	$874,616	$1,007,725	$1,183,790
Midwest	205	47	$955,806	$358,902	$694,333	$910,045	$1,147,735	$1,432,901
Southern	98	23	$1,116,295	$614,417	$817,224	$972,349	$1,183,142	$1,791,899
Western	128	27	$803,912	$289,520	$613,101	$747,962	$905,839	$1,168,463
Capitation								
No capitation	268	67	$937,267	$457,337	$672,351	$871,501	$1,100,005	$1,400,763
10% or less	115	25	$857,812	$278,486	$679,775	$847,564	$1,044,724	$1,205,237
11% to 50%	132	18	$945,651	$388,295	$697,304	$876,917	$1,074,275	$1,461,563
51% or more	23	5	$971,884	$375,428	$743,776	$888,339	$1,071,781	$1,675,229

Table 85C: Compensation to Gross Charges Ratio (TC/NPP Excluded)

	Physicians	Medical Practices	Mean	Std. Dev.	25th %tile	Median	75th %tile	90th %tile
Overall	526	114	.311	.092	.244	.302	.363	.422
1 to 2 Years in Specialty	26	21	.259	.052	.236	.254	.284	.334
Group Type								
Single-specialty	102	23	.301	.101	.232	.282	.345	.402
Multispecialty	424	91	.314	.089	.250	.307	.367	.426
Geographic Section								
Eastern	104	18	.291	.101	.222	.265	.338	.396
Midwest	205	47	.340	.098	.273	.330	.389	.460
Southern	89	22	.278	.081	.207	.263	.343	.386
Western	128	27	.306	.066	.251	.307	.350	.396
Capitation								
No capitation	262	66	.307	.091	.237	.297	.349	.412
10% or less	115	25	.342	.081	.282	.339	.387	.453
11% to 50%	126	18	.286	.075	.234	.266	.326	.401
51% or more	23	5	.348	.162	.263	.314	.367	.627

Obstetrics/Gynecology: Gyn only

Table 86A: Compensation

	Physicians	Medical Practices	Mean	Std. Dev.	25th %tile	Median	75th %tile	90th %tile
Overall	176	72	$224,273	$109,690	$146,714	$201,420	$270,286	$364,399
1 to 2 Years in Specialty	3	3	*	*	*	*	*	*
Group Type								
Single-specialty	47	24	$184,371	$81,712	$125,056	$167,301	$215,420	$330,118
Multispecialty	129	48	$238,810	$115,120	$165,659	$217,480	$276,419	$396,000
Geographic Section								
Eastern	34	16	$189,870	$79,378	$130,986	$180,008	$225,000	$311,580
Midwest	76	21	$259,282	$131,432	$170,959	$233,704	$287,848	$443,757
Southern	46	24	$205,154	$84,708	$134,829	$182,922	$275,229	$344,618
Western	20	11	$193,694	$76,179	$132,151	$184,369	$226,452	$306,833
Capitation								
No capitation	113	42	$232,205	$119,927	$153,273	$210,496	$275,431	$361,638
10% or less	34	14	$220,539	$100,598	$140,000	$183,644	$297,891	$401,591
11% to 50%	19	10	$204,088	$76,736	$133,533	$202,840	$240,000	$308,393
51% or more	10	6	$185,683	$52,258	$131,746	$178,049	$234,379	$276,004

Table 86B: Gross Charges (TC/NPP Excluded)

	Physicians	Medical Practices	Mean	Std. Dev.	25th %tile	Median	75th %tile	90th %tile
Overall	90	33	$781,265	$352,902	$489,832	$773,066	$986,809	$1,258,014
1 to 2 Years in Specialty	1	1	*	*	*	*	*	*
Group Type								
Single-specialty	9	5	*	*	*	*	*	*
Multispecialty	81	28	$799,571	$353,081	$509,730	$765,937	$1,041,789	$1,260,270
Geographic Section								
Eastern	10	6	$525,656	$238,976	$318,039	$598,723	$670,446	$887,903
Midwest	57	11	$892,542	$353,610	$663,301	$926,883	$1,128,573	$1,335,362
Southern	15	10	$636,596	$294,947	$374,158	$538,169	$891,120	$1,060,401
Western	8	6	*	*	*	*	*	*
Capitation								
No capitation	60	16	$860,475	$352,756	$590,232	$883,010	$1,106,491	$1,331,843
10% or less	17	9	$661,436	$290,245	$380,275	$705,699	$877,798	$1,035,517
11% to 50%	8	5	*	*	*	*	*	*
51% or more	5	3	*	*	*	*	*	*

Table 86C: Compensation to Gross Charges Ratio (TC/NPP Excluded)

	Physicians	Medical Practices	Mean	Std. Dev.	25th %tile	Median	75th %tile	90th %tile
Overall	89	33	.317	.155	.218	.256	.359	.515
1 to 2 Years in Specialty	1	1	*	*	*	*	*	*
Group Type								
Single-specialty	9	5	*	*	*	*	*	*
Multispecialty	80	28	.307	.139	.217	.245	.347	.501
Geographic Section								
Eastern	9	6	*	*	*	*	*	*
Midwest	57	11	.302	.152	.210	.231	.343	.505
Southern	15	10	.329	.097	.239	.301	.384	.512
Western	8	6	*	*	*	*	*	*
Capitation								
No capitation	60	16	.286	.136	.210	.233	.314	.428
10% or less	17	9	.369	.190	.234	.330	.427	.599
11% to 50%	7	5	*	*	*	*	*	*
51% or more	5	3	*	*	*	*	*	*

OCCUPATIONAL MEDICINE

Table 87A: Compensation

	Physicians	Medical Practices	Mean	Std. Dev.	25th %tile	Median	75th %tile	90th %tile
Overall	153	55	$197,461	$112,934	$141,282	$164,783	$206,796	$295,765
1 to 2 Years in Specialty	15	3	$156,907	$25,532	$144,478	$151,916	$164,203	$204,227
Group Type								
Single-specialty	8	3	*	*	*	*	*	*
Multispecialty	145	52	$194,961	$113,685	$140,906	$164,203	$201,435	$289,967
Geographic Section								
Eastern	13	7	$147,411	$33,032	$125,646	$137,767	$157,146	$217,931
Midwest	62	27	$222,506	$160,374	$138,845	$158,567	$211,060	$545,217
Southern	16	10	$215,814	$99,029	$107,113	$237,326	$292,688	$352,776
Western	62	11	$178,174	$42,393	$148,892	$168,753	$198,900	$227,425
Capitation								
No capitation	58	28	$235,409	$166,594	$129,544	$158,091	$282,460	$572,609
10% or less	20	8	$176,976	$55,401	$139,095	$180,774	$217,525	$227,993
11% to 50%	26	13	$174,974	$65,715	$132,431	$157,813	$194,980	$254,371
51% or more	21	5	$177,414	$44,530	$141,427	$168,264	$191,171	$267,180

Table 87B: Gross Charges (TC/NPP Excluded)

	Physicians	Medical Practices	Mean	Std. Dev.	25th %tile	Median	75th %tile	90th %tile
Overall	47	25	$408,614	$139,782	$281,161	$390,492	$525,102	$610,423
1 to 2 Years in Specialty	2	1	*	*	*	*	*	*
Group Type								
Multispecialty	47	25	$408,614	$139,782	$281,161	$390,492	$525,102	$610,423
Geographic Section								
Eastern	2	2	*	*	*	*	*	*
Midwest	30	15	$391,612	$137,894	$277,815	$367,878	$485,938	$622,828
Southern	3	3	*	*	*	*	*	*
Western	12	5	$453,329	$130,750	$347,062	$461,083	$586,529	$629,229
Capitation								
No capitation	21	10	$410,930	$118,031	$318,873	$390,492	$499,768	$619,082
10% or less	13	7	$405,848	$157,276	$264,727	$458,907	$551,995	$592,362
11% to 50%	10	6	$398,345	$173,101	$232,331	$350,374	$611,309	$639,905
51% or more	3	2	*	*	*	*	*	*

Table 87C: Compensation to Gross Charges Ratio (TC/NPP Excluded)

	Physicians	Medical Practices	Mean	Std. Dev.	25th %tile	Median	75th %tile	90th %tile
Overall	46	25	.427	.146	.340	.383	.521	.661
1 to 2 Years in Specialty	2	1	*	*	*	*	*	*
Group Type								
Multispecialty	46	25	.427	.146	.340	.383	.521	.661
Geographic Section								
Eastern	2	2	*	*	*	*	*	*
Midwest	29	15	.430	.152	.307	.421	.559	.664
Southern	3	3	*	*	*	*	*	*
Western	12	5	.398	.099	.338	.359	.404	.605
Capitation								
No capitation	21	10	.387	.117	.307	.364	.421	.600
10% or less	12	7	.419	.165	.340	.372	.435	.775
11% to 50%	10	6	.496	.169	.382	.444	.665	.765
51% or more	3	2	*	*	*	*	*	*

MEDICAL GROUP MANAGEMENT ASSOCIATION™

OPHTHALMOLOGY

Table 88A: Compensation

	Physicians	Medical Practices	Mean	Std. Dev.	25th %tile	Median	75th %tile	90th %tile
Overall	557	155	$301,761	$150,875	$200,000	$254,376	$375,057	$477,124
1 to 2 Years in Specialty	31	17	$169,721	$26,061	$157,000	$163,874	$183,710	$197,242
Group Type								
Single-specialty	179	34	$352,392	$172,188	$215,611	$344,000	$430,007	$569,253
Multispecialty	378	121	$277,784	$133,338	$196,102	$236,001	$336,605	$440,555
Geographic Section								
Eastern	90	22	$324,040	$146,150	$213,426	$291,504	$398,375	$537,285
Midwest	189	64	$327,574	$166,915	$207,655	$296,461	$404,138	$509,973
Southern	108	36	$291,127	$154,160	$168,723	$267,134	$367,574	$486,161
Western	170	33	$268,023	$123,994	$199,178	$234,704	$320,767	$402,824
Capitation								
No capitation	280	88	$331,069	$164,833	$211,156	$310,071	$410,442	$525,515
10% or less	90	31	$294,577	$130,439	$191,636	$267,928	$381,592	$449,712
11% to 50%	76	22	$291,267	$169,823	$197,149	$235,877	$336,148	$482,374
51% or more	46	13	$276,307	$112,139	$199,145	$231,694	$359,177	$457,307

Table 88B: Gross Charges (TC/NPP Excluded)

	Physicians	Medical Practices	Mean	Std. Dev.	25th %tile	Median	75th %tile	90th %tile
Overall	152	63	$1,302,468	$667,296	$852,996	$1,150,407	$1,633,727	$2,111,403
1 to 2 Years in Specialty	5	5	*	*	*	*	*	*
Group Type								
Single-specialty	13	4	$1,531,560	$1,057,119	$982,889	$1,300,000	$1,609,206	$3,731,787
Multispecialty	139	59	$1,281,042	$620,202	$842,204	$1,132,797	$1,641,411	$2,058,143
Geographic Section								
Eastern	28	8	$1,266,666	$511,875	$885,289	$1,222,620	$1,538,071	$2,058,405
Midwest	75	30	$1,344,429	$686,885	$889,968	$1,194,522	$1,747,541	$2,160,124
Southern	24	12	$1,434,043	$879,019	$880,757	$1,264,700	$1,847,094	$2,187,731
Western	25	13	$1,090,374	$490,316	$783,699	$976,107	$1,224,771	$1,981,700
Capitation								
No capitation	76	32	$1,201,917	$712,434	$791,857	$1,038,558	$1,404,181	$2,081,219
10% or less	31	16	$1,452,746	$474,047	$1,093,657	$1,360,440	$1,889,358	$2,057,510
11% to 50%	32	10	$1,506,520	$713,636	$993,782	$1,456,133	$1,851,673	$2,283,868
51% or more	13	5	$1,029,666	$489,319	$758,439	$900,234	$1,220,508	$1,975,259

Table 88C: Compensation to Gross Charges Ratio (TC/NPP Excluded)

	Physicians	Medical Practices	Mean	Std. Dev.	25th %tile	Median	75th %tile	90th %tile
Overall	133	60	.273	.093	.201	.257	.316	.406
1 to 2 Years in Specialty	5	5	*	*	*	*	*	*
Group Type								
Single-specialty	11	4	.362	.124	.274	.372	.434	.589
Multispecialty	122	56	.265	.086	.199	.252	.307	.389
Geographic Section								
Eastern	26	8	.275	.121	.187	.228	.381	.441
Midwest	65	29	.278	.091	.202	.269	.326	.398
Southern	18	10	.257	.092	.198	.234	.261	.469
Western	24	13	.267	.062	.212	.273	.306	.356
Capitation								
No capitation	71	31	.278	.093	.201	.257	.322	.425
10% or less	28	15	.245	.054	.199	.243	.275	.331
11% to 50%	22	9	.263	.127	.176	.210	.312	.494
51% or more	12	5	.320	.076	.274	.320	.394	.413

ORTHOPEDIC SURGERY

Table 89A: Compensation

	Physicians	Medical Practices	Mean	Std. Dev.	25th %tile	Median	75th %tile	90th %tile
Overall	904	226	$404,263	$186,004	$282,878	$364,060	$482,696	$626,991
1 to 2 Years in Specialty	58	36	$326,025	$139,321	$245,989	$286,192	$390,248	$541,551
Group Type	904	226	$404,263	$186,004	$282,878	$364,060	$482,696	$626,991
Single-specialty	403	105	$426,121	$188,308	$293,409	$411,375	$537,298	$662,832
Multispecialty	501	121	$386,681	$182,424	$278,885	$345,687	$450,231	$588,686
Geographic Section	904	226	$404,263	$186,004	$282,878	$364,060	$482,696	$626,991
Eastern	156	41	$390,019	$170,871	$251,635	$370,732	$483,360	$638,982
Midwest	307	83	$432,716	$205,535	$304,458	$389,650	$509,490	$647,107
Southern	193	50	$440,397	$216,527	$286,096	$403,053	$540,050	$678,030
Western	248	52	$349,881	$119,410	$274,398	$329,643	$392,250	$525,987
Capitation	904	226	$404,263	$186,004	$282,878	$364,060	$482,696	$626,991
No capitation	578	162	$430,182	$196,256	$292,557	$409,527	$531,969	$662,477
10% or less	89	30	$361,915	$146,111	$257,960	$318,762	$455,136	$591,340
11% to 50%	99	23	$382,316	$211,867	$260,722	$350,147	$414,550	$553,029
51% or more	45	9	$348,366	$90,537	$283,172	$328,480	$392,152	$520,446

Table 89B: Gross Charges (TC/NPP Excluded)

	Physicians	Medical Practices	Mean	Std. Dev.	25th %tile	Median	75th %tile	90th %tile
Overall	252	71	$1,521,862	$804,769	$1,072,485	$1,378,255	$1,750,987	$2,294,463
1 to 2 Years in Specialty	10	10	$1,507,400	$334,975	$1,257,105	$1,450,892	$1,637,696	$2,238,862
Group Type								
Single-specialty	47	13	$1,832,575	$1,341,631	$1,185,624	$1,380,350	$1,614,156	$3,753,272
Multispecialty	205	58	$1,450,626	$603,034	$1,052,398	$1,371,537	$1,818,207	$2,232,352
Geographic Section								
Eastern	26	7	$1,624,915	$588,717	$1,291,647	$1,508,895	$1,966,389	$2,273,237
Midwest	136	36	$1,476,150	$555,464	$1,091,308	$1,403,171	$1,746,501	$2,158,323
Southern	45	13	$1,906,156	$1,441,456	$899,087	$1,365,610	$2,469,718	$3,838,900
Western	45	15	$1,216,180	$462,441	$854,632	$1,202,314	$1,510,262	$1,782,832
Capitation								
No capitation	140	41	$1,533,095	$935,082	$1,050,552	$1,360,775	$1,726,234	$2,415,596
10% or less	47	16	$1,280,516	$520,651	$983,579	$1,144,542	$1,564,747	$2,171,738
11% to 50%	60	11	$1,675,263	$630,270	$1,267,432	$1,567,955	$2,015,699	$2,467,196
51% or more	5	3	*	*	*	*	*	*

Table 89C: Compensation to Gross Charges Ratio (TC/NPP Excluded)

	Physicians	Medical Practices	Mean	Std. Dev.	25th %tile	Median	75th %tile	90th %tile
Overall	236	69	.286	.092	.226	.274	.311	.417
1 to 2 Years in Specialty	7	7	*	*	*	*	*	*
Group Type								
Single-specialty	38	12	.338	.133	.259	.285	.465	.551
Multispecialty	198	57	.277	.078	.223	.273	.309	.357
Geographic Section								
Eastern	24	7	.230	.071	.179	.212	.270	.301
Midwest	132	36	.287	.090	.228	.275	.316	.406
Southern	36	12	.278	.058	.236	.282	.301	.349
Western	44	14	.322	.115	.235	.284	.382	.533
Capitation								
No capitation	129	40	.304	.093	.257	.283	.319	.456
10% or less	47	16	.282	.088	.223	.280	.317	.357
11% to 50%	56	11	.247	.082	.199	.225	.283	.327
51% or more	4	2	*	*	*	*	*	*

ORTHOPEDIC SURGERY: HAND

Table 90A: Compensation

	Physicians	Medical Practices	Mean	Std. Dev.	25th %tile	Median	75th %tile	90th %tile
Overall	140	79	$475,257	$237,377	$288,299	$419,676	$606,250	$774,989
1 to 2 Years in Specialty	4	4	*	*	*	*	*	*
Group Type								
Single-specialty	110	61	$486,647	$247,876	$286,245	$454,517	$620,555	$803,654
Multispecialty	30	18	$433,491	$191,951	$288,811	$401,339	$541,383	$692,887
Geographic Section								
Eastern	28	20	$439,600	$254,005	$259,414	$334,122	$617,245	$849,303
Midwest	41	22	$490,914	$225,378	$321,563	$462,523	$673,346	$772,447
Southern	46	19	$476,328	$244,900	$335,959	$433,967	$551,345	$765,624
Western	25	18	$487,543	$233,644	$313,418	$442,300	$607,082	$838,579
Capitation								
No capitation	112	63	$496,175	$253,323	$282,650	$462,579	$638,906	$832,527
10% or less	11	6	$401,982	$173,759	$290,446	$377,654	$531,437	$688,818
11% to 50%	15	8	$361,081	$75,899	$300,000	$378,604	$402,819	$482,270
51% or more	1	1	*	*	*	*	*	*

Table 90B: Gross Charges (TC/NPP Excluded)

	Physicians	Medical Practices	Mean	Std. Dev.	25th %tile	Median	75th %tile	90th %tile
Overall	30	20	$1,854,479	$983,492	$1,276,909	$1,515,303	$2,186,714	$2,929,992
1 to 2 Years in Specialty	1	1	*	*	*	*	*	*
Group Type								
Single-specialty	18	11	$2,060,877	$1,171,321	$1,358,546	$1,635,231	$2,373,410	$4,836,307
Multispecialty	12	9	$1,544,882	$505,384	$1,227,536	$1,374,585	$1,952,304	$2,378,953
Geographic Section								
Eastern	5	4	*	*	*	*	*	*
Midwest	15	10	$1,518,373	$448,920	$1,274,939	$1,471,605	$1,662,058	$2,375,973
Southern	3	1	*	*	*	*	*	*
Western	7	5	*	*	*	*	*	*
Capitation								
No capitation	23	15	$1,921,508	$1,093,928	$1,340,045	$1,555,276	$2,370,549	$4,079,276
10% or less	2	2	*	*	*	*	*	*
11% to 50%	4	2	*	*	*	*	*	*
51% or more	1	1	*	*	*	*	*	*

Table 90C: Compensation to Gross Charges Ratio (TC/NPP Excluded)

	Physicians	Medical Practices	Mean	Std. Dev.	25th %tile	Median	75th %tile	90th %tile
Overall	27	19	.319	.108	.256	.297	.360	.528
1 to 2 Years in Specialty	1	1	*	*	*	*	*	*
Group Type								
Single-specialty	15	10	.327	.107	.260	.319	.382	.515
Multispecialty	12	9	.309	.113	.237	.275	.329	.541
Geographic Section								
Eastern	5	4	*	*	*	*	*	*
Midwest	15	10	.305	.111	.240	.279	.335	.520
Western	7	5	*	*	*	*	*	*
Capitation								
No capitation	20	14	.322	.108	.257	.304	.376	.523
10% or less	2	2	*	*	*	*	*	*
11% to 50%	4	2	*	*	*	*	*	*
51% or more	1	1	*	*	*	*	*	*

ORTHOPEDIC SURGERY: SPINE

Table 91A: Compensation

	Physicians	Medical Practices	Mean	Std. Dev.	25th %tile	Median	75th %tile	90th %tile
Overall	134	81	$620,380	$332,373	$384,461	$545,412	$806,215	$1,100,000
1 to 2 Years in Specialty	12	10	$481,296	$167,610	$340,778	$495,517	$587,884	$726,349
Group Type								
Single-specialty	97	60	$633,646	$335,598	$385,441	$547,585	$824,888	$1,107,841
Multispecialty	37	21	$585,602	$325,694	$370,038	$538,982	$691,822	$1,085,626
Geographic Section								
Eastern	38	20	$625,748	$377,845	$384,461	$545,412	$770,562	$1,047,230
Midwest	48	28	$661,312	$359,070	$368,234	$590,223	$875,509	$1,183,615
Southern	20	13	$615,979	$313,780	$372,719	$536,250	$887,138	$1,126,229
Western	28	20	$546,067	$214,592	$410,510	$505,828	$633,006	$856,079
Capitation								
No capitation	110	68	$609,043	$345,135	$368,108	$497,220	$811,824	$1,091,643
10% or less	3	3	*	*	*	*	*	*
11% to 50%	9	6	*	*	*	*	*	*
51% or more	2	2	*	*	*	*	*	*

Table 91B: Gross Charges (TC/NPP Excluded)

	Physicians	Medical Practices	Mean	Std. Dev.	25th %tile	Median	75th %tile	90th %tile
Overall	34	22	$2,847,291	$1,706,175	$1,442,619	$2,479,173	$3,670,969	$6,174,830
1 to 2 Years in Specialty	2	2	*	*	*	*	*	*
Group Type								
Single-specialty	18	11	$2,991,083	$1,783,884	$1,583,179	$2,609,076	$3,711,289	$6,328,649
Multispecialty	16	11	$2,685,526	$1,656,805	$1,185,566	$2,186,873	$3,733,952	$5,552,011
Geographic Section								
Eastern	7	5	*	*	*	*	*	*
Midwest	21	11	$2,324,119	$958,636	$1,479,511	$2,005,745	$3,053,620	$3,740,250
Southern	1	1	*	*	*	*	*	*
Western	5	5	*	*	*	*	*	*
Capitation								
No capitation	25	16	$2,653,948	$1,647,575	$1,441,180	$2,116,900	$3,188,274	$6,155,221
10% or less	1	1	*	*	*	*	*	*
11% to 50%	6	3	*	*	*	*	*	*
51% or more	2	2	*	*	*	*	*	*

Table 91C: Compensation to Gross Charges Ratio (TC/NPP Excluded)

	Physicians	Medical Practices	Mean	Std. Dev.	25th %tile	Median	75th %tile	90th %tile
Overall	23	15	.268	.060	.226	.269	.289	.339
1 to 2 Years in Specialty	2	2	*	*	*	*	*	*
Group Type								
Single-specialty	11	6	.282	.065	.249	.269	.294	.429
Multispecialty	12	9	.256	.055	.202	.264	.288	.345
Geographic Section								
Eastern	1	1	*	*	*	*	*	*
Midwest	18	10	.268	.066	.225	.269	.290	.373
Western	4	4	*	*	*	*	*	*
Capitation								
No capitation	18	11	.269	.056	.242	.269	.282	.316
11% to 50%	3	2	*	*	*	*	*	*
51% or more	2	2	*	*	*	*	*	*

MEDICAL GROUP MANAGEMENT ASSOCIATION™

ORTHOPEDIC SURGERY: SPORTS MEDICINE

Table 92A: Compensation

	Physicians	Medical Practices	Mean	Std. Dev.	25th %tile	Median	75th %tile	90th %tile
Overall	260	102	$407,666	$249,561	$234,406	$344,229	$501,908	$717,599
1 to 2 Years in Specialty	30	19	$272,694	$169,120	$176,842	$201,041	$326,226	$514,274
Group Type								
Single-specialty	158	74	$494,559	$267,404	$325,138	$438,861	$611,789	$907,924
Multispecialty	102	28	$273,068	$135,835	$197,784	$240,211	$272,971	$450,287
Geographic Section								
Eastern	33	19	$469,784	$200,816	$326,032	$473,000	$619,772	$738,508
Midwest	63	32	$491,682	$298,597	$265,982	$403,753	$618,588	$929,594
Southern	72	26	$386,747	$213,008	$210,188	$364,246	$477,303	$649,107
Western	92	25	$344,224	$237,131	$226,485	$252,655	$378,824	$608,958
Capitation								
No capitation	178	82	$463,936	$264,521	$265,120	$405,181	$573,228	$830,895
10% or less	12	8	$356,303	$227,122	$219,177	$268,225	$501,779	$827,718
11% to 50%	11	7	$397,828	$124,246	$258,616	$428,493	$454,695	$575,601
51% or more	7	2	*	*	*	*	*	*

Table 92B: Gross Charges (TC/NPP Excluded)

	Physicians	Medical Practices	Mean	Std. Dev.	25th %tile	Median	75th %tile	90th %tile
Overall	55	28	$1,613,278	$769,165	$1,089,216	$1,587,659	$2,022,237	$2,440,954
1 to 2 Years in Specialty	4	4	*	*	*	*	*	*
Group Type								
Single-specialty	33	13	$1,752,674	$553,798	$1,311,967	$1,663,865	$2,163,656	$2,552,907
Multispecialty	22	15	$1,404,183	$988,746	$769,785	$1,120,796	$1,953,083	$2,472,323
Geographic Section								
Eastern	10	5	$2,199,840	$1,072,572	$1,224,342	$2,090,864	$2,793,486	$4,365,031
Midwest	25	14	$1,488,948	$708,742	$841,471	$1,638,852	$2,011,360	$2,336,463
Southern	10	3	$1,681,750	$523,348	$1,426,353	$1,523,107	$2,156,328	$2,634,001
Western	10	6	$1,269,067	$473,080	$1,014,925	$1,311,967	$1,685,489	$1,944,115
Capitation								
No capitation	38	17	$1,694,913	$579,690	$1,300,631	$1,665,606	$2,037,612	$2,409,538
10% or less	8	6	*	*	*	*	*	*
11% to 50%	5	3	*	*	*	*	*	*
51% or more	3	1	*	*	*	*	*	*

Table 92C: Compensation to Gross Charges Ratio (TC/NPP Excluded)

	Physicians	Medical Practices	Mean	Std. Dev.	25th %tile	Median	75th %tile	90th %tile
Overall	50	26	.272	.079	.215	.257	.304	.379
1 to 2 Years in Specialty	3	3	*	*	*	*	*	*
Group Type								
Single-specialty	29	12	.254	.064	.197	.254	.299	.359
Multispecialty	21	14	.295	.092	.229	.258	.340	.455
Geographic Section								
Eastern	8	4	*	*	*	*	*	*
Midwest	23	13	.301	.092	.224	.300	.359	.452
Southern	9	3	*	*	*	*	*	*
Western	10	6	.270	.054	.231	.262	.302	.372
Capitation								
No capitation	34	16	.255	.061	.202	.250	.300	.350
10% or less	8	6	*	*	*	*	*	*
11% to 50%	4	2	*	*	*	*	*	*
51% or more	3	1	*	*	*	*	*	*

OTORHINOLARYNGOLOGY

Table 93A: Compensation

	Physicians	Medical Practices	Mean	Std. Dev.	25th %tile	Median	75th %tile	90th %tile
Overall	424	146	$326,884	$177,842	$220,217	$277,585	$367,484	$545,954
1 to 2 Years in Specialty	19	16	$237,962	$88,076	$176,000	$226,877	$280,918	$399,696
Group Type								
Single-specialty	109	21	$314,175	$181,389	$201,712	$261,685	$348,216	$529,933
Multispecialty	315	125	$331,282	$176,677	$226,116	$278,307	$374,596	$550,472
Geographic Section								
Eastern	91	21	$336,231	$229,755	$206,109	$261,820	$353,472	$668,497
Midwest	134	56	$334,982	$137,707	$243,595	$301,647	$390,815	$542,159
Southern	118	38	$349,355	$206,742	$222,672	$288,926	$397,587	$592,693
Western	81	31	$270,249	$98,021	$209,228	$243,671	$307,150	$401,844
Capitation								
No capitation	244	80	$348,107	$199,512	$224,937	$286,645	$399,174	$597,015
10% or less	67	32	$300,661	$131,624	$214,604	$263,421	$346,199	$511,284
11% to 50%	79	23	$309,701	$154,642	$222,453	$275,255	$349,259	$460,949
51% or more	34	11	$266,175	$109,079	$215,991	$233,924	$295,171	$342,190

Table 93B: Gross Charges (TC/NPP Excluded)

	Physicians	Medical Practices	Mean	Std. Dev.	25th %tile	Median	75th %tile	90th %tile
Overall	195	76	$1,276,567	$620,772	$841,208	$1,122,047	$1,624,108	$2,037,970
1 to 2 Years in Specialty	8	7	*	*	*	*	*	*
Group Type								
Single-specialty	42	6	$1,246,486	$457,932	$916,003	$1,103,652	$1,615,462	$2,014,552
Multispecialty	153	70	$1,284,825	$659,511	$819,904	$1,131,272	$1,632,532	$2,040,339
Geographic Section								
Eastern	30	9	$1,112,438	$491,049	$787,206	$973,681	$1,236,064	$1,858,891
Midwest	97	40	$1,305,513	$495,841	$942,288	$1,265,686	$1,646,696	$1,958,275
Southern	32	14	$1,584,600	$1,005,677	$870,024	$1,457,037	$2,023,888	$3,146,979
Western	36	13	$1,061,542	$454,219	$728,975	$954,693	$1,235,096	$1,794,756
Capitation								
No capitation	95	40	$1,211,991	$595,948	$822,036	$1,103,531	$1,521,149	$1,967,168
10% or less	43	22	$1,032,488	$410,278	$744,906	$989,343	$1,186,161	$1,743,562
11% to 50%	53	12	$1,615,039	$682,847	$1,087,341	$1,547,970	$1,926,142	$2,401,401
51% or more	4	2	*	*	*	*	*	*

Table 93C: Compensation to Gross Charges Ratio (TC/NPP Excluded)

	Physicians	Medical Practices	Mean	Std. Dev.	25th %tile	Median	75th %tile	90th %tile
Overall	183	74	.270	.075	.210	.258	.317	.364
1 to 2 Years in Specialty	6	5	*	*	*	*	*	*
Group Type								
Single-specialty	39	6	.249	.084	.188	.216	.308	.345
Multispecialty	144	68	.276	.071	.221	.262	.327	.378
Geographic Section								
Eastern	26	9	.262	.055	.223	.263	.313	.342
Midwest	95	40	.275	.084	.204	.253	.341	.389
Southern	26	12	.281	.083	.223	.273	.313	.389
Western	36	13	.257	.053	.216	.245	.307	.348
Capitation								
No capitation	90	38	.277	.072	.216	.266	.317	.376
10% or less	43	22	.299	.070	.242	.295	.352	.387
11% to 50%	46	12	.223	.058	.186	.208	.237	.298
51% or more	4	2	*	*	*	*	*	*

PATHOLOGY: ANATOMIC AND CLINICAL

Table 94A: Compensation

	Physicians	Medical Practices	Mean	Std. Dev.	25th %tile	Median	75th %tile	90th %tile
Overall	233	44	$338,344	$173,094	$214,820	$285,087	$445,798	$531,028
1 to 2 Years in Specialty	16	7	$190,347	$37,084	$164,443	$172,595	$224,987	$255,448
Group Type								
Single-specialty	98	14	$461,112	$190,307	$350,140	$465,150	$528,400	$721,450
Multispecialty	135	30	$249,223	$81,442	$190,661	$222,923	$293,000	$343,599
Geographic Section								
Eastern	28	6	$304,686	$157,476	$205,985	$226,730	$410,095	$590,913
Midwest	73	16	$347,081	$131,624	$217,515	$333,958	$473,500	$525,584
Southern	47	10	$454,977	$261,941	$250,000	$349,210	$659,104	$839,600
Western	85	12	$277,437	$102,699	$206,422	$226,715	$344,976	$443,780
Capitation								
No capitation	115	25	$394,408	$152,586	$256,492	$415,251	$487,000	$579,959
10% or less	45	9	$391,237	$241,571	$250,000	$304,912	$414,543	$771,711
11% to 50%	20	5	$256,396	$68,273	$195,710	$224,185	$324,278	$355,600
51% or more	17	4	$195,933	$27,466	$171,363	$205,774	$222,305	$224,866

Table 94B: Gross Charges (TC/NPP Excluded)

	Physicians	Medical Practices	Mean	Std. Dev.	25th %tile	Median	75th %tile	90th %tile
Overall	48	15	$799,155	$427,265	$603,383	$754,221	$991,174	$1,074,398
1 to 2 Years in Specialty	3	2	*	*	*	*	*	*
Group Type								
Single-specialty	6	1	*	*	*	*	*	*
Multispecialty	42	14	$805,575	$457,092	$599,293	$735,707	$1,027,734	$1,083,714
Geographic Section								
Eastern	16	4	$872,343	$184,446	$725,762	$845,604	$1,066,013	$1,141,150
Midwest	14	5	$770,777	$225,271	$603,383	$611,238	$1,035,881	$1,071,524
Southern	14	4	$877,943	$693,788	$656,380	$754,221	$793,223	$2,116,374
Western	4	2	*	*	*	*	*	*
Capitation								
No capitation	22	8	$763,305	$220,561	$604,872	$754,221	$933,312	$1,106,657
10% or less	14	4	$939,882	$681,077	$603,383	$723,923	$1,052,348	$2,141,092
11% to 50%	9	2	*	*	*	*	*	*
51% or more	3	1	*	*	*	*	*	*

Table 94C: Compensation to Gross Charges Ratio (TC/NPP Excluded)

	Physicians	Medical Practices	Mean	Std. Dev.	25th %tile	Median	75th %tile	90th %tile
Overall	46	15	.389	.179	.262	.346	.466	.622
1 to 2 Years in Specialty	3	2	*	*	*	*	*	*
Group Type								
Single-specialty	6	1	*	*	*	*	*	*
Multispecialty	40	14	.386	.190	.242	.330	.495	.759
Geographic Section								
Eastern	16	4	.254	.067	.213	.236	.288	.391
Midwest	14	5	.461	.164	.331	.462	.528	.739
Southern	13	4	.444	.186	.293	.447	.467	.818
Western	3	2	*	*	*	*	*	*
Capitation								
No capitation	22	8	.407	.209	.272	.373	.466	.824
10% or less	13	4	.375	.137	.236	.388	.514	.548
11% to 50%	9	2	*	*	*	*	*	*
51% or more	2	1	*	*	*	*	*	*

PEDIATRIC: GENERAL

Table 95A: Compensation

	Physicians	Medical Practices	Mean	Std. Dev.	25th %tile	Median	75th %tile	90th %tile
Overall	2,215	321	$164,817	$56,005	$126,862	$153,098	$188,925	$241,844
1 to 2 Years in Specialty	158	76	$120,500	$22,267	$110,000	$119,907	$130,060	$146,332
Group Type								
Single-specialty	540	79	$174,362	$62,509	$126,772	$168,244	$211,910	$257,883
Multispecialty	1,675	242	$161,740	$53,398	$126,862	$150,507	$183,000	$230,282
Geographic Section								
Eastern	387	70	$159,716	$56,886	$120,000	$148,226	$188,366	$235,300
Midwest	736	116	$167,748	$54,560	$130,794	$155,758	$193,580	$243,756
Southern	411	64	$168,736	$68,676	$119,999	$150,046	$202,769	$258,826
Western	681	71	$162,183	$47,683	$131,900	$154,656	$178,810	$214,246
Capitation								
No capitation	921	162	$174,057	$61,048	$130,000	$165,011	$208,511	$256,837
10% or less	347	65	$160,125	$60,994	$120,000	$148,258	$183,000	$233,531
11% to 50%	498	66	$159,517	$54,195	$124,009	$147,239	$187,609	$238,857
51% or more	203	18	$156,723	$45,342	$126,520	$146,687	$172,270	$212,452

Table 95B: Gross Charges (TC/NPP Excluded)

	Physicians	Medical Practices	Mean	Std. Dev.	25th %tile	Median	75th %tile	90th %tile
Overall	925	148	$495,593	$178,520	$369,984	$465,456	$585,898	$732,941
1 to 2 Years in Specialty	51	36	$392,113	$133,062	$290,936	$402,162	$485,997	$583,335
Group Type								
Single-specialty	228	28	$504,977	$182,521	$370,257	$468,051	$609,418	$787,703
Multispecialty	697	120	$492,523	$177,216	$369,775	$465,198	$581,596	$717,783
Geographic Section								
Eastern	179	30	$483,443	$161,811	$355,902	$488,636	$577,533	$710,606
Midwest	427	65	$499,087	$191,710	$369,620	$450,044	$577,563	$773,320
Southern	126	23	$491,230	$199,075	$349,939	$473,561	$602,722	$783,916
Western	193	30	$501,978	$146,738	$390,778	$488,723	$599,050	$700,910
Capitation								
No capitation	473	78	$496,685	$178,932	$368,455	$460,177	$593,279	$738,259
10% or less	208	36	$466,522	$150,936	$353,168	$446,188	$559,746	$670,400
11% to 50%	207	27	$532,049	$204,508	$393,548	$491,745	$638,564	$825,073
51% or more	27	5	$469,383	$83,879	$409,587	$465,456	$525,089	$608,186

Table 95C: Compensation to Gross Charges Ratio (TC/NPP Excluded)

	Physicians	Medical Practices	Mean	Std. Dev.	25th %tile	Median	75th %tile	90th %tile
Overall	917	147	.352	.108	.272	.338	.399	.489
1 to 2 Years in Specialty	50	35	.337	.137	.246	.325	.378	.468
Group Type								
Single-specialty	225	28	.350	.113	.270	.321	.399	.523
Multispecialty	692	119	.353	.106	.272	.346	.400	.480
Geographic Section								
Eastern	178	30	.347	.122	.251	.337	.398	.507
Midwest	426	65	.363	.103	.298	.347	.402	.504
Southern	120	22	.358	.116	.275	.336	.421	.485
Western	193	30	.330	.095	.259	.312	.387	.448
Capitation								
No capitation	469	77	.354	.104	.290	.342	.397	.480
10% or less	208	36	.369	.115	.270	.366	.440	.529
11% to 50%	203	27	.324	.101	.253	.308	.379	.458
51% or more	27	5	.390	.118	.310	.348	.465	.607

PHYSIATRY

Table 96A: Compensation

	Physicians	Medical Practices	Mean	Std. Dev.	25th %tile	Median	75th %tile	90th %tile
Overall	178	81	$234,896	$137,062	$155,434	$192,490	$273,648	$357,265
1 to 2 Years in Specialty	18	11	$156,128	$67,241	$115,001	$145,222	$159,193	$303,026
Group Type								
Single-specialty	49	28	$311,237	$211,706	$159,385	$250,500	$361,293	$585,000
Multispecialty	129	53	$205,899	$78,049	$155,000	$186,061	$224,668	$306,926
Geographic Section								
Eastern	25	13	$251,470	$244,890	$135,000	$176,425	$273,365	$533,440
Midwest	68	36	$258,331	$119,983	$184,542	$220,246	$299,060	$418,726
Southern	25	16	$256,639	$133,621	$160,000	$210,244	$300,000	$460,472
Western	60	16	$192,373	$74,587	$151,279	$169,278	$196,990	$313,099
Capitation								
No capitation	99	53	$258,863	$169,793	$155,153	$207,430	$305,000	$496,428
10% or less	21	12	$233,464	$78,941	$184,274	$215,576	$298,920	$340,540
11% to 50%	27	13	$219,900	$79,641	$168,589	$201,668	$232,900	$341,710
51% or more	7	2	*	*	*	*	*	*

Table 96B: Gross Charges (TC/NPP Excluded)

	Physicians	Medical Practices	Mean	Std. Dev.	25th %tile	Median	75th %tile	90th %tile
Overall	51	28	$666,964	$369,586	$412,227	$597,948	$785,164	$1,111,239
1 to 2 Years in Specialty	1	1	*	*	*	*	*	*
Group Type								
Single-specialty	4	3	*	*	*	*	*	*
Multispecialty	47	25	$619,614	$271,223	$412,227	$589,360	$712,002	$1,101,413
Geographic Section								
Eastern	5	3	*	*	*	*	*	*
Midwest	36	19	$664,667	$420,483	$397,697	$556,877	$858,939	$1,123,846
Southern	2	2	*	*	*	*	*	*
Western	8	4	*	*	*	*	*	*
Capitation								
No capitation	30	16	$710,427	$429,330	$482,835	$597,680	$861,438	$1,117,603
10% or less	10	6	$547,304	$232,500	$339,655	$505,865	$695,702	$960,904
11% to 50%	9	5	*	*	*	*	*	*
51% or more	2	1	*	*	*	*	*	*

Table 96C: Compensation to Gross Charges Ratio (TC/NPP Excluded)

	Physicians	Medical Practices	Mean	Std. Dev.	25th %tile	Median	75th %tile	90th %tile
Overall	50	27	.390	.149	.280	.361	.482	.576
1 to 2 Years in Specialty	1	1	*	*	*	*	*	*
Group Type								
Single-specialty	3	2	*	*	*	*	*	*
Multispecialty	47	25	.390	.152	.274	.367	.481	.592
Geographic Section								
Eastern	5	3	*	*	*	*	*	*
Midwest	35	18	.432	.153	.337	.376	.513	.642
Southern	2	2	*	*	*	*	*	*
Western	8	4	*	*	*	*	*	*
Capitation								
No capitation	29	15	.379	.168	.253	.340	.421	.639
10% or less	10	6	.445	.109	.364	.440	.516	.635
11% to 50%	9	5	*	*	*	*	*	*
51% or more	2	1	*	*	*	*	*	*

PODIATRY

Table 97A: Compensation

	Physicians	Medical Practices	Mean	Std. Dev.	25th %tile	Median	75th %tile	90th %tile
Overall	127	72	$162,335	$57,982	$117,574	$151,328	$194,786	$239,272
1 to 2 Years in Specialty	10	9	$130,610	$36,820	$103,328	$118,000	$172,614	$192,749
Group Type								
Single-specialty	3	3	*	*	*	*	*	*
Multispecialty	124	69	$163,102	$58,114	$118,705	$151,638	$194,884	$239,527
Geographic Section								
Eastern	14	8	$158,349	$60,615	$108,373	$130,881	$235,167	$247,306
Midwest	62	35	$167,734	$60,338	$117,255	$161,013	$201,591	$255,988
Southern	22	13	$152,782	$53,912	$113,443	$135,720	$167,647	$260,413
Western	29	16	$159,961	$56,224	$130,570	$151,948	$178,849	$204,503
Capitation								
No capitation	55	36	$167,936	$60,664	$122,000	$160,229	$195,369	$239,442
10% or less	26	15	$158,213	$60,683	$106,889	$137,394	$213,777	$240,480
11% to 50%	27	14	$174,735	$60,727	$131,140	$167,205	$208,585	$264,655
51% or more	18	6	$134,034	$30,192	$110,284	$123,840	$162,674	$172,514

Table 97B: Gross Charges (TC/NPP Excluded)

	Physicians	Medical Practices	Mean	Std. Dev.	25th %tile	Median	75th %tile	90th %tile
Overall	69	40	$670,728	$262,759	$510,496	$614,746	$737,139	$1,080,044
1 to 2 Years in Specialty	3	3	*	*	*	*	*	*
Group Type								
Multispecialty	69	40	$670,728	$262,759	$510,496	$614,746	$737,139	$1,080,044
Geographic Section								
Eastern	3	2	*	*	*	*	*	*
Midwest	40	23	$676,506	$257,807	$507,327	$609,900	$734,819	$1,111,898
Southern	11	7	$620,776	$216,290	$429,032	$606,377	$789,786	$1,001,730
Western	15	8	$643,746	$275,012	$538,484	$634,612	$705,234	$1,054,184
Capitation								
No capitation	35	20	$648,460	$204,642	$534,000	$608,727	$705,234	$925,948
10% or less	13	8	$730,223	$311,860	$477,254	$647,602	$946,624	$1,299,747
11% to 50%	15	9	$755,008	$323,101	$489,587	$684,071	$1,051,792	$1,250,609
51% or more	6	3	*	*	*	*	*	*

Table 97C: Compensation to Gross Charges Ratio (TC/NPP Excluded)

	Physicians	Medical Practices	Mean	Std. Dev.	25th %tile	Median	75th %tile	90th %tile
Overall	67	38	.268	.059	.230	.259	.302	.349
1 to 2 Years in Specialty	2	2	*	*	*	*	*	*
Group Type								
Multispecialty	67	38	.268	.059	.230	.259	.302	.349
Geographic Section								
Eastern	3	2	*	*	*	*	*	*
Midwest	39	22	.275	.052	.237	.273	.310	.354
Southern	10	6	.274	.026	.256	.275	.287	.319
Western	15	8	.255	.085	.206	.220	.280	.438
Capitation								
No capitation	34	19	.260	.056	.212	.247	.311	.343
10% or less	13	8	.266	.037	.236	.273	.299	.309
11% to 50%	14	8	.252	.038	.236	.247	.284	.303
51% or more	6	3	*	*	*	*	*	*

PSYCHIATRY

Table 98A: Compensation

	Physicians	Medical Practices	Mean	Std. Dev.	25th %tile	Median	75th %tile	90th %tile
Overall	361	70	$163,906	$42,539	$135,942	$159,444	$184,536	$214,490
1 to 2 Years in Specialty	36	18	$152,499	$30,184	$135,512	$146,232	$159,476	$190,579
Group Type								
Single-specialty	10	3	$142,735	$15,690	$130,316	$140,193	$152,857	$173,943
Multispecialty	351	67	$164,509	$42,916	$136,243	$160,000	$185,566	$214,986
Geographic Section								
Eastern	86	14	$149,956	$41,927	$125,000	$144,999	$163,347	$195,775
Midwest	128	33	$161,522	$41,852	$134,117	$155,563	$183,718	$211,289
Southern	20	9	$167,805	$70,338	$122,702	$145,804	$190,324	$279,669
Western	127	14	$175,142	$34,705	$151,212	$171,351	$188,243	$221,161
Capitation								
No capitation	68	28	$178,754	$60,421	$137,182	$164,469	$199,033	$262,418
10% or less	82	16	$150,512	$46,531	$121,969	$140,169	$164,185	$207,814
11% to 50%	94	16	$153,372	$32,645	$130,223	$150,671	$171,948	$199,815
51% or more	40	9	$166,238	$31,539	$148,662	$165,345	$179,786	$211,001

Table 98B: Gross Charges (TC/NPP Excluded)

	Physicians	Medical Practices	Mean	Std. Dev.	25th %tile	Median	75th %tile	90th %tile
Overall	128	39	$359,497	$134,253	$269,633	$366,232	$439,668	$533,266
1 to 2 Years in Specialty	7	6	*	*	*	*	*	*
Group Type								
Single-specialty	3	1	*	*	*	*	*	*
Multispecialty	125	38	$358,406	$135,590	$267,550	$364,914	$439,614	$536,565
Geographic Section								
Eastern	21	6	$299,219	$154,280	$169,523	$265,871	$399,710	$542,183
Midwest	77	20	$380,814	$118,785	$296,836	$379,009	$449,804	$543,915
Southern	11	5	$347,320	$91,261	$270,846	$365,609	$425,873	$455,827
Western	19	8	$346,781	$173,424	$217,451	$340,885	$438,694	$633,050
Capitation								
No capitation	42	18	$380,910	$143,383	$277,221	$364,407	$449,890	$624,211
10% or less	34	10	$342,843	$133,421	$249,390	$332,870	$427,341	$534,407
11% to 50%	48	8	$357,459	$120,746	$258,940	$378,609	$442,338	$513,551
51% or more	4	3	*	*	*	*	*	*

Table 98C: Compensation to Gross Charges Ratio (TC/NPP Excluded)

	Physicians	Medical Practices	Mean	Std. Dev.	25th %tile	Median	75th %tile	90th %tile
Overall	119	36	.459	.156	.363	.425	.506	.664
1 to 2 Years in Specialty	6	6	*	*	*	*	*	*
Group Type								
Single-specialty	3	1	*	*	*	*	*	*
Multispecialty	116	35	.461	.157	.362	.426	.523	.669
Geographic Section								
Eastern	16	5	.506	.229	.365	.462	.587	.922
Midwest	76	20	.448	.133	.364	.426	.494	.586
Southern	10	5	.436	.103	.371	.395	.475	.668
Western	17	6	.480	.196	.326	.409	.605	.767
Capitation								
No capitation	39	17	.438	.113	.367	.409	.486	.567
10% or less	33	10	.515	.162	.416	.491	.606	.715
11% to 50%	45	8	.438	.177	.358	.379	.481	.725
51% or more	2	1	*	*	*	*	*	*

PULMONARY MEDICINE

Table 99A: Compensation

	Physicians	Medical Practices	Mean	Std. Dev.	25th %tile	Median	75th %tile	90th %tile
Overall	295	130	$230,983	$85,034	$175,084	$210,000	$277,140	$331,944
1 to 2 Years in Specialty	9	8	*	*	*	*	*	*
Group Type								
Single-specialty	33	11	$204,366	$47,726	$174,479	$196,504	$220,000	$286,232
Multispecialty	262	119	$234,336	$88,118	$175,481	$218,532	$280,031	$340,165
Geographic Section								
Eastern	53	22	$223,638	$103,631	$174,032	$192,000	$249,190	$292,149
Midwest	113	52	$248,977	$91,007	$181,761	$230,000	$305,018	$364,020
Southern	64	28	$219,872	$62,240	$173,728	$219,204	$260,609	$308,614
Western	65	28	$216,633	$72,349	$159,550	$204,244	$277,248	$311,745
Capitation								
No capitation	145	71	$239,787	$91,619	$176,005	$223,419	$296,666	$337,607
10% or less	72	31	$234,864	$80,645	$180,047	$219,438	$276,577	$350,048
11% to 50%	56	18	$213,925	$78,111	$164,686	$193,486	$257,435	$298,541
51% or more	18	9	$211,222	$62,405	$173,883	$193,216	$229,922	$341,502

Table 99B: Gross Charges (TC/NPP Excluded)

	Physicians	Medical Practices	Mean	Std. Dev.	25th %tile	Median	75th %tile	90th %tile
Overall	115	60	$799,620	$473,850	$595,007	$707,168	$865,272	$1,089,870
1 to 2 Years in Specialty	2	2	*	*	*	*	*	*
Group Type								
Single-specialty	1	1	*	*	*	*	*	*
Multispecialty	114	59	$799,870	$475,935	$593,682	$706,953	$874,580	$1,089,948
Geographic Section								
Eastern	20	8	$1,094,292	$986,367	$664,355	$762,376	$1,061,567	$3,388,232
Midwest	42	27	$744,116	$255,837	$587,498	$684,909	$833,030	$1,168,546
Southern	35	16	$777,476	$184,787	$663,181	$793,075	$902,965	$981,313
Western	18	9	$644,773	$236,654	$463,558	$548,774	$766,024	$1,036,103
Capitation								
No capitation	52	32	$848,228	$655,243	$595,505	$706,221	$863,797	$1,063,381
10% or less	36	16	$811,741	$250,401	$662,521	$778,004	$929,736	$1,184,161
11% to 50%	24	9	$686,602	$194,784	$519,984	$672,613	$795,061	$995,585
51% or more	3	3	*	*	*	*	*	*

Table 99C: Compensation to Gross Charges Ratio (TC/NPP Excluded)

	Physicians	Medical Practices	Mean	Std. Dev.	25th %tile	Median	75th %tile	90th %tile
Overall	110	57	.324	.096	.254	.311	.361	.443
1 to 2 Years in Specialty	2	2	*	*	*	*	*	*
Group Type								
Single-specialty	1	1	*	*	*	*	*	*
Multispecialty	109	56	.324	.097	.254	.311	.361	.444
Geographic Section								
Eastern	18	7	.297	.092	.242	.267	.309	.429
Midwest	42	27	.315	.082	.254	.314	.345	.432
Southern	32	14	.327	.081	.262	.314	.375	.452
Western	18	9	.364	.144	.279	.331	.416	.569
Capitation								
No capitation	47	29	.359	.095	.299	.336	.401	.496
10% or less	36	16	.293	.066	.242	.285	.331	.408
11% to 50%	24	9	.274	.046	.232	.286	.318	.335
51% or more	3	3	*	*	*	*	*	*

RADIOLOGY: DIAGNOSTIC-INVASIVE

Table 100A: Compensation

	Physicians	Medical Practices	Mean	Std. Dev.	25th %tile	Median	75th %tile	90th %tile
Overall	385	59	$412,515	$138,745	$313,604	$377,000	$510,110	$586,751
1 to 2 Years in Specialty	29	17	$248,564	$74,158	$197,160	$238,469	$301,403	$364,874
Group Type								
Single-specialty	238	31	$420,052	$152,500	$313,190	$435,000	$513,001	$601,598
Multispecialty	147	28	$400,313	$112,411	$315,000	$362,500	$491,039	$581,266
Geographic Section								
Eastern	43	9	$322,509	$77,260	$280,867	$317,053	$356,500	$450,773
Midwest	108	18	$474,487	$118,656	$371,762	$506,893	$550,000	$599,472
Southern	108	17	$433,300	$141,336	$322,475	$456,093	$555,366	$601,738
Western	126	15	$372,296	$140,965	$300,437	$341,264	$375,151	$497,816
Capitation								
No capitation	205	39	$427,124	$157,117	$315,942	$375,000	$542,205	$621,616
10% or less	80	10	$360,928	$101,490	$281,054	$350,000	$452,549	$473,322
11% to 50%	66	8	$470,632	$108,396	$386,485	$510,595	$542,564	$586,231
51% or more	6	1	*	*	*	*	*	*

Table 100B: Gross Charges (TC/NPP Excluded)

	Physicians	Medical Practices	Mean	Std. Dev.	25th %tile	Median	75th %tile	90th %tile
Overall	175	25	$1,444,019	$464,443	$1,120,530	$1,407,022	$1,744,226	$2,048,597
1 to 2 Years in Specialty	8	7	*	*	*	*	*	*
Group Type								
Single-specialty	106	10	$1,315,210	$391,442	$987,350	$1,321,230	$1,616,942	$1,769,858
Multispecialty	69	15	$1,641,900	$499,761	$1,278,906	$1,680,404	$2,024,051	$2,236,893
Geographic Section								
Eastern	22	5	$1,260,855	$498,351	$1,040,043	$1,252,182	$1,430,469	$1,760,193
Midwest	83	11	$1,460,333	$499,275	$1,046,961	$1,414,600	$1,788,558	$2,211,573
Southern	40	7	$1,673,570	$364,588	$1,458,357	$1,664,435	$1,906,584	$2,167,367
Western	30	2	$1,227,135	$288,512	$980,671	$1,244,531	$1,424,763	$1,627,481
Capitation								
No capitation	92	13	$1,478,157	$406,452	$1,217,590	$1,482,251	$1,747,027	$1,948,229
10% or less	23	5	$1,259,231	$273,009	$1,209,437	$1,278,906	$1,280,124	$1,682,613
11% to 50%	54	6	$1,465,643	$609,466	$950,919	$1,439,997	$1,935,804	$2,327,884
51% or more	6	1	*	*	*	*	*	*

Table 100C: Compensation to Gross Charges Ratio (TC/NPP Excluded)

	Physicians	Medical Practices	Mean	Std. Dev.	25th %tile	Median	75th %tile	90th %tile
Overall	164	25	.333	.132	.247	.301	.387	.508
1 to 2 Years in Specialty	3	3	*	*	*	*	*	*
Group Type								
Single-specialty	98	10	.377	.148	.271	.353	.441	.603
Multispecialty	66	15	.267	.063	.228	.260	.304	.342
Geographic Section								
Eastern	20	5	.291	.106	.209	.264	.336	.464
Midwest	79	11	.371	.158	.252	.319	.448	.627
Southern	36	7	.316	.080	.260	.306	.384	.434
Western	29	2	.279	.088	.210	.269	.313	.382
Capitation								
No capitation	83	13	.318	.084	.261	.309	.382	.431
10% or less	23	5	.284	.080	.246	.274	.304	.429
11% to 50%	52	6	.389	.190	.231	.314	.530	.675
51% or more	6	1	*	*	*	*	*	*

RADIOLOGY: DIAGNOSTIC-NONINVASIVE

Table 101A: Compensation

	Physicians	Medical Practices	Mean	Std. Dev.	25th %tile	Median	75th %tile	90th %tile
Overall	635	94	$367,754	$120,765	$278,822	$348,774	$446,049	$532,497
1 to 2 Years in Specialty	42	19	$266,834	$73,613	$228,399	$243,432	$275,098	$355,737
Group Type								
Single-specialty	244	28	$405,346	$140,526	$301,488	$392,525	$494,219	$601,337
Multispecialty	391	66	$344,296	$99,844	$272,433	$324,676	$403,646	$476,090
Geographic Section								
Eastern	83	10	$322,174	$88,348	$250,834	$300,000	$374,405	$477,885
Midwest	168	30	$418,693	$117,058	$345,350	$422,283	$498,748	$576,549
Southern	166	26	$398,651	$145,539	$295,564	$380,977	$490,796	$604,027
Western	218	28	$322,326	$86,039	$267,034	$305,559	$368,879	$432,098
Capitation								
No capitation	325	55	$408,348	$137,310	$306,606	$392,000	$496,255	$593,759
10% or less	79	17	$343,667	$91,128	$275,000	$349,291	$409,578	$455,335
11% to 50%	90	13	$334,326	$85,994	$264,014	$320,000	$416,684	$458,161
51% or more	56	7	$339,357	$80,453	$276,177	$321,159	$383,018	$479,071

Table 101B: Gross Charges (TC/NPP Excluded)

	Physicians	Medical Practices	Mean	Std. Dev.	25th %tile	Median	75th %tile	90th %tile
Overall	194	34	$1,345,207	$560,114	$1,021,512	$1,245,714	$1,600,279	$2,041,540
1 to 2 Years in Specialty	9	6	*	*	*	*	*	*
Group Type								
Single-specialty	97	10	$1,319,192	$413,728	$1,044,134	$1,324,922	$1,601,596	$1,969,847
Multispecialty	97	24	$1,371,223	$676,893	$942,190	$1,187,151	$1,567,252	$2,177,332
Geographic Section								
Eastern	49	4	$1,090,844	$311,587	$861,325	$1,032,511	$1,291,476	$1,512,736
Midwest	71	15	$1,441,435	$447,664	$1,108,474	$1,333,473	$1,704,293	$2,099,291
Southern	70	12	$1,433,190	$734,286	$1,090,590	$1,315,406	$1,660,374	$2,157,058
Western	4	3	*	*	*	*	*	*
Capitation								
No capitation	137	23	$1,281,969	$435,022	$984,732	$1,246,644	$1,556,081	$1,865,705
10% or less	17	6	$1,202,072	$428,533	$1,024,247	$1,024,247	$1,241,461	$2,139,843
11% to 50%	40	5	$1,622,631	$845,793	$1,027,457	$1,356,218	$2,041,540	$2,932,204

Table 101C: Compensation to Gross Charges Ratio (TC/NPP Excluded)

	Physicians	Medical Practices	Mean	Std. Dev.	25th %tile	Median	75th %tile	90th %tile
Overall	183	34	.335	.106	.240	.326	.423	.467
1 to 2 Years in Specialty	8	5	*	*	*	*	*	*
Group Type								
Single-specialty	93	10	.353	.107	.266	.364	.441	.494
Multispecialty	90	24	.316	.102	.237	.292	.413	.456
Geographic Section								
Eastern	47	4	.335	.104	.250	.333	.428	.461
Midwest	68	15	.319	.092	.239	.300	.412	.452
Southern	64	12	.348	.115	.222	.352	.420	.493
Western	4	3	*	*	*	*	*	*
Capitation								
No capitation	133	23	.355	.106	.271	.363	.440	.491
10% or less	17	6	.351	.090	.274	.374	.432	.440
11% to 50%	33	5	.245	.055	.223	.242	.264	.309

RHEUMATOLOGY

Table 102A: Compensation

	Physicians	Medical Practices	Mean	Std. Dev.	25th %tile	Median	75th %tile	90th %tile
Overall	268	131	$222,691	$97,884	$160,480	$193,410	$258,094	$357,635
1 to 2 Years in Specialty	10	8	$182,093	$62,544	$146,780	$159,088	$208,349	$298,858
Group Type								
Single-specialty	32	9	$260,071	$117,662	$158,514	$221,281	$340,308	$440,963
Multispecialty	236	122	$217,623	$94,041	$160,480	$191,670	$247,269	$339,481
Geographic Section								
Eastern	46	28	$203,747	$84,820	$145,719	$177,244	$235,852	$346,467
Midwest	87	49	$231,734	$94,048	$160,459	$201,823	$282,214	$395,837
Southern	63	26	$257,766	$124,453	$174,883	$215,172	$321,646	$389,195
Western	72	28	$193,178	$70,176	$161,417	$178,606	$202,814	$245,928
Capitation								
No capitation	132	66	$247,318	$114,051	$165,428	$212,205	$308,880	$395,837
10% or less	66	35	$212,258	$78,035	$159,925	$197,031	$233,018	$335,695
11% to 50%	34	18	$180,646	$56,680	$140,000	$168,537	$200,190	$266,036
51% or more	14	10	$187,185	$47,972	$145,609	$178,299	$242,474	$265,476

Table 102B: Gross Charges (TC/NPP Excluded)

	Physicians	Medical Practices	Mean	Std. Dev.	25th %tile	Median	75th %tile	90th %tile
Overall	120	60	$639,077	$346,176	$409,855	$546,275	$770,796	$987,897
1 to 2 Years in Specialty	5	5	*	*	*	*	*	*
Group Type								
Single-specialty	15	3	$828,112	$332,285	$678,055	$808,002	$1,006,138	$1,352,437
Multispecialty	105	57	$612,072	$341,128	$386,912	$540,258	$737,569	$930,906
Geographic Section								
Eastern	19	10	$606,928	$399,195	$342,647	$528,562	$823,547	$1,233,281
Midwest	52	26	$589,597	$363,891	$382,286	$497,513	$732,107	$934,369
Southern	30	14	$704,377	$304,011	$483,664	$648,888	$889,954	$1,251,468
Western	19	10	$703,543	$298,601	$536,117	$646,800	$802,741	$1,380,793
Capitation								
No capitation	56	26	$680,585	$330,026	$422,345	$609,451	$835,034	$994,580
10% or less	46	23	$631,317	$333,092	$410,662	$536,241	$756,982	$1,112,956
11% to 50%	14	7	$469,124	$186,252	$334,332	$502,074	$560,939	$739,088
51% or more	3	3	*	*	*	*	*	*

Table 102C: Compensation to Gross Charges Ratio (TC/NPP Excluded)

	Physicians	Medical Practices	Mean	Std. Dev.	25th %tile	Median	75th %tile	90th %tile
Overall	113	57	.382	.156	.259	.349	.480	.587
1 to 2 Years in Specialty	5	5	*	*	*	*	*	*
Group Type								
Single-specialty	14	3	.283	.098	.213	.257	.326	.473
Multispecialty	99	54	.397	.158	.269	.382	.485	.599
Geographic Section								
Eastern	18	10	.318	.084	.249	.293	.402	.432
Midwest	50	25	.428	.174	.297	.420	.497	.674
Southern	28	13	.374	.167	.233	.299	.535	.604
Western	17	9	.331	.090	.261	.300	.402	.498
Capitation								
No capitation	53	25	.365	.157	.240	.301	.476	.595
10% or less	44	22	.407	.173	.272	.384	.506	.605
11% to 50%	13	7	.378	.086	.304	.399	.426	.516
51% or more	2	2	*	*	*	*	*	*

SURGERY: GENERAL

Table 103A: Compensation

	Physicians	Medical Practices	Mean	Std. Dev.	25th %tile	Median	75th %tile	90th %tile
Overall	960	252	$286,670	$123,967	$205,782	$255,438	$334,847	$432,072
1 to 2 Years in Specialty	66	41	$224,364	$71,687	$181,510	$209,736	$246,001	$310,869
Group Type								
Single-specialty	187	43	$289,386	$139,053	$188,216	$254,250	$336,791	$515,162
Multispecialty	773	209	$286,013	$120,123	$210,378	$255,889	$333,464	$421,045
Geographic Section								
Eastern	151	40	$222,460	$73,035	$174,900	$213,211	$256,755	$304,182
Midwest	354	98	$318,642	$145,377	$211,188	$287,776	$389,356	$521,096
Southern	198	62	$300,739	$118,844	$222,000	$286,887	$356,492	$431,124
Western	257	52	$269,519	$100,691	$214,705	$247,170	$294,015	$369,624
Capitation								
No capitation	502	156	$304,176	$138,919	$208,276	$274,900	$355,981	$494,204
10% or less	187	50	$275,274	$122,035	$183,634	$241,877	$334,388	$419,035
11% to 50%	132	30	$276,450	$101,971	$209,968	$252,880	$314,505	$421,331
51% or more	58	12	$275,901	$81,851	$219,973	$252,297	$328,338	$381,865

Table 103B: Gross Charges (TC/NPP Excluded)

	Physicians	Medical Practices	Mean	Std. Dev.	25th %tile	Median	75th %tile	90th %tile
Overall	446	126	$1,138,140	$471,440	$816,346	$1,052,897	$1,351,551	$1,718,915
1 to 2 Years in Specialty	21	16	$892,645	$193,012	$731,352	$871,000	$984,818	$1,238,389
Group Type								
Single-specialty	78	16	$1,309,264	$538,978	$951,858	$1,161,840	$1,725,338	$2,062,680
Multispecialty	368	110	$1,101,869	$448,331	$808,229	$1,022,114	$1,314,122	$1,627,656
Geographic Section								
Eastern	74	20	$1,064,248	$376,230	$836,099	$1,005,644	$1,241,493	$1,477,061
Midwest	191	52	$1,151,795	$511,039	$807,887	$1,092,642	$1,421,891	$1,710,716
Southern	102	29	$1,320,120	$498,485	$968,913	$1,194,874	$1,679,973	$2,038,598
Western	79	25	$939,379	$297,735	$731,933	$877,599	$1,110,660	$1,333,638
Capitation								
No capitation	272	79	$1,165,833	$455,302	$837,894	$1,093,703	$1,385,340	$1,748,183
10% or less	93	28	$1,039,151	$412,055	$754,325	$975,940	$1,198,265	$1,645,502
11% to 50%	71	15	$1,188,385	$595,562	$820,850	$1,017,357	$1,473,209	$1,834,864
51% or more	10	4	$948,743	$262,112	$748,543	$854,743	$1,155,940	$1,383,130

Table 103C: Compensation to Gross Charges Ratio (TC/NPP Excluded)

	Physicians	Medical Practices	Mean	Std. Dev.	25th %tile	Median	75th %tile	90th %tile
Overall	434	125	.289	.108	.212	.265	.335	.413
1 to 2 Years in Specialty	21	16	.250	.056	.204	.221	.298	.331
Group Type								
Single-specialty	75	16	.287	.168	.191	.216	.311	.589
Multispecialty	359	109	.289	.092	.223	.277	.342	.403
Geographic Section								
Eastern	71	20	.228	.101	.177	.201	.245	.301
Midwest	188	52	.310	.093	.238	.297	.369	.436
Southern	96	28	.253	.065	.208	.241	.284	.352
Western	79	25	.336	.149	.227	.297	.360	.543
Capitation								
No capitation	263	78	.286	.117	.209	.253	.332	.415
10% or less	91	28	.298	.091	.239	.296	.351	.403
11% to 50%	70	15	.271	.083	.214	.254	.323	.368
51% or more	10	4	.401	.108	.304	.449	.488	.512

SURGERY: CARDIOVASCULAR

Table 104A: Compensation

	Physicians	Medical Practices	Mean	Std. Dev.	25th %tile	Median	75th %tile	90th %tile
Overall	187	51	$478,315	$210,015	$352,848	$433,353	$552,805	$770,677
1 to 2 Years in Specialty	11	8	$248,874	$93,803	$200,000	$233,613	$352,374	$375,818
Group Type								
Single-specialty	88	19	$537,272	$230,305	$390,153	$489,281	$614,442	$876,348
Multispecialty	99	32	$425,908	$175,298	$334,217	$390,500	$467,327	$686,913
Geographic Section								
Eastern	30	7	$462,801	$224,943	$369,200	$447,466	$482,017	$673,271
Midwest	44	17	$509,614	$234,831	$353,363	$405,577	$610,305	$906,502
Southern	74	17	$454,054	$197,924	$319,430	$430,140	$534,296	$716,519
Western	39	10	$500,970	$191,360	$362,418	$460,000	$600,000	$750,000
Capitation								
No capitation	125	31	$484,447	$229,443	$338,380	$439,919	$576,404	$782,530
10% or less	23	8	$481,707	$171,291	$354,909	$473,441	$527,793	$759,196
11% to 50%	29	10	$483,664	$179,708	$365,815	$417,440	$568,914	$750,000
51% or more	2	1	*	*	*	*	*	*

Table 104B: Gross Charges (TC/NPP Excluded)

	Physicians	Medical Practices	Mean	Std. Dev.	25th %tile	Median	75th %tile	90th %tile
Overall	102	30	$1,906,038	$678,614	$1,380,940	$1,886,190	$2,419,399	$2,840,865
1 to 2 Years in Specialty	4	4	*	*	*	*	*	*
Group Type								
Single-specialty	65	14	$2,010,836	$632,245	$1,543,984	$2,055,099	$2,471,842	$2,863,342
Multispecialty	37	16	$1,721,934	$725,743	$1,090,365	$1,518,199	$2,330,248	$2,806,143
Geographic Section								
Eastern	12	3	$2,305,953	$711,761	$1,735,157	$2,147,190	$2,991,176	$3,373,764
Midwest	29	11	$1,792,576	$805,577	$1,016,362	$1,551,620	$2,587,510	$2,841,556
Southern	41	11	$1,902,398	$508,856	$1,439,221	$2,030,341	$2,259,687	$2,516,741
Western	20	5	$1,838,073	$726,419	$1,366,146	$1,807,023	$2,290,611	$3,104,803
Capitation								
No capitation	74	19	$1,939,916	$637,551	$1,414,397	$1,968,745	$2,365,432	$2,840,405
10% or less	10	5	$1,747,234	$746,644	$1,186,304	$1,522,658	$2,375,202	$3,120,901
11% to 50%	16	5	$1,953,600	$818,041	$1,062,646	$2,029,165	$2,647,268	$3,059,262
51% or more	2	1	*	*	*	*	*	*

Table 104C: Compensation to Gross Charges Ratio (TC/NPP Excluded)

	Physicians	Medical Practices	Mean	Std. Dev.	25th %tile	Median	75th %tile	90th %tile
Overall	94	30	.287	.096	.208	.262	.340	.441
1 to 2 Years in Specialty	2	2	*	*	*	*	*	*
Group Type								
Single-specialty	61	14	.268	.082	.208	.250	.318	.397
Multispecialty	33	16	.321	.110	.205	.323	.393	.496
Geographic Section								
Eastern	9	3	*	*	*	*	*	*
Midwest	26	11	.306	.100	.206	.311	.387	.458
Southern	39	11	.284	.102	.208	.249	.325	.460
Western	20	5	.285	.071	.222	.269	.339	.398
Capitation								
No capitation	70	19	.278	.094	.208	.254	.324	.444
10% or less	9	5	*	*	*	*	*	*
11% to 50%	13	5	.281	.110	.192	.260	.388	.463
51% or more	2	1	*	*	*	*	*	*

SURGERY: NEUROLOGICAL

Table 105A: Compensation

	Physicians	Medical Practices	Mean	Std. Dev.	25th %tile	Median	75th %tile	90th %tile
Overall	201	66	$535,626	$316,926	$337,456	$470,476	$614,020	$855,159
1 to 2 Years in Specialty	13	11	$379,353	$117,321	$300,000	$388,075	$416,216	$597,186
Group Type								
Single-specialty	87	20	$582,702	$372,017	$349,000	$510,000	$637,144	$1,000,017
Multispecialty	114	46	$499,700	$263,508	$326,125	$443,633	$562,712	$802,004
Geographic Section								
Eastern	49	11	$460,291	$151,987	$325,750	$440,500	$601,049	$637,144
Midwest	72	27	$603,375	$355,158	$340,911	$531,292	$723,460	$995,578
Southern	43	17	$623,174	$437,388	$359,000	$528,324	$650,969	$1,293,160
Western	37	11	$401,815	$103,851	$317,578	$411,078	$466,678	$526,552
Capitation								
No capitation	127	40	$566,723	$296,641	$380,659	$510,000	$643,682	$874,069
10% or less	28	11	$508,611	$312,235	$303,652	$356,245	$597,496	$952,938
11% to 50%	29	13	$487,038	$459,913	$270,878	$375,000	$542,345	$1,000,000
51% or more	4	1	*	*	*	*	*	*

Table 105B: Gross Charges (TC/NPP Excluded)

	Physicians	Medical Practices	Mean	Std. Dev.	25th %tile	Median	75th %tile	90th %tile
Overall	97	31	$2,423,761	$1,265,495	$1,543,798	$2,133,091	$3,014,513	$4,410,126
1 to 2 Years in Specialty	8	7	*	*	*	*	*	*
Group Type								
Single-specialty	49	9	$3,011,121	$1,285,017	$2,059,854	$2,837,582	$3,446,152	$4,930,690
Multispecialty	48	22	$1,824,164	$926,210	$1,182,984	$1,661,478	$2,261,874	$3,129,738
Geographic Section								
Eastern	31	6	$2,481,883	$1,108,829	$1,722,275	$2,333,447	$3,077,438	$3,999,552
Midwest	45	15	$2,554,956	$1,535,525	$1,447,503	$1,967,585	$3,291,467	$4,870,535
Southern	13	6	$2,367,549	$601,433	$1,730,678	$2,301,246	$2,913,325	$3,152,084
Western	8	4	*	*	*	*	*	*
Capitation								
No capitation	75	19	$2,631,008	$1,307,063	$1,706,000	$2,297,215	$3,141,621	$4,736,222
10% or less	11	5	$1,340,613	$530,122	$910,174	$1,355,646	$1,689,025	$2,338,416
11% to 50%	11	7	$2,093,861	$847,661	$1,388,465	$2,133,091	$2,605,532	$3,293,482

Table 105C: Compensation to Gross Charges Ratio (TC/NPP Excluded)

	Physicians	Medical Practices	Mean	Std. Dev.	25th %tile	Median	75th %tile	90th %tile
Overall	77	31	.252	.077	.192	.229	.294	.377
1 to 2 Years in Specialty	4	4	*	*	*	*	*	*
Group Type								
Single-specialty	31	9	.220	.054	.184	.205	.260	.301
Multispecialty	46	22	.273	.083	.206	.249	.348	.416
Geographic Section								
Eastern	26	6	.237	.065	.192	.222	.263	.349
Midwest	31	15	.272	.091	.190	.262	.365	.409
Southern	12	6	.227	.050	.191	.215	.257	.322
Western	8	4	*	*	*	*	*	*
Capitation								
No capitation	56	19	.244	.071	.191	.218	.280	.364
10% or less	11	5	.289	.090	.225	.293	.388	.420
11% to 50%	10	7	.257	.087	.181	.249	.294	.422

SURGERY: VASCULAR

Table 106A: Compensation

	Physicians	Medical Practices	Mean	Std. Dev.	25th %tile	Median	75th %tile	90th %tile
Overall	140	53	$325,373	$135,237	$241,988	$303,517	$357,031	$465,179
1 to 2 Years in Specialty	13	6	$262,532	$91,795	$223,555	$256,770	$283,588	$438,253
Group Type								
Single-specialty	33	10	$344,637	$179,109	$223,288	$310,738	$372,997	$650,000
Multispecialty	107	43	$319,432	$118,942	$255,000	$303,083	$355,008	$434,378
Geographic Section								
Eastern	33	13	$309,007	$88,332	$225,944	$301,250	$354,431	$429,262
Midwest	33	16	$345,518	$185,844	$237,576	$328,670	$361,418	$448,952
Southern	29	12	$392,248	$155,032	$278,637	$353,905	$484,840	$650,000
Western	45	12	$279,505	$78,001	$240,000	$270,000	$315,869	$371,434
Capitation								
No capitation	73	29	$335,456	$145,062	$240,000	$309,260	$361,180	$557,797
10% or less	16	11	$366,701	$217,100	$230,095	$320,007	$412,701	$672,600
11% to 50%	23	10	$306,930	$83,191	$243,177	$311,250	$359,907	$432,540
51% or more	4	2	*	*	*	*	*	*

Table 106B: Gross Charges (TC/NPP Excluded)

	Physicians	Medical Practices	Mean	Std. Dev.	25th %tile	Median	75th %tile	90th %tile
Overall	50	26	$1,364,787	$733,139	$829,556	$1,241,860	$1,760,380	$2,489,975
1 to 2 Years in Specialty	3	3	*	*	*	*	*	*
Group Type								
Single-specialty	7	3	*	*	*	*	*	*
Multispecialty	43	23	$1,493,473	$707,655	$852,329	$1,350,966	$1,820,359	$2,539,675
Geographic Section								
Eastern	17	7	$1,340,922	$802,558	$655,380	$1,067,051	$1,934,074	$2,650,555
Midwest	20	11	$1,468,869	$753,500	$842,558	$1,299,213	$1,804,296	$2,520,565
Southern	3	3	*	*	*	*	*	*
Western	10	5	$1,058,177	$593,046	$750,585	$860,079	$1,319,671	$2,380,311
Capitation								
No capitation	25	13	$1,030,166	$492,383	$687,646	$852,329	$1,430,579	$1,783,954
10% or less	7	6	*	*	*	*	*	*
11% to 50%	18	7	$1,576,058	$684,076	$1,010,114	$1,419,949	$1,979,327	$2,617,186

Table 106C: Compensation to Gross Charges Ratio (TC/NPP Excluded)

	Physicians	Medical Practices	Mean	Std. Dev.	25th %tile	Median	75th %tile	90th %tile
Overall	44	25	.305	.139	.199	.265	.398	.505
1 to 2 Years in Specialty	3	3	*	*	*	*	*	*
Group Type								
Single-specialty	7	3	*	*	*	*	*	*
Multispecialty	37	22	.290	.136	.198	.233	.323	.459
Geographic Section								
Eastern	13	7	.396	.181	.225	.417	.505	.711
Midwest	19	10	.264	.092	.195	.233	.312	.444
Southern	3	3	*	*	*	*	*	*
Western	9	5	*	*	*	*	*	*
Capitation								
No capitation	24	13	.349	.162	.200	.316	.444	.563
10% or less	5	5	*	*	*	*	*	*
11% to 50%	15	7	.260	.092	.186	.233	.312	.445

URGENT CARE

Table 107A: Compensation

	Physicians	Medical Practices	Mean	Std. Dev.	25th %tile	Median	75th %tile	90th %tile
Overall	405	100	$172,269	$69,754	$131,653	$159,000	$200,779	$240,075
1 to 2 Years in Specialty	17	9	$151,507	$44,951	$128,242	$155,000	$179,977	$223,914
Group Type								
Single-specialty	40	5	$136,054	$34,366	$117,850	$131,747	$164,734	$184,964
Multispecialty	365	95	$176,238	$71,512	$136,163	$161,625	$205,562	$245,764
Geographic Section								
Eastern	35	10	$149,282	$42,495	$129,375	$140,000	$168,000	$186,800
Midwest	160	40	$175,771	$57,486	$137,571	$161,350	$206,080	$251,495
Southern	63	14	$180,538	$77,617	$118,808	$170,255	$228,643	$260,373
Western	147	36	$170,387	$81,933	$130,000	$157,162	$190,955	$234,418
Capitation								
No capitation	209	52	$176,669	$82,107	$136,901	$163,244	$195,782	$245,312
10% or less	72	21	$164,382	$57,033	$125,918	$143,953	$200,071	$246,947
11% to 50%	77	16	$162,657	$44,023	$130,321	$157,562	$189,102	$234,508
51% or more	45	10	$183,887	$59,256	$140,498	$180,317	$220,852	$262,001

Table 107B: Gross Charges (TC/NPP Excluded)

	Physicians	Medical Practices	Mean	Std. Dev.	25th %tile	Median	75th %tile	90th %tile
Overall	194	47	$492,241	$169,730	$375,057	$489,225	$586,088	$673,530
1 to 2 Years in Specialty	6	3	*	*	*	*	*	*
Group Type								
Single-specialty	22	2	$485,453	$105,698	$414,725	$483,315	$557,447	$621,275
Multispecialty	172	45	$493,109	$176,454	$370,452	$494,033	$588,915	$684,627
Geographic Section								
Eastern	2	2	*	*	*	*	*	*
Midwest	78	23	$441,134	$193,919	$299,300	$419,902	$534,927	$633,404
Southern	40	6	$518,740	$101,425	$460,952	$513,115	$585,860	$683,613
Western	74	16	$530,155	$158,789	$411,090	$542,914	$629,235	$682,983
Capitation								
No capitation	99	21	$513,977	$158,472	$409,579	$510,812	$603,681	$667,253
10% or less	52	14	$444,861	$203,788	$279,097	$419,732	$543,755	$733,951
11% to 50%	25	6	$488,737	$74,927	$450,448	$497,202	$555,384	$575,531
51% or more	16	5	$538,080	$198,753	$389,863	$522,535	$630,987	$867,945

Table 107C: Compensation to Gross Charges Ratio (TC/NPP Excluded)

	Physicians	Medical Practices	Mean	Std. Dev.	25th %tile	Median	75th %tile	90th %tile
Overall	193	47	.356	.105	.279	.340	.412	.495
1 to 2 Years in Specialty	6	3	*	*	*	*	*	*
Group Type								
Single-specialty	22	2	.248	.064	.194	.237	.283	.355
Multispecialty	171	45	.370	.101	.291	.352	.425	.506
Geographic Section								
Eastern	2	2	*	*	*	*	*	*
Midwest	77	23	.419	.114	.333	.405	.485	.597
Southern	40	6	.304	.091	.228	.292	.378	.440
Western	74	16	.322	.062	.277	.316	.360	.398
Capitation								
No capitation	99	21	.320	.087	.275	.305	.361	.444
10% or less	51	14	.424	.129	.316	.427	.521	.598
11% to 50%	25	6	.357	.058	.319	.363	.409	.417
51% or more	16	5	.369	.070	.306	.365	.400	.485

MEDICAL GROUP MANAGEMENT ASSOCIATION™

UROLOGY

Table 108A: Compensation

	Physicians	Medical Practices	Mean	Std. Dev.	25th %tile	Median	75th %tile	90th %tile
Overall	475	139	$333,712	$159,822	$224,173	$294,337	$401,456	$524,001
1 to 2 Years in Specialty	30	20	$202,905	$67,080	$169,007	$197,679	$213,307	$311,734
Group Type								
Single-specialty	156	30	$348,791	$160,832	$224,140	$316,151	$451,763	$549,876
Multispecialty	319	109	$326,338	$159,058	$224,173	$286,230	$392,092	$507,600
Geographic Section								
Eastern	76	21	$332,874	$181,356	$219,421	$298,678	$388,352	$544,392
Midwest	139	55	$355,213	$153,193	$235,919	$332,888	$430,141	$587,800
Southern	112	32	$369,511	$189,020	$240,562	$334,971	$437,091	$543,758
Western	148	31	$286,857	$113,793	$218,563	$255,779	$316,030	$428,613
Capitation								
No capitation	253	79	$364,456	$187,499	$224,466	$329,251	$462,452	$579,511
10% or less	78	30	$310,612	$108,260	$233,116	$302,857	$392,376	$445,269
11% to 50%	66	19	$343,335	$142,535	$272,075	$300,000	$401,978	$580,684
51% or more	34	10	$268,869	$59,385	$213,761	$272,297	$309,397	$354,568

Table 108B: Gross Charges (TC/NPP Excluded)

	Physicians	Medical Practices	Mean	Std. Dev.	25th %tile	Median	75th %tile	90th %tile
Overall	167	66	$1,323,482	$499,079	$1,028,802	$1,290,095	$1,547,929	$1,962,198
1 to 2 Years in Specialty	4	4	*	*	*	*	*	*
Group Type								
Single-specialty	37	9	$1,645,923	$395,015	$1,362,027	$1,544,169	$1,878,783	$2,328,287
Multispecialty	130	57	$1,231,711	$488,537	$948,697	$1,166,227	$1,421,989	$1,748,272
Geographic Section								
Eastern	32	9	$1,659,076	$681,596	$1,081,952	$1,583,905	$2,237,060	$2,645,165
Midwest	72	32	$1,234,406	$402,869	$987,395	$1,265,441	$1,407,159	$1,672,274
Southern	36	14	$1,367,758	$439,105	$1,099,531	$1,381,966	$1,563,325	$1,867,698
Western	27	11	$1,104,243	$346,955	$756,455	$1,076,205	$1,313,178	$1,666,783
Capitation								
No capitation	96	38	$1,388,512	$559,248	$1,038,651	$1,296,017	$1,590,196	$2,272,698
10% or less	39	16	$1,187,491	$413,917	$828,357	$1,176,142	$1,523,929	$1,645,868
11% to 50%	28	10	$1,362,237	$326,203	$1,121,922	$1,362,293	$1,564,601	$1,807,611
51% or more	4	2	*	*	*	*	*	*

Table 108C: Compensation to Gross Charges Ratio (TC/NPP Excluded)

	Physicians	Medical Practices	Mean	Std. Dev.	25th %tile	Median	75th %tile	90th %tile
Overall	147	63	.277	.088	.217	.258	.318	.407
1 to 2 Years in Specialty	3	3	*	*	*	*	*	*
Group Type								
Single-specialty	23	7	.299	.144	.195	.231	.365	.557
Multispecialty	124	56	.273	.074	.220	.259	.315	.379
Geographic Section								
Eastern	27	9	.259	.082	.201	.236	.285	.376
Midwest	70	32	.290	.099	.220	.268	.325	.412
Southern	25	11	.268	.071	.212	.260	.311	.374
Western	25	11	.268	.077	.205	.248	.326	.392
Capitation								
No capitation	79	35	.279	.098	.217	.255	.319	.420
10% or less	37	16	.283	.065	.238	.281	.317	.365
11% to 50%	27	10	.246	.068	.183	.232	.279	.363
51% or more	4	2	*	*	*	*	*	*

NOTES:

THIS PAGE INTENTIONALLY LEFT BLANK

PART-TIME PHYSICIANS

Table 109: Part-Time Physician Compensation (.7 Clinical FTE)

	Physicians	Medical Practices	Mean	Std. Dev.	25th %tile	Median	75th %tile	90th %tile
Allergy/Immunology	4	4	*	*	*	*	*	*
Anesthesiology	13	9	$273,348	$82,181	$202,440	$313,000	$333,058	$385,079
Anesth: Pain Management	1	1	*	*	*	*	*	*
Cardiology: Invasive	9	6	*	*	*	*	*	*
Cardiology: Inv-Intervntnl	4	3	*	*	*	*	*	*
Cardiology: Noninvasive	7	6	*	*	*	*	*	*
Dentistry	2	1	*	*	*	*	*	*
Dermatology	13	9	$182,757	$123,844	$102,010	$160,207	$195,149	$444,059
Emergency Medicine	23	16	$170,768	$66,440	$133,744	$149,891	$196,998	$284,982
Endocrinology/Metabolism	8	7	*	*	*	*	*	*
Family Practice (w/ OB)	43	29	$124,917	$37,912	$99,759	$120,000	$149,570	$180,205
Family Practice (w/o OB)	157	71	$113,751	$30,899	$89,838	$110,132	$132,802	$150,215
Family Practice: Sports Med	2	1	*	*	*	*	*	*
Gastroenterology	11	10	$220,447	$90,993	$185,794	$209,891	$263,452	$394,117
Gastroenterology: Hepatology	2	2	*	*	*	*	*	*
Hematology/Oncology	8	5	*	*	*	*	*	*
Infectious Disease	1	1	*	*	*	*	*	*
Internal Medicine: General	136	59	$111,193	$33,717	$92,631	$107,149	$131,452	$155,894
Internal Med: Hospitalist	3	3	*	*	*	*	*	*
Internal Med: Pediatric	10	5	$117,272	$16,476	$103,592	$110,870	$127,878	$151,008
Nephrology	1	1	*	*	*	*	*	*
Neurology	9	8	*	*	*	*	*	*
OBGYN: General	35	19	$189,015	$56,780	$144,500	$176,604	$234,466	$274,279
OBGYN: Gynecology (only)	10	8	$127,725	$54,312	$82,436	$131,114	$167,238	$208,556
OBGYN: Gyn Oncology	1	1	*	*	*	*	*	*
OBGYN: Maternal & Fetal Med	1	1	*	*	*	*	*	*
OBGYN: Repro Endocrinology	1	1	*	*	*	*	*	*
Occupational Medicine	5	5	*	*	*	*	*	*
Ophthalmology	10	7	$164,829	$82,621	$105,796	$170,414	$204,423	$305,053
Ophthalmology: Pediatric	2	2	*	*	*	*	*	*
Ophthalmology: Retina	2	2	*	*	*	*	*	*
Orthopedic (Non-surgical)	1	1	*	*	*	*	*	*
Orthopedic Surgery: General	3	2	*	*	*	*	*	*
Ortho Surg: Hip & Joint	1	1	*	*	*	*	*	*
Otorhinolaryngology	9	6	*	*	*	*	*	*
Pathology: Anatomic & Clinical	1	1	*	*	*	*	*	*
Pediatrics: General	114	59	$113,610	$29,544	$94,293	$111,337	$127,480	$145,854
Ped: Neonatal Medicine	1	1	*	*	*	*	*	*
Physiatry (Phys Med & Rehab)	4	4	*	*	*	*	*	*
Podiatry: General	2	2	*	*	*	*	*	*
Psychiatry: General	17	11	$97,327	$19,959	$88,484	$97,413	$110,400	$118,965
Pulmonary Medicine	4	4	*	*	*	*	*	*
Pulmonary Med: Critical Care	3	2	*	*	*	*	*	*
Radiation Oncology	3	3	*	*	*	*	*	*
Radiology: Diagnostic-Inv	15	7	$278,091	$77,549	$192,292	$293,368	$348,896	$363,272
Radiology: Diagnostic-Noninv	19	10	$310,280	$95,972	$245,938	$265,313	$424,284	$467,808
Rheumatology	5	5	*	*	*	*	*	*
Surgery: General	11	8	$181,965	$88,151	$93,124	$200,741	$261,930	$300,836
Surg: Cardiovascular	1	1	*	*	*	*	*	*
Surg: Neurological	3	1	*	*	*	*	*	*
Surg: Plastic & Reconstruction	1	1	*	*	*	*	*	*
Surg: Vascular (primary)	3	2	*	*	*	*	*	*
Urgent Care	16	10	$118,875	$30,347	$92,869	$114,979	$137,749	$171,379
Urology	6	6	*	*	*	*	*	*

Table 110: Part-Time Physician Compensation (.4-.6 Clinical FTE)

	Physicians	Medical Practices	Mean	Std. Dev.	25th %tile	Median	75th %tile	90th %tile
Anesthesiology	65	31	$155,222	$66,145	$102,150	$143,698	$188,214	$237,583
Cardiology: Invasive	14	8	$312,006	$113,620	$275,078	$298,250	$352,724	$507,112
Cardiology: Noninvasive	22	18	$143,584	$61,557	$103,893	$123,088	$186,549	$235,931
Dentistry	6	3	*	*	*	*	*	*
Dermatology	32	25	$142,050	$44,671	$103,482	$146,217	$173,464	$208,899
Emergency Medicine	27	15	$151,342	$51,909	$110,522	$141,998	$196,310	$218,096
Endocrinology/Metabolism	14	14	$114,133	$59,606	$67,218	$109,495	$132,003	$228,487
Family Practice (w/ OB)	60	35	$89,545	$40,528	$62,852	$80,481	$114,671	$142,058
Family Practice (w/o OB)	204	113	$82,664	$38,354	$57,916	$75,020	$93,145	$126,004
Internal Medicine: General	248	114	$88,447	$39,383	$65,584	$79,395	$100,177	$144,513
Internal Med: Hospitalist	8	6	*	*	*	*	*	*
Neurology	22	19	$117,301	$67,869	$67,274	$96,334	$174,924	$221,645
OBGYN: General	34	21	$110,988	$62,445	$73,847	$99,546	$123,290	$204,157
OBGYN: Gynecology (only)	16	12	$71,358	$21,499	$52,125	$70,762	$87,439	$105,593
Occupational Medicine	7	6	*	*	*	*	*	*
Ophthalmology	26	19	$133,118	$65,606	$83,777	$130,683	$168,057	$232,829
Ophthalmology: Pediatric	0	*	*	*	*	*	*	*
Orthopedic Surgery: General	17	13	$141,050	$45,438	$103,925	$148,366	$174,039	$214,163
Otorhinolaryngology	18	15	$135,386	$78,377	$83,815	$124,338	$152,523	$244,650
Pediatrics: General	162	88	$78,459	$28,331	$61,333	$76,192	$89,623	$107,187
Psychiatry: General	28	14	$89,797	$49,145	$57,463	$73,526	$98,254	$185,165
Pulmonary Medicine	4	4	*	*	*	*	*	*
Radiology: Diagnostic-Noninv	30	15	$172,288	$57,796	$123,141	$165,500	$219,196	$256,029
Surgery: General	16	15	$126,905	$69,621	$81,000	$112,019	$145,840	$257,705
Urgent Care	43	24	$90,573	$39,603	$64,800	$85,882	$105,742	$150,275

Table 111: Part-Time Physician Compensation (.4-.6 Clinical FTE) by Group Type

	Single-specialty			Multispecialty		
	Physicians	Medical Practices	Median	Physicians	Medical Practices	Median
Anesthesiology	52	23	$133,789	13	8	$157,500
Cardiology: Invasive	9	4	*	5	4	*
Cardiology: Noninvasive	11	9	$122,791	11	9	$161,654
Dentistry	1	1	*	5	2	*
Dermatology	8	6	*	24	19	$136,755
Emergency Medicine	13	5	$147,270	14	10	$134,385
Endocrinology/Metabolism	2	2	*	12	12	$109,626
Family Practice (w/ OB)	10	7	$79,486	50	28	$81,724
Family Practice (w/o OB)	30	22	$73,750	174	91	$75,020
Internal Medicine: General	12	7	$70,374	236	107	$79,739
Internal Med: Hospitalist	1	1	*	7	5	*
Neurology	6	4	*	16	15	$104,458
OBGYN: General	10	6	$76,056	24	15	$101,719
OBGYN: Gynecology (only)	9	6	*	7	6	*
Occupational Medicine	0	*	*	7	6	*
Ophthalmology	13	9	$103,711	13	10	$132,640
Ophthalmology: Pediatric	0	*	*	0	*	*
Orthopedic Surgery: General	8	6	*	9	7	*
Otorhinolaryngology	4	4	*	14	11	$124,338
Pediatrics: General	46	30	$69,346	116	58	$78,469
Psychiatry: General	1	1	*	27	13	$72,650
Pulmonary Medicine	1	1	*	3	3	*
Radiology: Diagnostic-Noninv	18	6	$165,500	12	9	$218,301
Surgery: General	2	2	*	14	13	$114,375
Urgent Care	0	*	*	43	24	$85,882

Table 112: Part-Time Physician Gross Charges (TC Excluded, .4-.6 Clinical FTE)

	Physicians	Medical Practices	Mean	Std. Dev.	25th %tile	Median	75th %tile	90th %tile
Anesthesiology	25	13	$487,016	$244,061	$310,541	$475,794	$552,830	$827,514
Cardiology: Invasive	8	3	*	*	*	*	*	*
Cardiology: Noninvasive	8	6	*	*	*	*	*	*
Dentistry	0	*	*	*	*	*	*	*
Dermatology	13	10	$488,122	$150,991	$375,232	$497,382	$560,479	$749,628
Emergency Medicine	17	9	$367,212	$143,331	$234,301	$325,000	$515,778	$602,243
Endocrinology/Metabolism	8	8	*	*	*	*	*	*
Family Practice (w/ OB)	32	18	$239,398	$99,526	$152,593	$209,209	$305,243	$411,864
Family Practice (w/o OB)	91	49	$212,267	$89,495	$153,757	$200,000	$263,000	$324,957
Internal Medicine: General	106	49	$236,220	$120,140	$151,627	$228,220	$308,264	$353,148
Internal Med: Hospitalist	5	4	*	*	*	*	*	*
Neurology	14	11	$362,528	$163,808	$234,596	$327,221	$451,123	$656,169
OBGYN: General	11	9	$423,914	$182,051	$345,133	$380,438	$563,296	$704,855
OBGYN: Gynecology (only)	10	8	$254,601	$72,455	$227,520	$264,443	$289,164	$368,671
Occupational Medicine	3	3	*	*	*	*	*	*
Ophthalmology	7	6	*	*	*	*	*	*
Ophthalmology: Pediatric	0	*	*	*	*	*	*	*
Orthopedic Surgery: General	6	5	*	*	*	*	*	*
Otorhinolaryngology	8	5	*	*	*	*	*	*
Pediatrics: General	66	42	$265,427	$113,710	$169,763	$266,501	$335,758	$416,392
Psychiatry: General	10	8	$200,026	$42,333	$194,934	$211,352	$221,392	$237,312
Pulmonary Medicine	2	2	*	*	*	*	*	*
Radiology: Diagnostic-Noninv	14	6	$830,249	$624,483	$409,294	$596,682	$1,135,866	$2,032,412
Surgery: General	11	10	$471,149	$245,216	$235,104	$393,600	$685,805	$837,642
Urgent Care	17	10	$278,383	$108,928	$176,224	$289,169	$336,062	$470,001

Table 113: Part-Time Physician Gross Charges (TC Excluded, .4-.6 Clinical FTE) by Group Type

	Single-specialty			Multispecialty		
	Physicians	Medical Practices	Median	Physicians	Medical Practices	Median
Anesthesiology	13	6	$457,303	12	7	$489,941
Cardiology: Invasive	7	2	*	1	1	*
Cardiology: Noninvasive	4	3	*	4	3	*
Dentistry	0	*	*	0	*	*
Dermatology	5	3	*	8	7	*
Emergency Medicine	11	4	$325,000	6	5	*
Endocrinology/Metabolism	1	1	*	7	7	*
Family Practice (w/ OB)	4	3	*	28	15	$199,205
Family Practice (w/o OB)	13	7	$205,000	78	42	$198,831
Internal Medicine: General	2	2	*	104	47	$230,756
Internal Med: Hospitalist	0	*	*	5	4	*
Neurology	4	2	*	10	9	$357,412
OBGYN: General	2	2	*	9	7	*
OBGYN: Gynecology (only)	6	4	*	4	4	*
Occupational Medicine	0	*	*	3	3	*
Ophthalmology	1	1	*	6	5	*
Ophthalmology: Pediatric	0	*	*	0	*	*
Orthopedic Surgery: General	1	1	*	5	4	*
Otorhinolaryngology	0	*	*	8	5	*
Pediatrics: General	18	12	$305,551	48	30	$263,541
Psychiatry: General	0	*	*	10	8	$211,352
Pulmonary Medicine	0	*	*	2	2	*
Radiology: Diagnostic-Noninv	6	1	*	8	5	*
Surgery: General	2	2	*	9	8	*
Urgent Care	0	*	*	17	10	$289,169

Table 114: Part-Time Physician Compensation to Gross Charges Ratio (TC Excluded, .4-.6 Clinical FTE)

	Physicians	Medical Practices	Mean	Std. Dev.	25th %tile	Median	75th %tile	90th %tile
Anesthesiology	25	13	.383	.132	.301	.361	.449	.613
Cardiology: Invasive	8	3	*	*	*	*	*	*
Cardiology: Noninvasive	8	6	*	*	*	*	*	*
Dentistry	0	*	*	*	*	*	*	*
Dermatology	13	10	.290	.083	.228	.273	.329	.452
Emergency Medicine	17	9	.434	.144	.352	.379	.565	.658
Endocrinology/Metabolism	8	8	*	*	*	*	*	*
Family Practice (w/ OB)	32	18	.400	.217	.276	.327	.416	.644
Family Practice (w/o OB)	91	49	.426	.172	.311	.395	.467	.661
Internal Medicine: General	106	49	.423	.199	.305	.376	.505	.627
Internal Med: Hospitalist	5	4	*	*	*	*	*	*
Neurology	14	11	.366	.163	.244	.335	.449	.653
OBGYN: General	11	9	.252	.070	.176	.264	.281	.370
OBGYN: Gynecology (only)	10	8	.281	.094	.222	.260	.307	.499
Occupational Medicine	3	3	*	*	*	*	*	*
Ophthalmology	7	6	*	*	*	*	*	*
Ophthalmology: Pediatric	0	*	*	*	*	*	*	*
Orthopedic Surgery: General	6	5	*	*	*	*	*	*
Otorhinolaryngology	8	5	*	*	*	*	*	*
Pediatrics: General	66	42	.356	.233	.232	.308	.403	.539
Psychiatry: General	10	8	.584	.290	.336	.557	.766	1.122
Pulmonary Medicine	2	2	*	*	*	*	*	*
Radiology: Diagnostic-Noninv	14	6	.298	.165	.181	.246	.404	.597
Surgery: General	11	10	.287	.082	.206	.281	.361	.423
Urgent Care	17	10	.335	.079	.289	.330	.367	.471

Table 115: Part-Time Physician Ambulatory Encounters (TC Excluded, .4-.6 Clinical FTE)

	Physicians	Medical Practices	Mean	Std. Dev.	25th %tile	Median	75th %tile	90th %tile
Anesthesiology	2	1	*	*	*	*	*	*
Cardiology: Invasive	9	4	*	*	*	*	*	*
Cardiology: Noninvasive	6	5	*	*	*	*	*	*
Dentistry	1	1	*	*	*	*	*	*
Dermatology	20	15	3,123	902	2,455	3,133	3,666	4,579
Emergency Medicine	11	6	1,609	353	1,306	1,584	1,778	2,290
Endocrinology/Metabolism	7	7	*	*	*	*	*	*
Family Practice (w/ OB)	38	23	2,255	997	1,369	2,137	2,929	3,463
Family Practice (w/o OB)	149	84	2,258	886	1,668	2,194	2,728	3,362
Internal Medicine: General	167	76	1,948	1,048	1,353	1,735	2,222	3,046
Internal Med: Hospitalist	4	3	*	*	*	*	*	*
Neurology	12	11	1,470	575	990	1,455	2,053	2,278
OBGYN: General	21	13	1,448	604	1,053	1,440	1,791	2,472
OBGYN: Gynecology (only)	12	9	2,304	2,534	777	1,776	2,562	7,821
Occupational Medicine	4	4	*	*	*	*	*	*
Ophthalmology	13	10	2,802	1,099	2,072	2,524	3,389	4,988
Ophthalmology: Pediatric	0	*	*	*	*	*	*	*
Orthopedic Surgery: General	9	6	*	*	*	*	*	*
Otorhinolaryngology	11	8	1,615	668	1,068	1,504	2,031	2,949
Pediatrics: General	94	58	2,563	1,211	1,898	2,434	3,147	3,948
Psychiatry: General	12	8	1,165	599	779	1,086	1,673	2,065
Pulmonary Medicine	4	4	*	*	*	*	*	*
Radiology: Diagnostic-Noninv	3	1	*	*	*	*	*	*
Surgery: General	12	11	917	417	642	828	1,091	1,752
Urgent Care	21	11	2,883	1,160	2,024	2,662	3,259	4,806

THIS PAGE INTENTIONALLY LEFT BLANK

NONPHYSICIAN PROVIDERS

Table 116: Nonphysician Provider Compensation

	Providers	Medical Practices	Mean	Std. Dev.	25th %tile	Median	75th %tile	90th %tile
Audiologist	104	47	$60,324	$21,675	$45,667	$56,110	$67,952	$100,232
Certified Diabetic Educator	6	4	*	*	*	*	*	*
Cert Reg Nurse Anesthetist	297	29	$112,665	$25,504	$98,936	$110,350	$126,357	$142,765
Chiropractor	23	11	$82,354	$42,399	$49,044	$80,425	$98,434	$166,356
Dietician/Nutritionist	19	11	$41,498	$11,976	$30,187	$39,811	$50,642	$54,902
Midwife-Out-/In-patient	116	56	$77,366	$17,661	$66,953	$74,542	$85,830	$96,879
Midwife-Outpatient (primary)	9	7	*	*	*	*	*	*
Midwife-Inpatient (primary)	9	5	*	*	*	*	*	*
Nurse Practitioner	921	314	$65,231	$15,483	$56,510	$64,377	$72,203	$81,396
NP: Adult	8	3	*	*	*	*	*	*
NP: Cardiology	19	9	$68,728	$10,189	$62,270	$68,989	$77,572	$80,928
NP: Family Practice	60	28	$70,846	$23,751	$58,006	$64,808	$74,276	$99,313
NP: Gerontology/Elder Health	11	3	$68,181	$11,761	$63,739	$68,841	$73,926	$88,266
NP: Internal Medicine	36	15	$61,496	$10,877	$54,842	$61,403	$67,704	$80,062
NP: Pediatric/Child Health	27	19	$63,020	$14,182	$52,318	$64,064	$69,325	$80,228
NP: OBGYN/Women's Health	40	23	$64,684	$17,092	$54,896	$60,314	$66,020	$89,186
Occupational Therapist	33	18	$54,204	$17,179	$45,310	$50,648	$61,999	$68,243
Optometrist	260	78	$105,638	$42,836	$82,126	$95,987	$116,113	$157,457
Orthotist/Prosthetist	2	1	*	*	*	*	*	*
Perfusionist	6	1	*	*	*	*	*	*
Pharmacist	57	9	$71,749	$11,988	$67,271	$73,191	$76,693	$86,901
Physical Therapist	196	44	$63,178	$21,734	$49,404	$57,057	$69,152	$91,291
Physician Asst (surgical)	280	100	$77,635	$21,576	$63,802	$73,335	$87,503	$108,430
Physician Asst (primary care)	676	219	$71,474	$18,178	$61,427	$69,294	$78,022	$90,728
Phys Asst (non-surg./non-prim care)	247	106	$71,262	$14,984	$61,522	$70,275	$79,526	$89,128
Physicist	2	1	*	*	*	*	*	*
Psychologist	208	51	$75,049	$28,059	$54,403	$71,886	$92,147	$114,060
Social Worker	86	27	$55,635	$17,197	$42,758	$54,041	$64,554	$77,185
Speech Therapist	10	6	$46,603	$9,876	$40,686	$43,988	$50,649	$68,139
Surgeon Assistant	15	9	$61,648	$19,222	$47,041	$56,867	$71,456	$98,701

Table 117: Nonphysician Provider Compensation by Group Type

	Single-specialty			Multispecialty		
	Providers	Medical Practices	Median	Providers	Medical Practices	Median
Audiologist	39	10	$49,363	65	37	$60,701
Certified Diabetic Educator	*	*	*	6	4	*
Cert Reg Nurse Anesthetist	192	13	$108,658	105	16	$116,261
Chiropractor	1	1	*	22	10	$80,753
Dietician/Nutritionist	1	1	*	18	10	$39,811
Midwife-Out-/In-patient	48	20	$73,503	68	36	$75,509
Midwife-Outpatient (primary)	4	3	*	5	4	*
Midwife-Inpatient (primary)	4	2	*	5	3	*
Nurse Practitioner	224	140	$66,327	697	174	$64,043
NP: Adult	1	1	*	7	2	*
NP: Cardiology	10	4	$74,482	9	5	*
NP: Family Practice	7	4	*	53	24	$65,000
NP: Gerontology/Elder Health	*	*	*	11	3	$68,841
NP: Internal Medicine	9	5	*	27	10	$60,622
NP: Pediatric/Child Health	14	9	$65,929	13	10	$63,479
NP: OBGYN/Women's Health	8	4	*	32	19	$60,314
Occupational Therapist	10	5	$54,391	23	13	$50,207
Optometrist	49	24	$106,631	211	54	$94,947
Orthotist/Prosthetist	*	*	*	2	1	*
Perfusionist	6	1	*	*	*	*
Pharmacist	*	*	*	57	9	$73,191
Physical Therapist	32	12	$59,620	164	32	$56,711
Physician Asst (surgical)	154	55	$74,275	126	45	$72,000
Physician Asst (primary care)	102	55	$70,164	574	164	$69,240
Phys Asst (non-surg./non-prim care)	124	61	$75,097	123	45	$65,301
Physicist	*	*	*	2	1	*
Psychologist	23	10	$75,000	185	41	$71,225
Social Worker	6	2	*	80	25	$54,409
Speech Therapist	2	1	*	8	5	*
Surgeon Assistant	6	3	*	9	6	*

MEDICAL GROUP MANAGEMENT ASSOCIATION™

Table 118: Nonphysician Provider Compensation by Geographic Section

	Eastern		Midwest		Southern		Western	
	Providers	Median	Providers	Median	Providers	Median	Providers	Median
Audiologist	15	$51,696	49	$62,440	34	$51,038	6	*
Certified Diabetic Educator	*	*	5	*	1	*	*	*
Cert Reg Nurse Anesthetist	34	$103,416	115	$117,170	135	$108,577	13	*
Chiropractor	3	*	15	$82,329	3	*	2	*
Dietician/Nutritionist	3	*	11	$34,213	4	*	1	*
Midwife-Out-/In-patient	28	$72,676	47	$75,015	13	$71,700	28	$77,986
Midwife-Outpatient (primary)	1	*	3	*	*	*	5	*
Midwife-Inpatient (primary)	*	*	5	*	3	*	1	*
Nurse Practitioner	233	$65,000	363	$61,582	166	$66,217	159	$67,962
NP: Adult	0	*	5	*	*	*	3	*
NP: Cardiology	4	*	11	$72,877	1	*	3	*
NP: Family Practice	4	*	37	$63,208	9	*	10	$67,787
NP: Gerontology/Elder Health	*	*	10	*	1	*	*	*
NP: Internal Medicine	12	$58,804	16	$63,520	2	*	6	*
NP: Pediatric/Child Health	3	*	15	$64,240	5	*	4	*
NP: OBGYN/Women's Health	9	*	19	$60,181	7	*	5	*
Occupational Therapist	8	*	17	$46,218	7	*	1	*
Optometrist	41	$91,037	120	$100,536	40	$95,001	59	$95,400
Orthotist/Prosthetist	*	*	*	*	*	*	2	*
Perfusionist	6	*	*	*	*	*	*	*
Pharmacist	40	$72,637	8	*	8	*	1	*
Physical Therapist	41	$55,566	98	$53,743	19	$60,800	38	$68,958
Physician Asst (surgical)	66	$75,365	85	$68,310	57	$72,434	72	$76,164
Physician Asst (primary care)	116	$67,303	296	$68,461	76	$71,322	188	$71,340
Phys Asst (non-surg./non-prim care)	107	$73,085	67	$67,858	31	$62,463	42	$73,043
Physicist	2	*	*	*	*	*	*	*
Psychologist	46	$61,107	112	$73,939	28	$79,794	22	$98,511
Social Worker	24	$55,779	46	$54,537	12	$41,730	4	*
Speech Therapist	2	*	5	*	2	*	1	*
Surgeon Assistant	*	*	2	*	6	*	7	*

Table 119: Nonphysician Provider Compensation by Percent of Capitation Revenue

	No capitation		10% or less		11% to 50%		51% or more	
	Providers	Median	Providers	Median	Providers	Median	Providers	Median
Audiologist	63	$53,845	15	$70,921	16	$58,314	10	$54,326
Certified Diabetic Educator	1	*	5	*	*	*	*	*
Cert Reg Nurse Anesthetist	225	$112,405	43	$109,135	23	$97,742	2	*
Chiropractor	17	$79,581	4	*	1	*	1	*
Dietician/Nutritionist	11	$49,055	6	*	2	*	0	*
Midwife-Out-/In-patient	55	$74,739	29	$72,409	19	$74,719	13	$80,076
Midwife-Outpatient (primary)	9	*	*	*	*	*	*	*
Midwife-Inpatient (primary)	6	*	2	*	*	*	1	*
Nurse Practitioner	489	$65,212	250	$60,922	111	$63,898	66	$72,883
NP: Adult	5	*	*	*	3	*	*	*
NP: Cardiology	13	$69,788	2	*	2	*	2	*
NP: Family Practice	31	$69,225	9	*	18	$63,346	1	*
NP: Gerontology/Elder Health	2	*	9	*	*	*	*	*
NP: Internal Medicine	18	$60,494	11	*	4	*	2	*
NP: Pediatric/Child Health	12	$66,352	8	*	5	*	2	*
NP: OBGYN/Women's Health	21	$60,181	5	*	12	$59,695	2	*
Occupational Therapist	19	$55,194	5	*	4	*	5	*
Optometrist	115	$99,968	47	$100,055	47	$95,635	50	$90,968
Orthotist/Prosthetist	*	*	2	*	*	*	*	*
Perfusionist	*	*	6	*	*	*	*	*
Pharmacist	14	$73,566	3	*	10	*	30	*
Physical Therapist	118	$56,432	28	$61,742	18	$55,505	32	$61,429
Physician Asst (surgical)	175	$75,000	60	$72,071	12	$67,798	33	$70,939
Physician Asst (primary care)	330	$69,923	170	$68,473	96	$68,112	67	$70,811
Phys Asst (non-surg./non-prim care)	157	$70,753	45	$69,547	30	$64,000	15	$73,290
Physicist	*	*	*	*	2	*	*	*
Psychologist	108	$68,713	54	$76,837	31	$78,794	15	$69,650
Social Worker	37	$51,085	20	$44,486	2	*	27	$57,070
Speech Therapist	8	*	0	*	2	*	*	*
Surgeon Assistant	11	$54,206	2	*	*	*	2	*

　　　MEDICAL GROUP MANAGEMENT ASSOCIATION™

Table 120: Nonphysician Provider Compensation by Years in Specialty

	1 to 2 years		3 to 7 years		8 to 17 years		18 years or more	
	Providers	Median	Providers	Median	Providers	Median	Providers	Median
Audiologist	9	*	28	$52,485	20	$57,656	23	$67,907
Certified Diabetic Educator	1	*	2	*	1	*	1	*
Cert Reg Nurse Anesthetist	9	*	36	$111,844	62	$105,556	66	$116,513
Chiropractor	4	*	6	*	10	$80,003	2	*
Dietician/Nutritionist	1	*	4	*	3	*	4	*
Midwife-Out-/In-patient	10	$61,286	32	$72,723	38	$80,498	18	$79,958
Midwife-Outpatient (primary)	2	*	2	*	4	*	1	*
Midwife-Inpatient (primary)	*	*	1	*	3	*	3	*
Nurse Practitioner	88	$58,250	312	$64,050	173	$65,511	115	$67,515
NP: Adult	3	*	4	*	*	*	1	*
NP: Cardiology	4	*	6	*	3	*	1	*
NP: Family Practice	6	*	29	$70,574	8	*	3	*
NP: Gerontology/Elder Health	1	*	5	*	1	*	2	*
NP: Internal Medicine	4	*	15	$60,622	7	*	4	*
NP: Pediatric/Child Health	2	*	7	*	10	$65,557	4	*
NP: OBGYN/Women's Health	5	*	11	$58,866	7	*	10	$70,055
Occupational Therapist	0	*	9	*	7	*	5	*
Optometrist	10	$73,685	53	$88,404	89	$95,400	83	$100,498
Perfusionist	*	*	*	*	1	*	5	*
Pharmacist	1	*	4	*	10	$76,504	5	*
Physical Therapist	7	*	49	$51,560	37	$63,732	28	$81,379
Physician Asst (surgical)	45	$62,025	95	$75,000	57	$77,000	26	$80,464
Physician Asst (primary care)	56	$59,096	213	$66,317	171	$70,271	85	$70,895
Phys Asst (non-surg./non-prim care)	35	$62,754	70	$68,143	40	$75,812	24	$71,937
Physicist	*	*	*	*	1	*	1	*
Psychologist	10	$63,497	27	$68,470	89	$69,000	73	$76,024
Social Worker	3	*	13	$42,874	19	$46,688	12	$54,264
Speech Therapist	1	*	2	*	1	*	4	*
Surgeon Assistant	*	*	3	*	2	*	5	*

Table 121: Nonphysician Provider Compensation by Gender

	Male			Female		
	Providers	Medical Practices	Median	Providers	Medical Practices	Median
Audiologist	26	19	$67,245	73	35	$52,117
Certified Diabetic Educator	*	*	*	6	4	*
Cert Reg Nurse Anesthetist	137	24	$118,895	150	27	$105,556
Chiropractor	11	10	$65,000	1	1	*
Dietician/Nutritionist	*	*	*	18	10	$40,006
Midwife-Out-/In-patient	*	*	*	113	55	$74,365
Midwife-Outpatient (primary)	2	2	*	7	6	*
Midwife-Inpatient (primary)	1	1	*	8	5	*
Nurse Practitioner	80	56	$70,724	771	290	$64,344
NP: Adult	*	*	*	8	3	*
NP: Cardiology	*	*	*	19	9	$68,989
NP: Family Practice	6	6	*	54	24	$64,104
NP: Gerontology/Elder Health	*	*	*	11	3	$68,841
NP: Internal Medicine	*	*	*	36	15	$61,403
NP: Pediatric/Child Health	0	*	*	26	18	$64,152
NP: OBGYN/Women's Health	7	3	*	33	21	$60,448
Occupational Therapist	11	7	$62,867	22	13	$48,099
Optometrist	176	65	$99,593	43	27	$85,000
Orthotist/Prosthetist	1	1	*	1	1	*
Perfusionist	6	1	*	*	*	*
Pharmacist	25	7	$73,940	29	7	$71,986
Physical Therapist	74	38	$62,259	98	32	$55,977
Physician Asst (surgical)	168	76	$77,944	108	55	$68,321
Physician Asst (primary care)	261	142	$74,274	362	160	$65,991
Phys Asst (non-surg./non-prim care)	102	59	$74,736	135	72	$66,683
Psychologist	96	39	$80,229	64	32	$62,476
Social Worker	27	14	$59,822	52	22	$51,152
Speech Therapist	1	1	*	6	5	*
Surgeon Assistant	4	3	*	11	8	$62,282

MEDICAL GROUP MANAGEMENT ASSOCIATION™

Table 122: Nonphysician Provider Retirement Benefits

	Providers	Medical Practices	Mean	Std. Dev.	25th %tile	Median	75th %tile	90th %tile
Audiologist	67	34	$4,565	$2,528	$2,765	$4,012	$5,440	$7,695
Certified Diabetic Educator	3	3	*	*	*	*	*	*
Cert Reg Nurse Anesthetist	234	24	$14,665	$5,363	$10,957	$15,281	$18,258	$21,183
Chiropractor	16	5	$6,724	$5,122	$3,809	$5,063	$5,678	$17,710
Dietician/Nutritionist	8	5	*	*	*	*	*	*
Midwife-Out-/In-patient	77	42	$5,659	$3,071	$3,310	$4,751	$7,575	$9,661
Midwife-Outpatient (primary)	7	5	*	*	*	*	*	*
Midwife-Inpatient (primary)	8	4	*	*	*	*	*	*
Nurse Practitioner	623	214	$5,186	$3,035	$3,150	$4,222	$6,312	$9,252
NP: Adult	8	3	*	*	*	*	*	*
NP: Cardiology	13	7	$4,857	$2,366	$2,538	$4,334	$7,309	$8,636
NP: Family Practice	47	22	$6,183	$3,133	$3,291	$5,694	$8,675	$10,692
NP: Gerontology/Elder Health	7	3	*	*	*	*	*	*
NP: Internal Medicine	21	13	$4,640	$2,707	$2,960	$3,928	$5,352	$7,363
NP: Pediatric/Child Health	16	12	$6,050	$3,514	$3,190	$5,505	$7,530	$11,641
NP: OBGYN/Women's Health	31	20	$5,895	$3,750	$2,930	$4,990	$7,736	$10,931
Occupational Therapist	22	12	$5,505	$3,496	$4,213	$5,063	$6,032	$7,973
Optometrist	191	62	$11,267	$7,185	$5,635	$8,770	$15,954	$20,563
Orthotist/Prosthetist	2	1	*	*	*	*	*	*
Perfusionist	6	1	*	*	*	*	*	*
Pharmacist	47	7	$4,730	$1,624	$2,897	$5,404	$5,809	$6,155
Physical Therapist	153	34	$5,239	$3,312	$2,974	$4,855	$6,222	$8,517
Physician Asst (surgical)	192	81	$7,285	$3,953	$4,332	$6,636	$9,403	$12,295
Physician Asst (primary care)	460	153	$5,703	$3,528	$3,270	$4,538	$7,166	$10,206
Phys Asst (non-surg./non-prim care)	191	84	$5,707	$2,894	$3,211	$5,087	$7,227	$9,913
Physicist	0	*	*	*	*	*	*	*
Psychologist	135	38	$6,651	$4,231	$3,529	$4,839	$8,900	$12,115
Social Worker	44	16	$5,458	$2,209	$3,866	$4,998	$6,920	$9,228
Speech Therapist	7	4	*	*	*	*	*	*
Surgeon Assistant	11	8	$6,603	$3,594	$4,597	$5,181	$7,291	$13,910

Table 123: Nonphysician Provider Retirement Benefits by Group Type

	Single-specialty			Multispecialty		
	Providers	Medical Practices	Median	Providers	Medical Practices	Median
Audiologist	19	6	$3,414	48	28	$4,036
Certified Diabetic Educator	*	*	*	3	3	*
Cert Reg Nurse Anesthetist	163	11	$15,913	71	13	$11,642
Chiropractor	0	*	*	16	5	$5,063
Dietician/Nutritionist	0	*	*	8	5	*
Midwife-Out-/In-patient	31	15	$3,367	46	27	$5,385
Midwife-Outpatient (primary)	2	1	*	5	4	*
Midwife-Inpatient (primary)	3	1	*	5	3	*
Nurse Practitioner	156	97	$5,016	467	117	$3,976
NP: Adult	1	1	*	7	2	*
NP: Cardiology	8	3	*	5	4	*
NP: Family Practice	5	3	*	42	19	$6,555
NP: Gerontology/Elder Health	*	*	*	7	3	*
NP: Internal Medicine	8	5	*	13	8	$3,928
NP: Pediatric/Child Health	8	5	*	8	7	*
NP: OBGYN/Women's Health	6	3	*	25	17	$4,990
Occupational Therapist	8	4	*	14	8	$5,073
Optometrist	36	20	$9,838	155	42	$8,482
Orthotist/Prosthetist	*	*	*	2	1	*
Perfusionist	6	1	*	*	*	*
Pharmacist	*	*	*	47	7	$5,404
Physical Therapist	21	9	$5,029	132	25	$4,799
Physician Asst (surgical)	112	48	$7,581	80	33	$5,072
Physician Asst (primary care)	61	36	$4,630	399	117	$4,490
Phys Asst (non-surg./non-prim care)	105	51	$5,719	86	33	$4,221
Physicist	*	*	*	0	*	*
Psychologist	11	6	$6,230	124	32	$4,757
Social Worker	5	1	*	39	15	$4,639
Speech Therapist	2	1	*	5	3	*
Surgeon Assistant	5	3	*	6	5	*

Table 124: Nonphysician Provider Gross Charges (TC Excluded)

	Providers	Medical Practices	Mean	Std. Dev.	25th %tile	Median	75th %tile	90th %tile
Audiologist	28	16	$221,082	$107,942	$156,078	$218,189	$259,731	$302,585
Certified Diabetic Educator	0	*	*	*	*	*	*	*
Cert Reg Nurse Anesthetist	56	11	$365,366	$201,857	$216,438	$376,276	$525,111	$662,405
Chiropractor	14	3	$233,077	$128,853	$141,073	$205,135	$300,107	$465,040
Dietician/Nutritionist	1	1	*	*	*	*	*	*
Midwife-Out-/In-patient	55	23	$292,952	$106,494	$228,298	$291,269	$357,150	$417,270
Midwife-Outpatient (primary)	5	4	*	*	*	*	*	*
Midwife-Inpatient (primary)	5	2	*	*	*	*	*	*
Nurse Practitioner	392	115	$256,107	$128,852	$164,799	$237,982	$319,125	$410,563
NP: Adult	4	2	*	*	*	*	*	*
NP: Cardiology	6	3	*	*	*	*	*	*
NP: Family Practice	38	17	$246,062	$75,697	$188,473	$228,418	$285,511	$342,370
NP: Gerontology/Elder Health	11	3	$134,756	$40,860	$101,501	$129,798	$153,448	$214,012
NP: Internal Medicine	23	9	$192,235	$73,184	$130,183	$160,768	$258,828	$297,938
NP: Pediatric/Child Health	20	13	$357,598	$167,630	$238,733	$301,339	$497,262	$645,324
NP: OBGYN/Women's Health	14	9	$248,527	$109,831	$150,552	$258,421	$322,411	$420,849
Occupational Therapist	9	7	*	*	*	*	*	*
Optometrist	107	38	$355,603	$154,333	$257,200	$344,843	$424,284	$546,368
Orthotist/Prosthetist	0	*	*	*	*	*	*	*
Perfusionist	0	*	*	*	*	*	*	*
Pharmacist	1	1	*	*	*	*	*	*
Physical Therapist	62	12	$317,250	$141,339	$195,060	$298,760	$431,716	$526,293
Physician Asst (surgical)	109	43	$347,338	$241,689	$194,869	$275,450	$438,058	$666,263
Physician Asst (primary care)	303	86	$320,649	$142,885	$217,997	$287,045	$392,975	$519,989
Phys Asst (non-surg./non-prim care)	89	39	$296,198	$190,503	$155,634	$252,077	$418,125	$507,278
Physicist	0	*	*	*	*	*	*	*
Psychologist	154	37	$182,139	$93,529	$118,479	$161,354	$219,382	$286,172
Social Worker	39	14	$130,130	$35,542	$102,756	$130,747	$149,240	$168,730
Speech Therapist	5	2	*	*	*	*	*	*
Surgeon Assistant	7	4	*	*	*	*	*	*

Table 125: Nonphysician Provider Gross Charges (TC Excluded) by Group Type

	Single-specialty			Multispecialty		
	Providers	Medical Practices	Median	Providers	Medical Practices	Median
Audiologist	7	2	*	21	14	$182,330
Certified Diabetic Educator	*	*	*	0	*	*
Cert Reg Nurse Anesthetist	29	4	$366,122	27	7	$426,942
Chiropractor	0	*	*	14	3	$205,135
Dietician/Nutritionist	0	*	*	1	1	*
Midwife-Out-/In-patient	24	8	$304,970	31	15	$259,764
Midwife-Outpatient (primary)	1	1	*	4	3	*
Midwife-Inpatient (primary)	3	1	*	2	1	*
Nurse Practitioner	63	44	$230,951	329	71	$238,446
NP: Adult	1	1	*	3	1	*
NP: Cardiology	4	2	*	2	1	*
NP: Family Practice	4	2	*	34	15	$214,042
NP: Gerontology/Elder Health	*	*	*	11	3	$129,798
NP: Internal Medicine	1	1	*	22	8	$159,455
NP: Pediatric/Child Health	10	6	$480,978	10	7	$267,035
NP: OBGYN/Women's Health	1	1	*	13	8	$248,131
Occupational Therapist	5	4	*	4	3	*
Optometrist	14	6	$409,143	93	32	$336,009
Orthotist/Prosthetist	*	*	*	0	*	*
Perfusionist	0	*	*	*	*	*
Pharmacist	*	*	*	1	1	*
Physical Therapist	12	4	$478,662	50	8	$257,087
Physician Asst (surgical)	64	20	$261,181	45	23	$298,851
Physician Asst (primary care)	35	19	$317,466	268	67	$284,994
Phys Asst (non-surg./non-prim care)	36	17	$305,413	53	22	$222,727
Physicist	*	*	*	0	*	*
Psychologist	22	10	$117,353	132	27	$163,929
Social Worker	6	2	*	33	12	$134,272
Speech Therapist	2	1	*	3	1	*
Surgeon Assistant	4	2	*	3	2	*

Table 126: Nonphysician Provider Gross Charges (TC Excluded) by Geographic Section

	Eastern		Midwest		Southern		Western	
	Providers	Median	Providers	Median	Providers	Median	Providers	Median
Audiologist	12	$258,203	13	$185,840	1	*	2	*
Certified Diabetic Educator	*	*	0	*	0	*	*	*
Cert Reg Nurse Anesthetist	1	*	28	$344,786	22	$494,369	5	*
Chiropractor	1	*	13	*	0	*	0	*
Dietician/Nutritionist	1	*	0	*	0	*	0	*
Midwife-Out-/In-patient	10	$343,451	33	$263,587	3	*	9	*
Midwife-Outpatient (primary)	0	*	3	*	*	*	2	*
Midwife-Inpatient (primary)	*	*	2	*	3	*	0	*
Nurse Practitioner	102	$231,659	178	$230,362	51	$264,911	61	$253,802
NP: Adult	0	*	1	*	*	*	3	*
NP: Cardiology	0	*	6	*	0	*	0	*
NP: Family Practice	3	*	24	$203,741	5	*	6	*
NP: Gerontology/Elder Health	*	*	10	*	1	*	*	*
NP: Internal Medicine	5	*	14	$169,061	0	*	4	*
NP: Pediatric/Child Health	3	*	11	$282,694	4	*	2	*
NP: OBGYN/Women's Health	2	*	8	*	2	*	2	*
Occupational Therapist	3	*	4	*	1	*	1	*
Optometrist	9	*	70	$344,492	10	$304,135	18	$424,009
Orthotist/Prosthetist	*	*	*	*	*	*	0	*
Perfusionist	0	*	*	*	*	*	*	*
Pharmacist	1	*	0	*	0	*	0	*
Physical Therapist	10	$494,581	27	$198,187	1	*	24	$343,021
Physician Asst (surgical)	15	$323,487	22	$268,886	33	$262,858	39	$308,241
Physician Asst (primary care)	52	$280,492	145	$269,348	20	$314,742	86	$318,885
Phys Asst (non-surg./non-prim care)	34	$344,748	30	$196,909	10	$303,045	15	$306,977
Physicist	0	*	*	*	*	*	*	*
Psychologist	34	$157,063	86	$158,904	15	$167,215	19	$201,518
Social Worker	9	*	23	$134,145	3	*	4	*
Speech Therapist	0	*	3	*	2	*	0	*
Surgeon Assistant	*	*	0	*	3	*	4	*

Table 127: Nonphysician Provider Gross Charges (TC Excluded) by Percent of Capitation Revenue

	No capitation		10% or less		11% to 50%		51% or more	
	Providers	Median	Providers	Median	Providers	Median	Providers	Median
Audiologist	15	$210,026	8	*	4	*	1	*
Certified Diabetic Educator	0	*	0	*	*	*	*	*
Cert Reg Nurse Anesthetist	46	$349,328	10	$629,313	0	*	0	*
Chiropractor	13	*	1	*	0	*	0	*
Dietician/Nutritionist	1	*	0	*	0	*	0	*
Midwife-Out-/In-patient	27	$306,175	22	$251,194	5	*	1	*
Midwife-Outpatient (primary)	5	*	*	*	*	*	*	*
Midwife-Inpatient (primary)	5	*	0	*	*	*	0	*
Nurse Practitioner	191	$259,564	153	$218,638	38	$224,929	8	*
NP: Adult	1	*	*	*	3	*	*	*
NP: Cardiology	4	*	0	*	0	*	2	*
NP: Family Practice	17	$275,726	3	*	16	$202,050	1	*
NP: Gerontology/Elder Health	2	*	9	*	*	*	*	*
NP: Internal Medicine	5	*	11	*	4	*	2	*
NP: Pediatric/Child Health	5	*	8	*	5	*	2	*
NP: OBGYN/Women's Health	3	*	4	*	7	*	0	*
Occupational Therapist	6	*	1	*	0	*	2	*
Optometrist	60	$360,548	21	$373,299	21	$332,725	4	*
Orthotist/Prosthetist	*	*	0	*	*	*	*	*
Perfusionist	*	*	0	*	*	*	*	*
Pharmacist	1	*	0	*	0	*	0	*
Physical Therapist	44	$245,348	10	*	0	*	8	*
Physician Asst (surgical)	73	$276,196	32	$265,345	2	*	2	*
Physician Asst (primary care)	161	$330,892	91	$265,552	27	$304,858	23	$275,544
Phys Asst (non-surg./non-prim care)	62	$276,184	15	$172,697	8	*	4	*
Physicist	*	*	*	*	0	*	*	*
Psychologist	89	$158,417	35	$156,088	23	$180,472	7	*
Social Worker	29	$134,145	9	*	0	*	1	*
Speech Therapist	5	*	0	*	0	*	*	*
Surgeon Assistant	5	*	2	*	*	*	0	*

MEDICAL GROUP MANAGEMENT ASSOCIATION™

Table 128: Nonphysician Provider Compensation to Gross Charges Ratio (TC Excluded)

	Providers	Medical Practices	Mean	Std. Dev.	25th %tile	Median	75th %tile	90th %tile
Audiologist	26	15	.349	.161	.201	.345	.414	.568
Certified Diabetic Educator	0	*	*	*	*	*	*	*
Cert Reg Nurse Anesthetist	45	8	.339	.146	.234	.322	.351	.631
Chiropractor	13	2	*	*	*	*	*	*
Dietician/Nutritionist	1	1	*	*	*	*	*	*
Midwife-Out-/In-patient	53	22	.301	.119	.230	.280	.337	.389
Midwife-Outpatient (primary)	5	4	*	*	*	*	*	*
Midwife-Inpatient (primary)	5	2	*	*	*	*	*	*
Nurse Practitioner	348	109	.315	.136	.221	.275	.368	.493
NP: Adult	4	2	*	*	*	*	*	*
NP: Cardiology	4	2	*	*	*	*	*	*
NP: Family Practice	37	17	.298	.072	.241	.283	.363	.390
NP: Gerontology/Elder Health	11	3	.554	.187	.482	.593	.720	.801
NP: Internal Medicine	23	9	.359	.137	.247	.360	.424	.601
NP: Pediatric/Child Health	14	10	.234	.065	.193	.220	.255	.368
NP: OBGYN/Women's Health	13	9	.296	.111	.205	.241	.393	.485
Occupational Therapist	7	6	*	*	*	*	*	*
Optometrist	105	38	.331	.149	.224	.280	.397	.520
Orthotist/Prosthetist	0	*	*	*	*	*	*	*
Perfusionist	0	*	*	*	*	*	*	*
Pharmacist	1	1	*	*	*	*	*	*
Physical Therapist	54	11	.263	.068	.213	.241	.296	.360
Physician Asst (surgical)	92	37	.320	.150	.206	.273	.409	.562
Physician Asst (primary care)	257	82	.275	.087	.215	.264	.318	.382
Phys Asst (non-surg./non-prim care)	72	35	.323	.165	.203	.268	.385	.533
Physicist	0	*	*	*	*	*	*	*
Psychologist	150	36	.420	.134	.352	.420	.489	.573
Social Worker	37	14	.394	.120	.319	.377	.411	.556
Speech Therapist	5	2	*	*	*	*	*	*
Surgeon Assistant	7	4	*	*	*	*	*	*

Table 129: Nonphysician Provider Compensation to Gross Charges Ratio (TC Excluded) by Group Type

	Single-specialty			Multispecialty		
	Providers	Medical Practices	Median	Providers	Medical Practices	Median
Audiologist	6	2	*	20	13	.384
Certified Diabetic Educator	*	*	*	0	*	*
Cert Reg Nurse Anesthetist	22	2	*	23	6	.256
Chiropractor	0	*	*	13	2	*
Dietician/Nutritionist	0	*	*	1	1	*
Midwife-Out-/In-patient	23	8	.267	30	14	.291
Midwife-Outpatient (primary)	1	1	*	4	3	*
Midwife-Inpatient (primary)	3	1	*	2	1	*
Nurse Practitioner	55	39	.281	293	70	.274
NP: Adult	1	1	*	3	1	*
NP: Cardiology	4	2	*	0	*	*
NP: Family Practice	3	2	*	34	15	.299
NP: Gerontology/Elder Health	*	*	*	11	3	.593
NP: Internal Medicine	1	1	*	22	8	.362
NP: Pediatric/Child Health	4	3	*	10	7	.226
NP: OBGYN/Women's Health	1	1	*	12	8	.265
Occupational Therapist	3	3	*	4	3	*
Optometrist	14	6	.214	91	32	.288
Orthotist/Prosthetist	*	*	*	0	*	*
Perfusionist	0	*	*	*	*	*
Pharmacist	*	*	*	1	1	*
Physical Therapist	6	4	*	48	7	.241
Physician Asst (surgical)	54	16	.268	38	21	.283
Physician Asst (primary care)	26	16	.261	231	66	.265
Phys Asst (non-surg./non-prim care)	27	14	.245	45	21	.303
Physicist	*	*	*	0	*	*
Psychologist	20	9	.444	130	27	.419
Social Worker	6	2	*	31	12	.384
Speech Therapist	2	1	*	3	1	*
Surgeon Assistant	4	2	*	3	2	*

Table 130: Nonphysician Provider Ambulatory Encounters

	Providers	Medical Practices	Mean	Std. Dev.	25th %tile	Median	75th %tile	90th %tile
Audiologist	34	19	1,909	1,563	973	1,543	2,206	4,094
Certified Diabetic Educator	1	1	*	*	*	*	*	*
Cert Reg Nurse Anesthetist	0	*	*	*	*	*	*	*
Chiropractor	16	5	4,408	2,579	2,254	4,813	5,185	7,849
Dietician/Nutritionist	4	4	*	*	*	*	*	*
Midwife-Out-/In-patient	48	28	1,892	993	1,147	1,706	2,522	3,235
Midwife-Outpatient (primary)	7	5	*	*	*	*	*	*
Midwife-Inpatient (primary)	7	3	*	*	*	*	*	*
Nurse Practitioner	515	186	2,708	1,263	1,768	2,668	3,452	4,213
NP: Adult	4	2	*	*	*	*	*	*
NP: Cardiology	11	4	1,108	895	597	928	1,148	3,195
NP: Family Practice	48	21	3,351	1,072	2,771	3,254	3,928	4,718
NP: Gerontology/Elder Health	1	1	*	*	*	*	*	*
NP: Internal Medicine	24	10	2,391	853	1,666	2,469	3,262	3,636
NP: Pediatric/Child Health	17	12	3,770	1,227	2,914	3,978	4,496	5,537
NP: OBGYN/Women's Health	18	12	2,051	716	1,749	2,064	2,402	2,993
Occupational Therapist	13	8	2,551	991	1,847	2,463	3,320	4,185
Optometrist	126	48	3,895	1,576	2,797	3,811	4,855	6,038
Orthotist/Prosthetist	0	*	*	*	*	*	*	*
Perfusionist	0	*	*	*	*	*	*	*
Pharmacist	2	2	*	*	*	*	*	*
Physical Therapist	73	16	3,179	1,463	2,128	2,685	4,271	5,627
Physician Asst (surgical)	70	37	1,571	1,098	565	1,353	2,356	2,974
Physician Asst (primary care)	410	147	3,428	1,244	2,597	3,337	4,119	4,937
Phys Asst (non-surg./non-prim care)	104	57	2,901	1,800	1,457	2,715	4,111	5,015
Physicist	0	*	*	*	*	*	*	*
Psychologist	127	30	1,241	576	927	1,193	1,397	1,738
Social Worker	44	14	1,239	357	979	1,227	1,453	1,693
Speech Therapist	7	4	*	*	*	*	*	*
Surgeon Assistant	1	1	*	*	*	*	*	*

Table 131: Nonphysician Provider Ambulatory Encounters by Group Type

	Single-specialty			Multispecialty		
	Providers	Medical Practices	Median	Providers	Medical Practices	Median
Audiologist	4	1	*	30	18	1,643
Certified Diabetic Educator	*	*	*	1	1	*
Cert Reg Nurse Anesthetist	0	*	*	0	*	*
Chiropractor	0	*	*	16	5	4,813
Dietician/Nutritionist	1	1	*	3	3	*
Midwife-Out-/In-patient	18	9	1,753	30	19	1,706
Midwife-Outpatient (primary)	3	2	*	4	3	*
Midwife-Inpatient (primary)	3	1	*	4	2	*
Nurse Practitioner	100	73	2,837	415	113	2,606
NP: Adult	1	1	*	3	1	*
NP: Cardiology	9	3	*	2	1	*
NP: Family Practice	5	3	*	43	18	3,245
NP: Gerontology/Elder Health	*	*	*	1	1	*
NP: Internal Medicine	7	3	*	17	7	2,543
NP: Pediatric/Child Health	9	6	*	8	6	*
NP: OBGYN/Women's Health	1	1	*	17	11	2,081
Occupational Therapist	7	4	*	6	4	*
Optometrist	30	14	4,071	96	34	3,750
Orthotist/Prosthetist	*	*	*	0	*	*
Perfusionist	0	*	*	*	*	*
Pharmacist	*	*	*	2	2	*
Physical Therapist	8	4	*	65	12	2,692
Physician Asst (surgical)	36	17	1,170	34	20	1,589
Physician Asst (primary care)	70	39	3,724	340	108	3,304
Phys Asst (non-surg./non-prim care)	53	35	2,779	51	22	2,478
Physicist	*	*	*	0	*	*
Psychologist	19	7	886	108	23	1,257
Social Worker	6	2	*	38	12	1,253
Speech Therapist	2	1	*	5	3	*
Surgeon Assistant	0	*	*	1	1	*

Table 132: Nonphysician Provider Surgical/Anesthesia Encounters

	Providers	Medical Practices	Mean	Std. Dev.	25th %tile	Median	75th %tile	90th %tile
Audiologist	1	1	*	*	*	*	*	*
Certified Diabetic Educator	0	*	*	*	*	*	*	*
Cert Reg Nurse Anesthetist	97	12	308	313	96	130	491	870
Chiropractor	0	*	*	*	*	*	*	*
Dietician/Nutritionist	0	*	*	*	*	*	*	*
Midwife-Out-/In-patient	32	18	361	529	62	123	384	1,222
Midwife-Outpatient (primary)	3	2	*	*	*	*	*	*
Midwife-Inpatient (primary)	7	3	*	*	*	*	*	*
Nurse Practitioner	135	66	251	338	63	124	332	589
NP: Adult	0	*	*	*	*	*	*	*
NP: Cardiology	0	*	*	*	*	*	*	*
NP: Family Practice	24	10	291	319	71	96	442	909
NP: Gerontology/Elder Health	0	*	*	*	*	*	*	*
NP: Internal Medicine	13	5	156	179	48	76	232	524
NP: Pediatric/Child Health	4	2	*	*	*	*	*	*
NP: OBGYN/Women's Health	12	6	334	340	81	207	524	1,036
Occupational Therapist	1	1	*	*	*	*	*	*
Optometrist	28	15	181	336	32	74	107	774
Orthotist/Prosthetist	0	*	*	*	*	*	*	*
Perfusionist	0	*	*	*	*	*	*	*
Pharmacist	0	*	*	*	*	*	*	*
Physical Therapist	8	1	*	*	*	*	*	*
Physician Asst (surgical)	84	34	383	376	190	253	447	790
Physician Asst (primary care)	157	63	289	284	86	185	417	618
Phys Asst (non-surg./non-prim care)	28	16	245	263	77	142	328	576
Physicist	0	*	*	*	*	*	*	*
Psychologist	0	*	*	*	*	*	*	*
Social Worker	0	*	*	*	*	*	*	*
Speech Therapist	0	*	*	*	*	*	*	*
Surgeon Assistant	2	2	*	*	*	*	*	*

Table 133: Nonphysician Provider Surgical/Anesthesia Encounters by Group Type

	Single-specialty			Multispecialty		
	Providers	Medical Practices	Median	Providers	Medical Practices	Median
Audiologist	0	*	*	1	1	*
Certified Diabetic Educator	*	*	*	0	*	*
Cert Reg Nurse Anesthetist	61	5	123	36	7	491
Chiropractor	0	*	*	0	*	*
Dietician/Nutritionist	0	*	*	0	*	*
Midwife-Out-/In-patient	8	5	*	24	13	148
Midwife-Outpatient (primary)	1	1	*	2	1	*
Midwife-Inpatient (primary)	3	1	*	4	2	*
Nurse Practitioner	23	19	127	112	47	124
NP: Adult	0	*	*	0	*	*
NP: Cardiology	0	*	*	0	*	*
NP: Family Practice	4	2	*	20	8	90
NP: Gerontology/Elder Health	*	*	*	0	*	*
NP: Internal Medicine	1	1	*	12	4	66
NP: Pediatric/Child Health	0	*	*	4	2	*
NP: OBGYN/Women's Health	0	*	*	12	6	207
Occupational Therapist	0	*	*	1	1	*
Optometrist	4	3	*	24	12	72
Orthotist/Prosthetist	*	*	*	0	*	*
Perfusionist	0	*	*	*	*	*
Pharmacist	*	*	*	0	*	*
Physical Therapist	0	*	*	8	1	*
Physician Asst (surgical)	53	21	244	31	13	401
Physician Asst (primary care)	18	12	129	139	51	197
Phys Asst (non-surg./non-prim care)	3	2	*	25	14	145
Physicist	*	*	*	0	*	*
Psychologist	0	*	*	0	*	*
Social Worker	0	*	*	0	*	*
Speech Therapist	0	*	*	0	*	*
Surgeon Assistant	1	1	*	1	1	*

THIS PAGE INTENTIONALLY LEFT BLANK

APPENDICES

APPENDICES

MEDICAL GROUP MANAGEMENT ASSOCIATION™

APPENDIX A: ABBREVIATIONS, ACRONYMS AND GEOGRAPHIC SECTIONS

Abbrev	Definition
%tile	percentile
anesth	anesthesiology / anesthesia
asst	assistant
cert	certified
CMS	Centers for Medicare & Medicaid Services
comp	compensation
DO	Doctor of Osteopathy
FTE	full-time equivalent
gyn	gynecology
intervntnl	interventional
inv	invasive
MD	Doctor of Medicine
med	medicine / medical
MSO	Management Services Organization
NPP	nonphysician provider
noninv	noninvasive
non-surg	non-surgical

Abbrev	Definition
non-prim	non-primary
NP	nurse practitioner
OB/gyn	obstetrics / gynecology
ortho	orthopedic
ped	pediatrics
PhD	Doctor of Philosophy
PPMC	Physician Practice Management Company
RBRVS	Resource Based Relative Value Scale
recon	reconstruction
reg	registered
rehab	rehabilitation
repro	reproductive
RVU	relative value unit(s)
std dev	standard deviation
surg	surgery
TC	technical component
w/	with
w/o	without

GEOGRAPHIC SECTIONS

Eastern Section: Connecticut, Delaware, District of Columbia, Maine, Maryland, Massachusetts, New Hampshire, New Jersey, New York, North Carolina, Pennsylvania, Rhode Island, Vermont, Virginia and West Virginia.

Midwest Section: Illinois, Indiana, Iowa, Michigan, Minnesota, Nebraska, North Dakota, Ohio, South Dakota and Wisconsin.

Southern Section: Alabama, Arkansas, Florida, Georgia, Kansas, Kentucky, Louisiana, Mississippi, Missouri, Oklahoma, South Carolina, Tennessee and Texas.

Western Section: Alaska, Arizona, California, Colorado, Hawaii, Idaho, Montana, Nevada, New Mexico, Oregon, Utah, Washington and Wyoming.

APPENDIX B: TERMS USED IN REPORT

A

Adjusted charges

The total amounts expected to be paid by patients or third-party payers. This figure can be calculated by taking gross charges and subtracting the adjustments from third-party payer's and charge restrictions from Medicare/Medicaid.

Administrative or governance responsibility

Administrative or governance responsibility that encompasses non-clinical administrative, or strategic, leadership or oversight for the practice. Typically, this term is used to help describe the non-clinical activities of physicians.

Ambulatory encounters (see also "Encounters")

Ambulatory encounters are a documented face-to-face contact between a patient and a provider who exercises independent judgment in the provision of services to the individual. If the patient with the same diagnosis sees two different providers on the same day, it is one encounter. If the patient sees two different providers on the same day for two different diagnoses, then it is considered two encounters. Ambulatory encounters are those performed in the following Centers for Medicare and Medicaid Services (CMS) place of service codes:
11 Office
12 Home
22 Outpatient Hospital
23 Emergency Room
24 Ambulatory Surgical Center
31 Skilled Nursing Facility
32 Nursing Facility*
33 Custodial Care Facility
34 Hospice
50 Federally Qualified Health Center
52 Psychiatric Facility Partial Hospitalization
53 Community Mental Health Facility
54 Intermediate Care Facility for Mentally Retarded
55 Residential Substance Abuse Treatment Facility
56 Psychiatric Residential Treatment Center
62 Comprehensive Outpatient Rehabilitation Facility
65 End Stage Renal Disease Treatment Facility
71 State or Local Public Health Clinic
72 Rural Health Clinic
81 Independent Laboratory

B

Business corporation

A for-profit organization recognized by law as a business entity separate and distinct from its shareholders. Shareholders need not be licensed in the profession practiced by the corporation.

C

Capitation contract

A contract in which the practice agrees to provide medical services to a defined population for a fixed price per beneficiary per month, regardless of actual services provided. Capitation contracts, which always contain an element of risk, include HMO, Medicare and Medicaid capitation contracts.

Clinical activities

Those activities performed by the physician in which patients are seen in the office, outpatient clinic, emergency room, nursing home, operating room, or labor and delivery; any time spent on hospital rounds, telephone conversations with patients, consultations with providers, interpretation of diagnostic tests and chart review. Should also include "on-call" hours if the physician is required to be present in the medical facility such as a medical clinic or hospital.

Clinical full-time equivalent (FTE)

The clinical full-time equivalent for each provider based upon the number of hours worked on clinical activities. A provider cannot be more than 1.0 FTE, but may be less. For example: a physician administrator who is 80% clinical and 20% administrative would be 0.8 clinical FTE; a physician with a normal workweek of 32 hours (4 days) working in a clinic or hospital for 32 hours would be 1.0 clinical FTE; a physician with a normal workweek of 50 hours (5 days) working 32 clinical or hospital hours would be a 0.64 clinical FTE (32 divided by 50 hours).

Clinical science department

A unit of organization in a medical school with an independent chair and single budget. The department's mission is to conduct teaching, research and/or clinical activities related to the entire spectrum of health care delivery to humans, from prevention through treatment. Residents in training or fellows may be present.

Appendix B: Terms Used in Report

Collections for professional charges

The actual dollars collected that can be attributed to a physician for all professional services. Includes fee-for-service collections, allocated capitation payments, administration of chemotherapy drugs, administration of immunizations. However, should not include, collections on drug charges, including vaccinations, allergy injections, and immunizations, as well as chemotherapy and antinauseant drugs, the technical component associated with any laboratory, radiology, medical diagnostic or surgical procedure collections, collections attributed to nonphysician providers, infusion-related collections, facility fees, supplies, revenue associated with the sale of hearing aids, eyeglasses, contact lenses, etc.

Community outreach

Direct involvement in community service activities to promote a better public health and build rapport between health providers and members of their communities.

E

Encounters

A documented, face-to-face contact between a patient and a provider who exercises independent judgment in the provision of services to the individual in an ambulatory or hospital setting. If the patient with the same diagnosis sees two different providers on the same day, it is one encounter. If patient sees two different providers on the same day for two different diagnoses, then it is considered two encounters. Encounters should include only procedures from the evaluation and management chapter (CPT codes 99201-99499) or the medicine chapter (CPT codes 90800-99199) of the Physicians' Current Procedural Terminology, Fourth Edition, copyrighted by the American Medical Association (AMA).

See also "ambulatory encounters" *and* "hospital encounters"

Equal shares option

Each shareholder in the practice is paid an equal share of compensation based upon overall practice performance (i.e., equal distribution of practice profits).

Established primary care physician

A physician with over two years in a primary care specialty. Primary care is comprised of Family Practice, Geriatrics, Internal Medicine and Pediatrics. The count of the number of years should begin at the time the physician completes the latter of the residency or fellowship.

Established specialist

A physician with over two years in a specialty other than primary care. The count of the number of years should begin at the time the physician completes the latter of the residency or fellowship.

F

Faculty practice plan

A formal organizational framework that structures the clinical practice activities of medical school faculty. The plan performs a range of services including billing, collections, contract negotiations and the distribution of income. Plans may form a separate legal organization or may be affiliated with the medical school through a clinical science department or teaching hospital. Faculty associated with the plan must provide patient care as part of a teaching or research program.

Fiscal year

The corporate year established by the practice for business purposes. For many practices, this is January 2002 through December 2002.

Freestanding Ambulatory Surgery Center (ASC)

A freestanding entity that is specifically licensed to provide surgery services that are performed on a same-day outpatient basis. A freestanding ambulatory surgery center does not employ physicians.

Appendix B: Terms Used in Report

Full-time equivalent (FTE) physician

A full-time equivalent physician works whatever number of hours the practice considers to be the minimum for a normal workweek, which could be 37.5, 40, 50 hours or some other standard. To compute the FTE of a part-time physician divide the total hours worked by the physician by the number of hours that your medical practice considers to be a normal workweek. For example, a physician working in a clinic or hospital on behalf of the practice for 30 hours compared to a normal workweek of 40 hours would be 0.75 FTE (30 divided by 40 hours). A physician working full-time for three months during a year would be 0.25 FTE (3 divided by 12 months). A medical director devoting 50% effort to clinical activity would be 0.5 FTE. A physician cannot exceed more than 1.0 FTE regardless of the number of hours worked.

G

Government

A governmental organization at the federal, state or local level. Government funding is not a sufficient criterion. Government ownership is the key factor. An example would be a medical clinic at a federal, state or county correctional facility.

Guaranteed or base salary option

A specific portion of the provider's total compensation that the practice or employing entity agrees to pay. The balance of compensation is determined by other factors (e.g., productivity, bonus, capitation, performance).

H

Health Maintenance Organization (HMO)

An HMO is an insurance company that accepts responsibility for providing and delivering a predetermined set of comprehensive health maintenance and treatment services to a voluntarily enrolled population for a negotiated and fixed periodic premium.

Hospital

A hospital is an inpatient facility that admits patients for overnight stays, incurs nursing care costs and generates bed-day revenues.

Hospital encounters (*see also* "Encounters")

Hospital encounters are a documented face-to-face contact between a patient and a provider who exercises independent judgment in the provision of services to the individual. If the patient with the same diagnosis sees two different providers on the same day, it is one encounter. If the patient sees two different providers on the same day for two different diagnoses, then it is considered two encounters

Hospital encounters should be reported only if performed in the following Centers for Medicare & Medicaid Services (CMS) place of service codes:

21 Inpatient Hospital
25 Birthing Center
26 Military Treatment Facility
51 Inpatient Psychiatric Facility
61 Comprehensive Inpatient Rehabilitation Facility

Hours worked per week

The number of hours an individual (e.g., physician) works during a normal (typical) workweek engaged in professional activities.

I

Insurance company

An insurance company is an organization that indemnifies an insured party against a specified loss in return for premiums paid, as stipulated by a contract.

Integrated Delivery System (IDS)

An IDS is a network of organizations that provide or coordinate and arrange for the provision of a continuum of health care services to consumers and are willing to be held clinically and fiscally responsible for the outcomes and the health status of the populations served. Generally consisting of hospitals, physician groups, health plans, home health agencies, hospices, skilled nursing facilities, or other provider entities, these networks may be built through "virtual" integration processes encompassing contractual arrangements and strategic alliances as well as through direct ownership. An emerging description of this same type of entity is Integradted Delivery Network (IDN).

Independent Practice Association (IPA)

An association or network of licensed providers and/or medical practices. An IPA is usually a unique legal entity, most often operating on a for-profit basis. Typically, the primary purpose of the IPA is to secure and maintain contractual relationships between providers and health plans.

Appendix B: Terms Used in Report

L

Limited liability company

A legal entity that is a hybrid between a corporation and a partnership, because it provides limited liability to owners like a corporation while passing profits and losses through to owners like a partnership.

M

Management Services Organization (MSO)

An MSO is an entity organized to provide various forms of practice management and administrative support services to health care providers. These services may include centralized billing and collections services, management information services and other components of the managed care infrastructure. MSOs do not actually deliver health care services. MSOs may be jointly or solely owned and sponsored by physicians, hospitals or other parties. Some MSOs also purchase assets of affiliated physicians and enter into long-term management service arrangements with a provider network. Some expand their ownership base by involving outside investors to help capitalize the development of such practice infrastructure.

Medical school

A medical school is an institution that trains physicians and awards medical and osteopathic degrees.

Metropolitan area (50,000 to 250,000)

The community in which the practice is located is an MSA or Census Bureau defined urbanized area of 50,000 to 250,000 population.

Metropolitan area (250,001 to 1,000,000)

The community in which the practice is located is an MSA or Census Bureau defined urbanized area of 250,001 to 1,000,000 population.

Metropolitan area (over 1,000,000)

The community in which the practice is located is a "primary metropolitan statistical area" (PMSA) having over 1,000,000 population.

Multispecialty practice with primary and specialty care

A medical practice which consists of physicians practicing in different specialties, including at least one primary care specialty listed below.
Family practice: general
Family practice: sports medicine
Family practice: urgent care
Family practice: with obstetrics
Family practice: without obstetrics
Geriatrics
Internal medicine: general
Pediatrics: adolescent medicine
Pediatrics: general
Pediatrics: sports medicine

Multispecialty practice with primary care only

A medical practice that consists of physicians practicing in more than one of the following primary care specialties listed above or the surgical specialties of obstetrics/gynecology, gynecology (only), obstetrics (only).

Multispecialty with specialty care only

A medical practice, which consists of physicians practicing in different specialties, none of which are the primary care specialties listed above.

N

New physician

A physician with less than two years in a specialty. The count of the number of years should begin at the time the physician completes the latter of the residency or fellowship.

Non-metropolitan area (under 50,000)

The community in which the practice is located is generally referred to as "rural." It is located outside of a "metropolitan statistical area" (MSA), as defined by the United States Office of Management and Budget, and has a population under 50,000.

Nonphysician providers (NPP)

Specially trained and licensed providers who can provide medical care and billable services. Examples of nonphysician providers include audiologists, Certified Registered Nurse Anesthetists (CRNAs), dieticians/nutritionists, midwives, nurse practitioners, occupational therapists, optometrists, physical therapists, physician assistants, psychologists, social workers, speech therapists and surgeon's assistants.

APPENDIX B: TERMS USED IN REPORT

Not-for-profit corporation/foundation

An organization that has obtained special exemption under Section 501(c) of the Internal Revenue code that qualifies the organization to be exempt from federal income taxes. To qualify as a tax-exempt organization, a practice or faculty practice plan would have to provide evidence of a charitable, educational or research purpose.

P

Part-time physician

To compute the FTE of a part-time physician divide the total hours worked by the physician by the number of hours that your medical practice considers to be a normal workweek. For example, a physician working in a clinic or hospital on behalf of the practice for 30 hours compared to a normal workweek of 40 hours would be 0.75 FTE (30 divided by 40 hours). A physician working full-time for three months during a year would be 0.25 FTE (3 divided by 12 months). A medical director devoting 50% effort to clinical activity would be 0.5 FTE.

See also "Full-time equivalent physician"

Partnership

An organization where two or more individuals have agreed that they will share profits, losses, assets and liabilities, although not necessarily on an equal basis. The partnership agreement may or may not be formalized in writing.

Peer review

A review process of physician clinical performance provided by a panel of other physicians.

Physician

Any doctor of medicine (MD) or doctor of osteopathy (DO) who is duly licensed and qualified under the law of jurisdiction in which treatment is received.

Physician patient panel

The number of patients, regardless of payer, assigned to a physician.

Physician Practice Management Company (PPMC)

PPMCs are usually publicly held or entrepreneurial directed enterprises that acquire total or partial ownership interests in physician organizations. PPMCs are a type of MSO, however the motivations, goals, strategies, and structures arising from their unequivocal ownership character - development of growth and profits for their investors, not for participating providers — differentiate them from other MSO models.

Physician Work RVUs (*see also* "Relative Value Units")

Physician Work RVUs refer the physician work component of the total RVU.

Productivity-based option

Provider compensation based wholly or partially upon individual physician output measurements.

Professional activities

Those services performed by the physician including both clinical and non-clinical time.

Professional corporation/association

A for-profit organization recognized by law as a business entity separate and distinct from its shareholders. Shareholders must be licensed in the profession practiced by the organization.

Professional gross charges

Gross patient charges are the full dollar value, at the practice's established undiscounted rates, of services provided to all patients, before reduction by charitable adjustments, professional courtesy adjustments, contractual adjustments, employee discounts, bad debts, etc. For both Medicare participating and nonparticipating providers, gross charges should include the practice's full, undiscounted charge and not the Medicare limiting charge.

Include:
1. Fee-for-service charges.
2. In-house equivalent gross fee-for-service charges for capitated patients.
3. Administration of chemotherapy drugs.
4. Administration of immunizations.

APPENDIX B: TERMS USED IN REPORT

Do not include:
1. Charges for drugs, including vaccinations, allergy, injections, and immunizations as well as chemotherapy and antinauseant drugs.
2. The technical component associated with any laboratory, radiology, medical diagnostic or surgical procedure.
3. Charges attributed to nonphysician providers.
4. Infusion-related charges.
5. Facility fees.
6. Supplies.
7. Charges associated with the sale of hearing aids, eyeglasses, contact lenses, etc.

R

Retirement benefit contributions (exclude FICA)

All employer contributions to retirement plans including defined benefit and contribution plans, 401(k), 403(b) and Keogh Plans, and any non-qualified funded retirement plan. For defined benefit plans, estimate the employer's contribution made on behalf of each plan participant by multiplying the employer's total contribution by each plan participant's compensation divided by the total compensation of all plan participants.

Do not include:
1. Employer contributions to social security mandated by the Federal Insurance Contributions Act (FICA).
2. Voluntary employee contributions that are an allocation of salary to a 401(k), 403(b), or Keogh Plan.
3. The dollar value of any other fringe benefits paid by the practice, such as life and health insurance, automobile allowances, etc.

Relative Value Units (RVUs)

Relative value units are nonmonetary, relative units of measure that indicate the value of health care services and relative difference in resources consumed when providing different procedures and services. RVUs assign relative values or weights to medical procedures primarily for the purpose of the reimbursement of services performed. They are used as a standardized method of analyzing resources involved in the provision of services or procedures.

S

Single-specialty practice

Classifying the type of specialty is the focus of clinical work and not necessarily the specialties of the physicians in the practice. For example, a single-specialty neurosurgery practice may include a neurologist and a radiologist.

Sole proprietorship

An organization with a single owner who is responsible for all profits, losses, assets and liabilities.

Specialty code

A provider should be classified in the specialty or subspecialty where the provider spends 50% or more time.

Straight salary

100% of provider compensation is attributed to a fixed salary.

Structured incentive/bonus

Compensation incentives that may be based on individual characteristics, corporate goals, overall practice performance, or other factors. A formula may be used to determine the amount.

Surgery/anesthesia cases

A case between a provider and a patient where at least one procedure performed is a procedure from the surgery chapter (CPT codes 10040-69979) or anesthesia chapter (CPT codes 00100-01999) of the Physicians' Current Procedural Terminology, Fourth Edition, copyrighted by the American Medical Association (AMA). Surgery/anesthesia cases include cases performed on an inpatient or outpatient basis, regardless of facility or site. For anesthesia care teams, anesthesiologist supervises one or more CRNAs, include total care team cases.

APPENDIX B: TERMS USED IN REPORT

T

Technical component (TC)

Modifier-TC, when attached to an appropriate CPT code, represents the technical component of the procedure and includes the cost of equipment and supplies to perform that procedure. This modifier corresponds to the equipment / facility part of a given procedure.

See also "RVUs"

Total compensation

The amount reported as direct compensation on a W2, 1099, or K1 (for partnerships) plus all voluntary salary reductions (e.g., 401(k), 403(b), Section 125 Tax Savings Plan, Medical Savings Plan). The amount should include salary, bonus and/or incentive payments, research stipends, honoraria and distribution of profits. However, it does not include the dollar value of expense reimbursements, fringe benefits paid by the medical practice (i.e., retirement plan contributions, life and health insurance, or automobile allowances), or any employer contributions to a 401(k), 403(b) or Keogh Plan.

Total medical revenue (collections)

The sum of fee-for-service collections, capitation payments, and other medical activity revenues.

U

Undiscounted rates

The full retail prices before Medicare/Medicaid charge restrictions, third-party payer (such as commercial insurance and/or managed care organization) contractual adjustments, and other charitable, professional courtesy or employee adjustments.

University

An institution of higher learning with teaching and research facilities comprising undergraduate, graduate and professional schools.

W

Weeks worked per year

The number of weeks the physician works during the year engaged in professional activities.

Y

Years in specialty

The number of years each physician and nonphysician provider has practiced in a specialty . The count of the number of years should begin at the time the physician completes the latter of the residency or fellowship.

APPENDIX C:
COMPENSATION AND PRODUCTION SURVEY: 2003 QUESTIONNAIRE BASED ON 2002 DATA

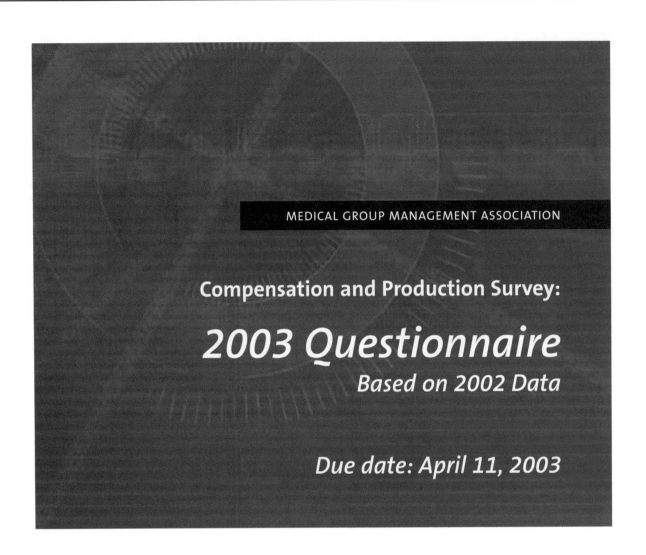

MEDICAL GROUP MANAGEMENT ASSOCIATION

Compensation and Production Survey:

2003 Questionnaire
Based on 2002 Data

Due date: April 11, 2003

E-Questionnaire:
To respond electronically, go to
www.mgma.com/surveys and
download the questionnaire.

toll-free 877.ASK.MGMA
www.mgma.com/surveys

Medical Group
Management
Association
✳ MGMA™

APPENDIX C:
COMPENSATION AND PRODUCTION SURVEY: 2003 QUESTIONNAIRE BASED ON 2002 DATA

MEDICAL GROUP MANAGEMENT ASSOCIATION
Compensation and Production Survey: 2003 Questionnaire Based on 2002 Data

Instructions

Please refer to the *Compensation and Production Survey: 2003 Guide to the Questionnaire Based on 2002 Data* (Guide) for definitions and instructions for completing the questionnaire.

If your organization is a Management Services Organization (MSO), Physician Practice Management Company (PPMC), hospital, integrated health care system, and/or a medical practice consisting of more than one legal entity, please read the instructions on page 3 of the Guide.

2002 Fiscal Year Definition

All the questions on this questionnaire refer to the 2002 fiscal year. This is typically January 2002 through December 2002. If your practice uses an alternative fiscal year, you are encouraged to use it in your responses.

1. For the purposes of reporting the information in this questionnaire, what fiscal year was used?

    Beginning month$_a$ ☐　Beginning year$_b$ ☐　*through* Ending month$_c$ ☐　Ending year$_d$ ☐

Medical Practice Information

Please answer the following questions in the way that best describes your practice at the end of the 2002 fiscal year. Pages 4 to 8 in the Guide contain additional information for answering questions in this section.

2. What was your practice type? (check only one)

    Single specialty .... $_1$ ☐

    Multispecialty with primary and specialty care .... $_2$ ☐

    Multispecialty with primary care only .... $_3$ ☐

    Multispecialty with specialty care only .... $_4$ ☐

3. If you answered "Single specialty" for question 2, what specialty was your practice?

    _____

4. Was your organization a freestanding ambulatory surgery center only? Answer "No" if the ambulatory surgery center was a unit of the medical practice.

    Yes .... $_1$ ☐

    No .... $_2$ ☐

5. Was your practice a medical school faculty practice plan and/or clinical science department?

    Yes .... $_1$ ☐

    No .... $_2$ ☐

6. Did an MSO or a PPMC provide services to your practice?

    Yes .... $_1$ ☐

    No .... $_2$ ☐

7. What was the legal organization of your practice? (check only one)

    Business corporation .... $_1$ ☐

    Limited liability company .... $_2$ ☐

    Not-for-profit corporation/foundation .... $_3$ ☐

    Partnership .... $_4$ ☐

    Professional corporation/association .... $_5$ ☐

    Sole proprietorship .... $_6$ ☐

    Other .... $_7$ ☐

8. Who was the majority owner of your practice? (check only one)

    Government .... $_1$ ☐

    *Hospital/integrated delivery system .... $_2$ ☐

    Insurance company or health maintenance organization (HMO) .... $_3$ ☐

    *MSO or PPMC .... $_4$ ☐

    Physicians .... $_5$ ☐

    *University or medical school .... $_6$ ☐

    *Other _____ $_7$ ☐

    *Please indicate the name and location of your parent organization (owner) on lines 44 through 47 on page 8.

Need Help? Call Survey Operations at 877.275.6462, ext. 895.　2

MEDICAL GROUP MANAGEMENT ASSOCIATION™

APPENDIX C:
COMPENSATION AND PRODUCTION SURVEY: 2003 QUESTIONNAIRE BASED ON 2002 DATA

MEDICAL GROUP MANAGEMENT ASSOCIATION
Compensation and Production Survey: 2003 Questionnaire Based on 2002 Data

Medical Practice Information (continued)

9. Which population designation best describes the area surrounding the primary location of your practice? If your practice had multiple sites, choose the option that represents the location with the largest number of FTE physicians. (check only one)

   Non-metropolitan (under 50,000) .... ₁ ☐

   Metropolitan (50,000 to 250,000) .... ₂ ☐

   Metropolitan (250,001 to 1,000,000) .... ₃ ☐

   Metropolitan (over 1,000,000) .... ₄ ☐

10. Did your practice derive revenue from capitation contracts?

   Yes .... ₁ ☐

   No .... ₂ ☐

11. If you answered "Yes" to question 10, what percentage of your practice's total medical revenue was derived from capitation contracts?

   _____ % capitation

12. What was the total medical revenue (collections) for your practice?

   _____total medical revenue

13. How many full-time equivalent (FTE) physicians were in your practice?

   _____physicians

14. How many FTE nonphysician providers were in your practice?

   _____ nonphysician providers

15. Does your practice intend to change its physician compensation method within the next year?

   Yes.. ₁ ☐

   No .... ₂ ☐

Please report the percentage of compensation attributed to the following options. If the option does not apply, please enter zero as your answer in the space provided. The percentage total should equal 100%.

	New Physician (1-2 yrs in specialty)ₐ	Established Primary Care Physician_b	Established Specialist_c
16. Productivity-based....................	%	%	%
17. Guaranteed or base salary	%	%	%
18. Straight salary..........................	%	%	%
19. Equal shares	%	%	%
20. Capitation	%	%	%
21. Structured incentive/bonus	%	%	%
22. Other _____	%	%	%
	100 %	100 %	100 %

23. If compensation is productivity-based, please indicate how production is measured. (check all that apply)

   Gross charges ....ₐ ☐

   Adjusted charges ...._b ☐

   Collections for professional charges ...._c ☐

   Number of patient encounters ...._d ☐

   Size of physician's patient panel....................._e ☐

   Number of RVUs ...._f ☐

   Other _____ _g ☐

24. If compensation is based on a structured incentive/bonus, please indicate the basis for the incentive/bonus. (check all that apply)

   Patient satisfaction ....ₐ ☐

   Peer review ...._b ☐

   Administrative/governance responsibility ...._c ☐

   Service quality ...._d ☐

   Seniority in the medical practice ...._e ☐

   Community outreach.._f ☐

   Other _____ _g ☐

3

APPENDIX C:
COMPENSATION AND PRODUCTION SURVEY: 2003 QUESTIONNAIRE BASED ON 2002 DATA

MEDICAL GROUP MANAGEMENT ASSOCIATION
Compensation and Production Survey: 2003 Questionnaire Based on 2002 Data

Physician Compensation and Production Matrix

Please refer to pages 8 to 9 in the Guide before completing the following matrix. The matrix should be completed only for providers who have worked the entire 12-month period reported in question 1. If your practice has more than 15 providers, you are encouraged to submit responses using the electronic version of the questionnaire available at www.mgma.com/surveys.

	1 Provider Tracking Number	2 Specialty Code (use codes below)	3 Total Compensation	4 Retirement Benefits (exclude FICA)	5 Years in Specialty	6 Gender	7 Hours Worked per Week	8 Weeks Worked per Year	9 Clinical FTE	10 Collections for Professional Charges
1	_____	_____	$_____	$_____	_____	M F	_____	_____	_____	$_____
2	_____	_____	$_____	$_____	_____	M F	_____	_____	_____	$_____
3	_____	_____	$_____	$_____	_____	M F	_____	_____	_____	$_____
4	_____	_____	$_____	$_____	_____	M F	_____	_____	_____	$_____
5	_____	_____	$_____	$_____	_____	M F	_____	_____	_____	$_____
6	_____	_____	$_____	$_____	_____	M F	_____	_____	_____	$_____
7	_____	_____	$_____	$_____	_____	M F	_____	_____	_____	$_____
8	_____	_____	$_____	$_____	_____	M F	_____	_____	_____	$_____
9	_____	_____	$_____	$_____	_____	M F	_____	_____	_____	$_____
10	_____	_____	$_____	$_____	_____	M F	_____	_____	_____	$_____
11	_____	_____	$_____	$_____	_____	M F	_____	_____	_____	$_____
12	_____	_____	$_____	$_____	_____	M F	_____	_____	_____	$_____
13	_____	_____	$_____	$_____	_____	M F	_____	_____	_____	$_____
14	_____	_____	$_____	$_____	_____	M F	_____	_____	_____	$_____
15	_____	_____	$_____	$_____	_____	M F	_____	_____	_____	$_____

For each provider, select one specialty code where they spent 50% or more time.

Physician Specialty List

1	Allergy/Immunology	24	Hematology/Oncology: Oncology (only)	47	Ortho Surg: Spine
2*	Anesthesiology	25	Infectious Disease	48	Ortho Surg: Trauma
3*	Anesthesiology: Pain Management	26	Internal Medicine: General	49	Ortho Surg: Sports Medicine
4*	Anesthesiology: Pediatric	27	Internal Medicine: Hospitalist	50	Otorhinolaryngology
5	Cardiology: Electrophysiology	28	Internal Medicine: Pediatrics	51	Otorhinolaryngology: Pediatric
6	Cardiology: Invasive	29	Nephrology	52	Pathology: Anatomic and Clinical
7	Cardiology: Inv-Intervntnl	30	Neurology	53	Pathology: Anatomic
8	Cardiology: Noninvasive	31	Obstetrics/Gynecology: General	54	Pathology: Clinical
9	Critical Care: Intensivist	32	Ob/Gyn: Gynecology (only)	55	Pediatrics: General
10	Dentistry	33	Ob/Gyn: Gynecological Oncology	56	Ped: Adolescent Medicine
11	Dermatology	34	Ob/Gyn: Maternal & Fetal Medicine	57	Ped: Allergy/Immunology
12	Dermatology: MOHS Surgery	35	Ob/Gyn: Reproductive Endocrinology	58	Ped: Cardiology
13	Emergency Medicine	36	Occupational Medicine	59	Ped: Child Development
14	Endocrinology/Metabolism	37	Ophthalmology	60	Ped: Clinical & Lab Immunology
15	Family Practice (with OB)	38	Ophthalmology: Pediatric	61	Ped: Critical Care/Intensivist
16	Family Practice (without OB)	39	Ophthalmology: Retina	62	Ped: Emergency Medicine
17	Family Practice: Sports Medicine	40	Orthopedic (Nonsurgical)	63	Ped: Endocrinology
18	Family Practice: Urgent Care	41	Ortho Surg: General	64	Ped: Gastroenterology
19	Gastroenterology	42	Ortho Surg: Foot & Ankle	65	Ped: Genetics
20	Gastroenterology: Hepatology	43	Ortho Surg: Hand	66	Ped: Hematology/Oncology
21	Genetics	44	Ortho Surg: Hip & Joint	67	Ped: Hospitalist
22	Geriatrics	45	Ortho Surg: Oncology	68	Ped: Infectious Disease
23	Hematology/Oncology	46	Ortho Surg: Pediatric	69	Ped: Neonatal Medicine

* Please refer to page 8, column 2 in the Guide for more information.

Need Help? Call Survey Operations at 877.275.6462, ext. 895.   4

MEDICAL GROUP MANAGEMENT ASSOCIATION™

APPENDIX C:
COMPENSATION AND PRODUCTION SURVEY: 2003 QUESTIONNAIRE BASED ON 2002 DATA

MEDICAL GROUP MANAGEMENT ASSOCIATION
Compensation and Production Survey: 2003 Questionnaire Based on 2002 Data

Physician Compensation and Production Matrix (continued)

For column 10A, 11A and 15A, TC = Technical Component for laboratory, radiology, medical diagnostic and surgical procedures. Column 17 refers to columns 10 through 16.

10A Level of TC included in col 10 (circle one)	11 Professional Gross Charges	11A Level of TC included in col 11 (circle one)	12 Ambulatory Encounters	13 Hospital Encounters	14 Surgery/ Anesthesia Cases	15 Total RVUs	15A TC included in col 15	16 Physician Work RVUs	17 Nonphysician Provider Productivity (included in col 11-16)	
0% 1-10% >10%	$_____	0% 1-10% >10%	_____	_____	_____	_____	Y N	_____	Y N	1
0% 1-10% >10%	$_____	0% 1-10% >10%	_____	_____	_____	_____	Y N	_____	Y N	2
0% 1-10% >10%	$_____	0% 1-10% >10%	_____	_____	_____	_____	Y N	_____	Y N	3
0% 1-10% >10%	$_____	0% 1-10% >10%	_____	_____	_____	_____	Y N	_____	Y N	4
0% 1-10% >10%	$_____	0% 1-10% >10%	_____	_____	_____	_____	Y N	_____	Y N	5
0% 1-10% >10%	$_____	0% 1-10% >10%	_____	_____	_____	_____	Y N	_____	Y N	6
0% 1-10% >10%	$_____	0% 1-10% >10%	_____	_____	_____	_____	Y N	_____	Y N	7
0% 1-10% >10%	$_____	0% 1-10% >10%	_____	_____	_____	_____	Y N	_____	Y N	8
0% 1-10% >10%	$_____	0% 1-10% >10%	_____	_____	_____	_____	Y N	_____	Y N	9
0% 1-10% >10%	$_____	0% 1-10% >10%	_____	_____	_____	_____	Y N	_____	Y N	10
0% 1-10% >10%	$_____	0% 1-10% >10%	_____	_____	_____	_____	Y N	_____	Y N	11
0% 1-10% >10%	$_____	0% 1-10% >10%	_____	_____	_____	_____	Y N	_____	Y N	12
0% 1-10% >10%	$_____	0% 1-10% >10%	_____	_____	_____	_____	Y N	_____	Y N	13
0% 1-10% >10%	$_____	0% 1-10% >10%	_____	_____	_____	_____	Y N	_____	Y N	14
0% 1-10% >10%	$_____	0% 1-10% >10%	_____	_____	_____	_____	Y N	_____	Y N	15

Physician Specialty List (continued)

70	Ped: Nephrology	93	Surg: Colon and Rectal
71	Ped: Neurology	94	Surg: Neurological
72	Ped: Pulmonology	95	Surg: Oncology
73	Ped: Rheumatology	96	Surg: Oral
74	Ped: Sports Medicine	97	Surg: Pediatric
75	Physiatry (Physical Med & Rehab)	98	Surg: Plastic & Reconstruction
76	Podiatry: General	99	Surg: Plastic & Reconstr-Hand
77	Podiatry: Surg-Foot & Ankle	100	Surg: Plastic & Reconstr-Pediatric
78	Podiatry: Surg-Forefoot Only	101	Surg: Thoracic (primary)
79	Psychiatry: General	102	Surg: Transplant
80	Psychiatry: Child & Adolescent	103	Surg: Trauma
81	Psychiatry: Forensic	104	Surg: Trauma-Burn
82	Psychiatry: Geriatric	105	Surg: Vascular (primary)
83	Pulmonary Medicine	106	Urgent Care
84	Pumonary Medicine: Critical Care	107	Urology
85	Radiation Oncology	108	Urology: Pediatric
86	Radiology: Diagnostic-Invasive	109	Other Physician Specialty (write in column 2)
87	Radiology: Diagnostic-Noninvasive		
88	Radiology: Nuclear Medicine		
89	Rheumatology		
90	Surgery: General		
91	Surg: Cardiovascular		
92	Surg: Cardiovascular-Pediatric		

Nonphysician Provider List

115	Audiologist
116	Certified Reg. Nurse Anesthetist
117	Dietician/Nutritionist
118	Nurse Midwife: Outpatient/inpatient deliveries
119	Nurse Midwife: Outpatient (only)
120	Nurse Midwife: Inpatient (only)
121*	Nurse Practitioner
122	Occupational Therapist
123	Optometrist
124	Orthotist/Prosthetist
125	Perfusionist
126	Pharmacist
127	Physical Therapist
128	Physician Assistant (surgical)
129	Physician Assistant (primary care)
130	Physician Assistant (non-surg, non-primary care)
131	Physicist
132	Psychologist
133	Social Worker
134	Speech Therapist
135	Surgeon Assistant
136	Other nonphysician provider (write in column 2)

* Please refer to page 8, column 2 in the Guide for more information.

5

APPENDIX C:
COMPENSATION AND PRODUCTION SURVEY: 2003 QUESTIONNAIRE BASED ON 2002 DATA

MEDICAL GROUP MANAGEMENT ASSOCIATION
Compensation and Production Survey: 2003 Questionnaire Based on 2002 Data

Management Compensation Matrix

CHANGES HAVE BEEN MADE TO SOME POSITION DESCRIPTIONS. Please refer to pages 12 to 20 in the Guide before completing the following matrix. The matrix requests information for executives, managerial staff, specialists and supervisors that held the same position for the entire 12-month reporting period and were employed

	1 Employee Tracking Code	2 Position Title (use codes below)	3 Total Compensation (include amount from column 4)	4 Bonus/Incentive Amount	5 Retirement Benefits (exclude FICA)	6 Compensation Method (use codes on pg. 7)
1	_____	_____	$_____	$_____	$_____	_____
2	_____	_____	$_____	$_____	$_____	_____
3	_____	_____	$_____	$_____	$_____	_____
4	_____	_____	$_____	$_____	$_____	_____
5	_____	_____	$_____	$_____	$_____	_____
6	_____	_____	$_____	$_____	$_____	_____
7	_____	_____	$_____	$_____	$_____	_____
8	_____	_____	$_____	$_____	$_____	_____
9	_____	_____	$_____	$_____	$_____	_____
10	_____	_____	$_____	$_____	$_____	_____

Select one position that best describes each individual's responsibilities from the list below, and place the corresponding number in column 2. Pages 12 to 20 in the Guide contain position descriptions.

Physician Executive Positions
1   Physician Chief Executive Officer (CEO)/President
2   Medical Director
3   Associate/Assistant Medical Director

Executive Management Positions
4   Chief Executive Officer (CEO)/Executive Director
5   Administrator
6   MSO Administrator/Executive Director
7   Chief Operating Officer (COO)
8   Chief Financial Officer (CFO)
9   Assistant Administrator

Senior Management Positions (formerly General Managers)
10   Ambulatory/Clinical Services Director (formerly Director, Ambulatory/Clinical Services)
11   Building and Grounds Director (formerly Director, Facilities Management)
12   Business Services Director (formerly Director, Business Services/Business Office Manager)
13   Clinical Research Director (formerly Director, Clinical Research)
14   Compliance Director (formerly Compliance Officer)
15   Education and Training Director (formerly Director, Education and Training/Training Manager)
16   Finance Director (new)
17   Human Resources Director (formerly Director, Human Resources)
18   Information Systems Director (formerly Director, Management Information Services (MIS)/Information Systems Manager)

19   Laboratory Services Director (formerly Director, Laboratory Services/Laboratory Manager)
20   Managed Care Director (formerly Director, Managed Care)
21   Marketing and Sales Director (formerly Director, Marketing & Sales)
22   Medical Records Director (formerly Director, Medical Records/Medical Records Manager)
23   Nursing Services Director (formerly Director, Nursing Services/Nursing Supervisor)
24   Quality Improvement/Quality Assurance Director (formerly Director, Quality Improvement/Quality Assurance)
25   Radiology Services Director (formerly Director, Radiology Services/Radiology Manager)
26   Reimbursement Director (formerly Director, Reimbursement)

General Management Positions
27   Benefits Manager (formerly Compensation/Benefits Manager)
28   Branch/Satellite Clinic Manager
29   Business Office Manager (formerly part of Director, Business Services/Business Office Manager)
30   Clinical Department Manager
31   Clinic Research Manager (new)
32   General Accounting Manager (formerly Controller)
33   Laboratory Services Manager (formerly part of Director, Laboratory Services/Laboratory Services Manager)
34   Materials Management Manager (formerly Director, Purchasing)
35   Medical Records Manager (formerly part of Director, Medical Records/Medical Records Manager)
36   Nursing Manager (new)

6

APPENDIX C:
COMPENSATION AND PRODUCTION SURVEY: 2003 QUESTIONNAIRE BASED ON 2002 DATA

MEDICAL GROUP MANAGEMENT ASSOCIATION
Compensation and Production Survey: 2003 Questionnaire Based on 2002 Data

on a full-time basis. If your practice has more than 10 management staff, you are encouraged to submit responses using the electronic version of the questionnaire available at www.mgma.com/surveys.

7 Formal Education (use codes below)	8 Years of Management Experience	9 Gender	10 ACMPE Status (use codes below)	11 MGMA National Member (circle one)	Positions 1 thru 26 ONLY 12 Professional Organization Fees	Positions 1 thru 3 ONLY 13 Physician Executive Time Percentage Admin/Clinical	
_____	_____	M F	_____	Y N	$_____	_____% _____%	1
_____	_____	M F	_____	Y N	$_____	_____% _____%	2
_____	_____	M F	_____	Y N	$_____	_____% _____%	3
_____	_____	M F	_____	Y N	$_____	_____% _____%	4
_____	_____	M F	_____	Y N	$_____	_____% _____%	5
_____	_____	M F	_____	Y N	$_____	_____% _____%	6
_____	_____	M F	_____	Y N	$_____	_____% _____%	7
_____	_____	M F	_____	Y N	$_____	_____% _____%	8
_____	_____	M F	_____	Y N	$_____	_____% _____%	9
_____	_____	M F	_____	Y N	$_____	_____% _____%	10

37 Office Manager
38 Operations Manager
39 Patient Accounting Manager (formerly Professional Fee
     Billing Coordinator/Billing Manager)
40 Radiology Services Manager (formerly part of Director,
     Radiology Services/Radiology Manager)
41 Training/Education Manager (formerly part of Director,
     Education and Training/Training Manager)
     Director of Education and Training Services)

Specialists
42 Benefits/Payroll Specialist (new)
43 Marketing/Communication Specialist (formerly Director,
     Public Relations/Communications)
Supervisors
44 Business Office Supervisor (new)
45 Clinic Supervisor (new)
46 Nursing Supervisor (formerly part of Director, Nursing
     Services/Nursing Supervisor)
47 Other - (describe the position title in column 2)

Select the choice that best describes the compensation method for each individual listed in column 2, and place the corresponding number in column 6.

1 Hourly
2 Straight salary only (no bonus)
3 Base salary + discretionary bonus (e.g., Christmas bonus)
4 Base salary + percentage of practice productivity and/or physician income (formula bonus)
5 Base salary + percentage of practice's net profit (formula bonus)
6 Base salary + other formula bonus (e.g., number of patient visits, patient satisfaction)
7 Base salary + deferred compensation (e.g., trusts, stock options)
8 Base salary + combination of discretionary and formula bonuses + deferred compensation
9 Other (describe the compensation method in column 6)

Select the highest level of formal education attained by each individual, and place the corresponding number in column 7.

1 High school diploma or the equivalent
2 Associate degree or other two-year degree
3 Bachelor's degree or other four-year degree
4 Master's degree
5 PhD, JD, EdD
6 MD, DO
7 MD or DO (with Master's Degree)
8 Other (describe the education level in column 7)

Select each individual's status in the American College of Medical Practice Executives (ACMPE), the professional credentialing arm of MGMA, and place the corresponding number in column 10.

1 Not affiliated
2 Nominee
3 Certified (CMPE)
4 Fellow (FACMPE)

7   *Need Help? Call Survey Operations at 877.275.6462, ext. 895.*

APPENDIX C:
COMPENSATION AND PRODUCTION SURVEY: 2003 QUESTIONNAIRE BASED ON 2002 DATA

MEDICAL GROUP MANAGEMENT ASSOCIATION
Compensation and Production Survey: 2003 Questionnaire Based on 2002 Data

Questionnaire Contact

Please provide contact information for the individual who completed this questionnaire, as well as the name of the observed practice for which data is reported.

25. Name _____
26. Title _____
27. Telephone number (____) _____
28. Fax number (____) _____
29. E-mail address _____
30. Observed Practice Name _____
31. Please provide the Federal Tax ID# for the observed practice. _____
32. Please report the total number of hours required to complete all parts of this survey questionnaire by all personnel working on it. _____

Organizations will be mailed a **Respondent Ranking Report** and a complimentary copy of the survey report as a benefit of participation. To ensure this confidential information reaches the appropriate individual, please indicate below the recipient's name, organization, and mailing address in the spaces provided, if different from the information appearing on the mailing label. Please provide complete information.

33. Name _____
34. Title _____
35. Organization _____
36. Address _____
37. City _____
38. State _____
39. Zip _____
40. Telephone number (____) _____
41. E-mail address _____
42. MGMA member # _____
43. MGMA Use Only _____

Parent Organization Information

The observed medical practice is the medical practice for which data has been reported on this questionnaire. If you indicated in question 8 on page 2, ownership of the observed practice by a 'hospital/integrated delivery system', 'MSO', 'PPMC', 'University' or 'other' type of organization, please provide the name of the parent organization (owner) and their location in the spaces provided below.

44. Parent Name _____
45. Address _____
46. City _____
47. State _____

Comments

Thank you for participating, and remember to keep a copy of this questionnaire for your records.

8

APPENDIX D:
COMPENSATION AND PRODUCTION SURVEY: 2003 GUIDE TO THE QUESTIONNAIRE BASED ON 2002 DATA

MEDICAL GROUP MANAGEMENT ASSOCIATION

Compensation and Production Survey:

2003 Guide
to the Questionnaire Based on 2002 Data

Due date: April 11, 2003

APPENDIX D:
COMPENSATION AND PRODUCTION SURVEY: 2003 GUIDE TO THE QUESTIONNAIRE BASED ON 2002 DATA

MEDICAL GROUP MANAGEMENT ASSOCIATION
Compensation and Production Survey: 2003 Guide to the Questionnaire Based on 2002 Data

Frequently Asked Questions

What is the purpose of this survey questionnaire?
This survey questionnaire collects data for the *Physician Compensation and Production Survey: 2003 Report Based on 2002 Data* and the *Management Compensation Survey: 2003 Report Based on 2002 Data*. These reports provide comparison data on physician and nonphysician provider compensation and production, as well as managerial compensation to help evaluate decisions in a medical practice.

Who is conducting this survey?
The Medical Group Management Association (MGMA) Survey Operations Department.

Who should complete this survey?
One questionnaire should be completed by the medical practice.

If your organization is an Integrated Delivery System (IDS), hospital, Management Services Organization (MSO), Physician Practice Management Company (PPMC), Independent Practice Association (IPA), or other entity that owns, manages, or provides services to medical practices, one questionnaire should be completed for each medical practice that you own, manage, or service. See the Instructions on page 3 for definitions.

Academic practices, faculty practice plans, and clinical science departments associated with medical schools should not participate in this survey. Freestanding ambulatory surgery centers should not participate in this survey. See questions 4 and 5 on page 4 for definitions. Instead, they should participate respectively in the *Academic Practice Compensation and Production Survey Questionnaire* or the *Ambulatory Surgery Center Performance Survey Questionnaire*.

Questionnaires should not be submitted for departments within multispecialty practices. A questionnaire must represent a complete medical practice.

Why should I participate?
Please see the enclosed postcard for information.

Do I need to answer all of the questions on the survey?
We would appreciate receiving the requested information on your organization, to the extent you can provide it. The quality of our reported results depends upon the completeness and accuracy of every response.

What if I am unsure about how to answer a question properly?
Please refer to the Definitions section of this Guide. For any questions about the survey questionnaire, please call the MGMA Survey Operations Department toll-free, 877.275.6462, ext. 895, or e-mail surveys@mgma.com.

Are all survey data confidential?
Yes. The MGMA and the MGMA Center for Research Policy on Data Confidentiality states: All data submitted to the MGMA or to the MGMA Center for Research will be kept confidential. All submitted data and related materials that identify a specific organization or individual will be safeguarded and will not be published or voluntarily released within the public domain without written permission.

Only summary statistics will be published. A summary statistic will be reported only if there are sufficient responses and if the anonymity of those submitting data is protected.

When is my response due?
The due date is April 11, 2003. The survey results will be much more useful to you if we can report the results on a timely basis. We have a very tight schedule for obtaining responses, processing the data and publishing the *2003 Physician Compensation and Production Survey Report* and the *2003 Management Compensation Survey Report*. Therefore, we would sincerely appreciate your giving this survey a high priority and returning your completed questionnaire as soon as you can.

Can the data be submitted electronically?
Yes. Please go to www.mgma.com/surveys and follow the directions on the screen.

Where do I send a completed questionnaire?
Use the enclosed reply envelope and mail the completed questionnaire to the MGMA Survey Operations Department, 104 Inverness Terrace East, Englewood, CO 80112-5306. Or you may fax your response to 303.643.9567, Attention: Survey Operations. If you used the electronic version of the questionnaire, you may e-mail your response to surveys@mgma.com. Be sure to keep a photocopy of the completed questionnaire for your reference.

2

MEDICAL GROUP MANAGEMENT ASSOCIATION™

APPENDIX D:
COMPENSATION AND PRODUCTION SURVEY: 2003 GUIDE TO THE QUESTIONNAIRE BASED ON 2002 DATA

MEDICAL GROUP MANAGEMENT ASSOCIATION
Compensation and Production Survey: 2003 Guide to the Questionnaire Based on 2002 Data

Instructions

There are three units of observation for this survey: the medical practice, the individual provider, and managerial personnel. For the purpose of this survey, a medical practice is defined as a single legal entity or collection of legal entities consisting of at least one physician and/or nonphysician provider who delivers health care services. An individual provider is defined as being one of two types, a physician or nonphysician provider. Managerial personnel include physician executives, executive management, senior managment, general management, specialists and supervisors.

Integrated Delivery System (IDS)/Hospital
An IDS is a network of organizations that provide or coordinate and arrange for the provision of a continuum of health care services to consumers and are willing to be held clinically and fiscally responsible for the outcomes and the health status of the populations served. Generally consisting of hospitals, physician groups, health plans, home health agencies, hospices, skilled nursing facilities, or other provider entities, these networks may be built through "virtual" integration processes encompassing contractual arrangements and strategic alliances as well as through direct ownership.

A hospital is an inpatient facility that admits patients for overnight stays, incurs nursing care costs and generates bed-day revenues.

If your organization is an IDS or hospital that owns and/or manages medical practices, you should complete one questionnaire for each practice that you own or manage. Also, complete the *Cost Survey for Integrated Delivery System Practices: 2003 Questionnaire Based on 2002 Data*.

When completing a questionnaire on behalf of an owned practice, please identify the parent organization (owner) by completing the Parent Organization Information section on page 8 of the questionnaire.

Management Services Organizations, Physician Practice Management Companies, etc.
If your organization is a Management Services Organization (MSO), Physician Practice Management Company (PPMC) or other type of management organization, you may also participate in the *Management Services Organization Performance Survey: 2003 Questionnaire Based on 2002 Data*, available in July 2003.

If you would like to receive a copy of the *2003 Management Services Organization Performance Survey Ques-tionnaire*, you can call the MGMA Survey Operations Department toll-free, 877.275.6462, ext. 895, or e-mail surveys@mgma.com.

An MSO is an entity organized to provide various forms of practice management and administrative support services to health care providers. These services may include centralized billing and collections services, management information services and other components of the managed care infrastructure. MSOs do not actually deliver health care services. MSOs may be jointly or solely owned and sponsored by physicians, hospitals or other parties. Some MSOs also purchase assets of affiliated physicians and enter into long-term manage-ment service arrangements with a provider network. Some expand their ownership base by involving outside investors to help capitalize the development of such practice infrastructure.

PPMCs are usually publicly held or entrepreneurial directed enterprises that acquire total or partial owner-ship interests in physician organizations. PPMCs are a type of MSO, however the motivations, goals, strategies, and structures arising from their unequivocal ownership character - development of growth and profits for their investors, not for participating providers — differentiate them from other MSO models.

An IPA is an association or network of licensed providers and/or medical practices. An IPA is usually a unique legal entity, most often operating on a for-profit basis. Typically, the primary purpose of the IPA is to secure and maintain contractual relationships between providers and health plans.

If your organization is an MSO, PPMC, IPA or other type of management organization, you should complete one questionnaire for each medical practice that you manage or service. You may make as many photocopies of this questionnaire as necessary or call MGMA to receive additional copies.

When completing a questionnaire on behalf of a man-aged practice, please identify the parent organization (owner) by completing the Parent Organization Informa-tion section on page 8 of the questionnaire.

Hospitals or health systems
If your organization is a hospital or health system that owns and/or manages medical practices, you should complete one questionnaire for each practice that you own or manage.

3

APPENDIX D:
COMPENSATION AND PRODUCTION SURVEY: 2003 GUIDE TO THE QUESTIONNAIRE BASED ON 2002 DATA

MEDICAL GROUP MANAGEMENT ASSOCIATION
Compensation and Production Survey: 2003 Guide to the Questionnaire Based on 2002 Data

Definitions

2002 Fiscal Year Definition

1. **For the purposes of reporting the information in this questionnaire, what fiscal year was used?**
   For many practices, this is January 2002 through December 2002. If your practice uses an alternative fiscal year, you are encouraged to use it in your responses. Do not report data for periods less than 12 months.

   If your medical practice was involved in a merger or acquisition during 2002 and you cannot assemble 12 months of practice data, you may not be able to participate this year. Please call the MGMA Survey Operations Department if you are uncertain about your eligibility to participate.

Medical Practice Information

2. **What was your practice type? (check only one)**
   Single-specialty: A medical practice that focuses its clinical work in one specialty. The determining factor for classifying the type of specialty is the focus of clinical work and not necessarily the specialties of the physicians in the practice. For example, a single-specialty neurosurgery practice may include a neurologist and a radiologist.

   Practices that include only the subspecialties of internal medicine should be classified as a single-specialty internal medicine practice. Internal medicine subspecialties include:
   Allergy and immunology
   Cardiology
   Endocrinology/metabolism
   Gastroenterology
   Hematology/oncology
   Infectious disease
   Nephrology
   Pulmonary disease
   Rheumatology

Multispecialty with primary and specialty care: A medical practice which consists of physicians practicing in different specialties, including at least one primary care specialty listed below.
Family practice: general
Family practice: sports medicine
Family practice: urgent care
Family practice: with obstetrics
Family practice: without obstetrics
Geriatrics
Internal medicine: general
Internal medicine: urgent care
Pediatrics: adolescent medicine
Pediatrics: general
Pediatrics: sports medicine

Multispecialty with primary care only: A medical practice that consists of physicians practicing in more than one of the following primary care specialties listed above or the surgical specialties of
Obstetrics/gynecology
Gynecology (only)
Obstetrics (only)

Multispecialty with specialty care only: A medical practice, which consists of physicians practicing in different specialties, none of which are the primary care specialties listed above.

3. **If you answered "Single-specialty" for question 2, what specialty was your practice?**
   State the name of the single-specialty that most closely describes your practice.

4. **Was your organization a freestanding ambulatory surgery center only? Answer "No" if the ambulatory surgery center was a unit of the medical practice.**
   An ambulatory surgery center is a freestanding entity that is specifically licensed to provide surgery services that are performed on a same-day outpatient basis. A freestanding ambulatory surgery center does not employ physicians.

5. **Was your practice a medical school faculty practice plan and/or clinical science department?**
   A faculty practice plan is a formal framework that structures the clinical practice activities of medical school faculty. The plan performs a range of services

4

    MEDICAL GROUP MANAGEMENT ASSOCIATION™

APPENDIX D:
COMPENSATION AND PRODUCTION SURVEY: 2003 GUIDE TO THE QUESTIONNAIRE BASED ON 2002 DATA

MEDICAL GROUP MANAGEMENT ASSOCIATION
Compensation and Production Survey: 2003 Guide to the Questionnaire Based on 2002 Data

including billing, collections, contract negotiations and the distribution of income. Plans may form a separate legal organization or may be affiliated with the medical school through a clinical science department or teaching hospital. Faculty associated with the plan must provide patient care as part of a teaching or research program.

A clinical science department is a unit of organization in a medical school with an independent chair and single budget. The department's mission is to conduct teaching, research and/or clinical activities related to the entire spectrum of health care delivery to humans, from prevention through treatment.

6. **Did an MSO or a PPMC provide services to your practice?**
Answer "Yes" if your practice had a contract with an MSO or a PPMC to provide services to your practice. See page 3 for a definition of MSO and/or PPMC.

7. **What was the legal organization of your practice? (check only one)**
Business corporation: A for-profit organization recognized by law as a business entity separate and distinct from its shareholders. Shareholders need not be licensed in the profession practiced by the corporation.
Limited liability company: A legal entity that is a hybrid between a corporation and a partnership, because it provides limited liability to owners like a corporation while passing profits and losses through to owners like a partnership.
Not-for-profit corporation/foundation: An organization that has obtained special exemption under Section 501(c) of the Internal Revenue Service code that qualifies the organization to be exempt from federal income taxes. To qualify as a tax-exempt organization, a practice or faculty practice plan would have to provide evidence of a charitable, educational or research purpose.
Partnership: An unincorporated organization where two or more individuals have agreed that they will share profits, losses, assets and liabilities, although not necessarily on an equal basis. The partnership agreement may or may not be formalized in writing.
Professional corporation/association: A for-profit organization recognized by law as a business entity separate and distinct from its shareholders. Share-

holders must be licensed in the profession practiced by the organization.
Sole proprietorship: An organization with a single owner who is responsible for all profit, losses, assets and liabilities.

8. **Who was the majority owner of your practice? (check only one)**
Government: A governmental organization at the federal, state or local level. Government funding is not a sufficient criterion. Government ownership is the key factor. An example would be a medical clinic at a federal, state or county correctional facility.
Hospital/integrated delivery system (IDS): See page 3 in the Guide for a definition of a hospital and IDS. If your practice is owned by a hospital/IDS, please indicate the name of your parent organization (owner) on lines 44-47, on page 8.
Insurance company or health maintenance organization (HMO): An insurance company is an organization that indemnifies an insured party against a specified loss in return for premiums paid, as stipulated by a contract. An HMO is an insurance company that accepts responsibility for providing and delivering a predetermined set of comprehensive health maintenance and treatment services to a voluntarily enrolled population for a negotiated and fixed periodic premium.
MSO or PPMC: See page 3 in the Guide for a definition of an MSO or a PPMC. If your practice is owned by an MSO or PPMC, please indicate the name and location of your parent organization (owner) on lines 44-47, on page 8.
Physicians: Any doctor of medicine (MD) or doctor of osteopathy (DO) who is duly licensed and qualified under the law of jurisdiction in which treatment is received.
University or medical school: A university is an institution of higher learning with teaching and research facilities comprising undergraduate, graduate and professional schools. A medical school is an institution that trains physicians and awards medical and osteopathic degrees. If your practice is owned by a university or medical school, please indicate the name and location of your parent organization (owner) on lines 44-47, on page 8.
Other: If your practice is owned by an entity other than the options provided, please indicate the type of entity and location of your parent organization (owner) on lines 44-47, on page 8.

5

APPENDIX D:
COMPENSATION AND PRODUCTION SURVEY: 2003 GUIDE TO THE QUESTIONNAIRE BASED ON 2002 DATA

MEDICAL GROUP MANAGEMENT ASSOCIATION
Compensation and Production Survey: 2003 Guide to the Questionnaire Based on 2002 Data

9. **Which population designation best describes the area surrounding the primary location of your practice? If your practice had multiple sites, choose the option that represents the location with the largest number of FTE physicians. (check only one)**
    Non-metropolitan (under 50,000): The community in which the practice is located is generally referred to as "rural." It is located outside of a "metropolitan statistical area" (MSA), as defined by the United States Office of Management and Budget, and has a population under 50,000.
    Metropolitan (50,000 to 250,000): The community in which the practice is located is an MSA or Census Bureau defined urbanized area of 50,000 to 250,000 population.
    Metropolitan (250,001 to 1,000,000): The community in which the practice is located is an MSA or Census Bureau defined urbanized area of 250,001 to 1,000,000 population.
    Metropolitan (over 1,000,000): The community in which the practice is located is a "primary metropolitan statistical area" (PMSA) having over 1,000,000 population.

10. **Did your practice derive revenue from capitation contracts?**
    A capitation contract is a contract in which the practice agrees to provide medical services to a defined population for a fixed price per beneficiary per month, regardless of actual services provided. Capitation contracts, which always contain an element of risk, include HMO, Medicare and Medicaid capitation contracts.

11. **If you answered "Yes" to question 10, what percentage of your practice's total medical revenue was derived from capitation contracts?**
    Report the percentage of your total medical revenue that was from capitation contracts. See question 10 above for a definition of capitation contracts.

12. **What was the total medical revenue (collections) for your practice?**
    In general, net of gross practice revenue, refunds, returned checks, contractual discounts and allowances, bad debts and write-offs. Total medical revenue is the sum of fee-for-service collections, capitation payments, and other medical activity revenues.

13. **How many full-time equivalent (FTE) physicians were in your practice?**
    A full-time physician works whatever number of hours the practice considers to be the minimum for a normal workweek, which could be 37.5, 40, 50 hours or some other standard. To compute the FTE of a part-time physician divide the total hours worked by the physician by the number of hours that your medical practice considers to be a normal workweek. For example, a physician working in a clinic or hospital on behalf of the practice for 30 hours compared to a normal workweek of 40 hours would be 0.75 FTE (30 divided by 40 hours). A physician working full-time for three months during a year would be 0.25 FTE (3 divided by 12 months). A medical director devoting 50% effort to clinical activity would be 0.5 FTE. **Do not report a physician as more than 1.0 FTE regardless of the number of hours worked.**
    Include:
    1. Practice physicians such as shareholders/partners, salaried associates, employed and contracted physicians and locum tenens.
    2. Only physicians involved in clinical care.
    Do not include:
    1. Full-time physician administrators

14. **How many FTE nonphysician providers were in your practice?**
    Nonphysician providers (midlevels) are specially trained and licensed providers who can provide medical care and billable services. Examples of nonphysician providers include audiologists, Certified Registered Nurse Anesthetists (CRNAs), dieticians/nutritionists, midwives, nurse practitioners, occupational therapists, optometrists, physical therapists, physician assistants, psychologists, social workers, speech therapists and surgeon's assistants. To compute the number of nonphysician providers see the definition for FTE physicians given in question 13 on this page.

15. **Does your practice intend to change its physician compensation method within the next year?**
    Answer "Yes" if the current method of determining your physician's compensation will change in the next year.

The following definitions should be used for questions 16 through 22.

6

APPENDIX D:
COMPENSATION AND PRODUCTION SURVEY: 2003 GUIDE TO THE QUESTIONNAIRE BASED ON 2002 DATA

MEDICAL GROUP MANAGEMENT ASSOCIATION
Compensation and Production Survey: 2003 Guide to the Questionnaire Based on 2002 Data

a. **New physician.**
A physician with less than two years in a specialty. The count of the number of years should begin at the time the physician completes the latter of the residency or fellowship.

b. **Established primary care physician.**
A physician with over two years in a primary care specialty as defined in question 2 on page 4. The count of the number of years should begin at the time the physician completes the latter of the residency or fellowship.

c. **Established specialist.**
A physician with over two years in a specialty other than a primary care specialty as defined in question 2 on page 4. The count of the number of years should begin at the time the physician completes the latter of the residency or fellowship.

Please report the percentage of compensation attributed to the following options. If the option does not apply, please enter zero as your answer in the space provided. The percentage total should equal 100%.

16. **Productivity-based.**
Provider compensation is based wholly or partially upon individual physician productivity measurements.

17. **Guaranteed or base salary.**
A portion of the provider's compensation is a guaranteed or base salary. The balance of compensation is determined by other factors (e.g., productivity, bonus, capitation).

18. **Straight salary.**
100% of provider compensation is attributed to a fixed salary.

19. **Equal shares.**
The provider in the practice is paid equal shares based upon overall practice performance.

20. **Capitation.**
The provider is paid an established dollar amount per patient panel member per month.

21. **Structured incentive/bonus.**
The incentive may be based on individual characteristics, corporate goals, overall practice performance, or other factors. A formula may be used to determine the amount.

22. **Other.**
Please describe.

23. **If compensation is productivity-based, please indicate how production is measured. (check all that apply)**
a. **Gross charges.**
Gross charges are the full value, at the practice's undiscounted rates, of all services provided. Undiscounted rates are the full retail prices before Medicare/Medicaid charge restrictions, third-party payer (such as commercial insurance and/or managed care organization) contractual adjustments, and other charitable, professional courtesy or employee adjustments. See page 9, column 11 for more information on gross charges.

b. **Adjusted charges. (gross charges *minus* contractual discounts/allowances)**
Adjusted charges are the total amounts expected to be paid by patients or third-party payers. This figure can be calculated by taking gross charges and subtracting the adjustments from third-party payer's and charge restrictions from Medicare/Medicaid.

c. **Collections for professional charges.**
Amount of revenue attributed to a physician for their professional services to patients. See page 9, column 10 for more information on collections.

d. **Number of patient encounters.**
A documented, face-to-face contact between a patient and a provider who exercises independent judgment in the provision of services to the individual. If the patient with the same diagnosis sees two different providers on the same day, it is one encounter. If patient sees two different providers on the same day for two different diagnoses, then it is considered two encounters.

e. **Size of physician's patient panel.**
The number of patients, regardless of payer, assigned to a primary care physician.

f. **Number of RVUs.**
The number of relative value units, as measured by the Resource Based Relative Value Scale (RBRVS). The RBRVS units may be measured either as physician work units or total units.

g. **Other.**
Please describe.

7

APPENDIX D:
COMPENSATION AND PRODUCTION SURVEY: 2003 GUIDE TO THE QUESTIONNAIRE BASED ON 2002 DATA

MEDICAL GROUP MANAGEMENT ASSOCIATION
Compensation and Production Survey: 2003 Guide to the Questionnaire Based on 2002 Data

24. If compensation is based on a structured incentive/bonus, please indicate the basis for the incentive/bonus. (check all that apply)

a. Patient satisfaction.
Evaluation of clinical services by patients who assess their degree of satisfaction.

b. Peer review.
An internal review process of practice providers by a panel of group physicians.

c. Administrative or governance responsibility.
If a physician holds administrative or governance responsibility, and receives a bonus or incentive payment for their non-clinical administrative and governance work.

d. Service quality.
Some measurement decided by the practice on the quality of a physician's service to patients.

e. Seniority in the medical practice.
The length of time a physician has been with the practice.

f. Community outreach.
Direct involvement in community service activities.

g. Other.
Please describe.

Physician Compensation and Production Matrix

The matrix requests information for Columns 1 through 17. Instructions for completing each column follows. Please complete the matrix for all providers who worked for your medical practice during the 12 months indicated in question 1. Please make sure that all physician administrators are also reported in the Management Matrix on pages 6 and 7 of the questionnaire, if 50% or more of their time is spent administratively.

Column 1 - Provider tracking number

Indicate your medical practice's internal tracking number (i.e., last four numbers of SSN or initials) for each individual. This number may be numeric, alpha or a combination of both and may be up to 6 digits long. This number will make it easier to interpret the Respondent Ranking Report.

Column 2 - Specialty code

Select only one specialty for each physician and nonphysician provider using the specialty codes listed below the matrix. A provider should be classified in the specialty or subspecialty where the provider spends 50% or more time. If a provider falls under "Other," write his/her specialty in column 2.

For <u>anethesiologists</u>, when completing column 15, total RVUs, please provide American Society of Anethesiologists (ASA) units. Use time measured in 15-minute increments.

For <u>nurse practitioners</u>, select code 121 and provide the specialty area where at least 50% of their time is being spent, such as acute care, adult, emergency, family practice, gerontologic/elder health, neonatal/perinatal, occupational health, oncology, pediatric/child health, psychiatric/mental health, school/college health or women's health.

Column 3 - Total compensation

State the amount reported as direct compensation on a W2, 1099, or K1 (for partnerships) plus all voluntary salary reductions (e.g., 401(k), 403(b), Section 125 Tax Savings Plan, Medical Savings Plan). The amount reported should include salary, bonus and/or incentive payments, research stipends, honoraria and distribution of profits.

Do not include:
1. the dollar value of expense reimbursements, fringe benefits paid by the medical practice (i.e., retirement plan contributions, life and health insurance, or automobile allowances), or any employer contributions to a 401(k), 403(b) or Keogh Plan.

Column 4 - Retirement benefits (exclude FICA)

Report all employer contributions to retirement plans including defined benefit and contribution plans, 401(k), 403(b) and Keogh Plans, and any non-qualified funded retirement plan. For defined benefit plans, estimate the employer's contribution made on behalf of each plan participant by multiplying the employer's total contribution by each plan participant's compensation divided by the total compensation of all plan participants.

Do not include:
1. Employer contributions to social security mandated by the Federal Insurance Contributions Act (FICA).

8

Appendix D:
Compensation and Production Survey: 2003 Guide to the Questionnaire Based on 2002 Data

Medical Group Management Association
Compensation and Production Survey: 2003 Guide to the Questionnaire Based on 2002 Data

2. Voluntary employee contributions that are an allocation of salary to a 401(k), 403(b), or Keogh Plan.
3. The dollar value of any other fringe benefits paid by the practice, such as life and health insurance, automobile allowances, etc.

Column 5 - Years in specialty
Report the number of years each physician and nonphysician provider has practiced in the specialty reported in column 2. The count of the number of years should begin at the time the physician completes the latter of the residency or fellowship.

Column 6 - Gender
Report gender by circling M for "Male" or F for "Female."

Column 7 - Hours worked per week
Indicate the number of hours the physician works during a normal (typical) workweek engaged in professional activities. Professional activities include both clinical and non-clinical time.

Clinical activities include patients seen in the office, outpatient clinic, emergency room, nursing home, operating room, or labor and delivery: time spent on hospital rounds, telephone conversations with patients, consultations with providers, interpretation of diagnostic tests and chart review. Include "on-call" hours if the physician is required to be present in the medical facility such as a medical clinic or hospital. Non-clinical activities include teaching, research, writing, and administration.

Column 8 - Weeks worked per year
Estimate to the nearest week the number of weeks the provider was engaged in professional activities in the practice. Refer to the definition of professional activities under column 7, above. Exclude vacation, sick leave, and medical or continuing education.

Column 9 - Clinical FTE
Report the clinical full-time equivalent for each provider based upon the number of hours worked on clinical activities. See column 7 for the definition of clinical activities. A provider cannot be more than 1.0 FTE. Example: a physician administrator who is 80% clinical and 20% administrative would be 0.8 clinical FTE; a physician with a normal workweek of 32 hours (4 days) working in a clinic or hospital for 32 hours would be 1.0 clinical FTE; a physician with a normal workweek of 50 hours (5 days) working 32

clinical or hospital hours would be a 0.64 clinical FTE (32 divided by 50 hours).

Column 10 - Collections for professional charges
Report amount of collections attributed to a physician for all professional services.
Include:
1. Fee-for-service collections.
2. Allocated capitation payments.
3. Administration of chemotherapy drugs.
4. Administration of immunizations.
Do not include:
1. Collections on drug charges, including vaccinations, allergy injections, and immunizations, as well as chemotherapy and antinauseant drugs.
2. The technical component associated with any laboratory, radiology, medical diagnostic or surgical procedure collections.
3. Collections attributed to nonphysician providers.
4. Infusion-related collections.
5. Facility fees.
6. Supplies.
7. Revenue associated with the sale of hearing aids, eyeglasses, contact lenses, etc.

Important: If collections in column 10 are reported, respondents must complete columns 10A and 17.

Column 10A - Level of technical component (TC) included in professional collections
If collections in column 10 do not include the technical component (referred to as professional services only billing), circle "0%." If collections does include the technical component (referred to as global fee billing), indicate the approximate percentage of charges represented by the technical component by circling either "1-10%" or ">10%."

Column 11 - Professional gross charges
Report the total gross patient charges attributed to a physician for all professional services. Gross patient charges are the full dollar value, at the practice's established undiscounted rates, of services provided to all patients, before reduction by charitable adjustments, professional courtesy adjustments, contractual adjustments, employee discounts, bad debts, etc. For both Medicare participating and nonparticipating providers, gross charges should include the practice's full, undiscounted charge and not the Medicare limiting charge.
Include:
1. Fee-for-service charges.

9

APPENDIX D:
COMPENSATION AND PRODUCTION SURVEY: 2003 GUIDE TO THE QUESTIONNAIRE BASED ON 2002 DATA

MEDICAL GROUP MANAGEMENT ASSOCIATION
Compensation and Production Survey: 2003 Guide to the Questionnaire Based on 2002 Data

2. In-house equivalent gross fee-for-service charges for capitated patients.
3. Administration of chemotherapy drugs.
4. Administration of immunizations.

Do not include:
1. Charges for drugs, including vaccinations, allergy, injections, and immunizations as well as chemo- therapy and antinauseant drugs.
2. The technical component associated with any laboratory, radiology, medical diagnostic or surgical procedure. If your practice cannot break this out, report gross charges and answer the appropriate response in column 11A.
3. Charges attributed to nonphysician providers. If your practice cannot break this out, report gross charges and answer Y for "Yes" in column 17.
4. Infusion-related charges.
5. Facility fees.
6. Supplies.
7. Charges associated with the sale of hearing aids, eyeglasses, contact lenses, etc.

Important: If gross charges in column 11 are reported, respondents must complete columns 11A and 17.

Column 11A - Level of technical component (TC) included in professional gross charges

Gross charges for laboratory, radiology, medical diagnostic and surgical procedures may have two components: the physician's professional charge (e.g., interpretation) and the technical charge for the operation and use of the equipment. If gross charges in column 11 do not include the technical component (referred to as professional services only billing), circle "0%." If gross charges does include the technical component (referred to as global fee billing), indicate the approximate percentage of charges represented by the technical component by circling either "1-10%" or ">10%."

Columns 12 and 13 – Encounters

A documented, face-to-face contact between a patient and a provider who exercises independent judgment in the provision of services to the indi- vidual. If the patient with the same diagnosis sees two different providers on the same day, it is one encounter. If patient sees two different providers on the same day for two different diagnoses, then it is considered two encounters. Columns 12 and 13 request encounters and should include only proce- dures from the evaluation and management chapter (CPT codes 99201-99499) or the medicine chapter

(CPT codes 90800-99199) of the Physicians' Current Procedural Terminology, Fourth Edition, copyrighted by the American Medical Association (AMA).

Include:
1. Pre- and post-operative visits and other visits associated with a global charge.
2. For diagnostic radiologists, report the total number of procedures or reads, regardless of place of service.
3. For obstetrics care, where a single CPT-4 code is used for a global service, count each ambulatory contact as a separate ambulatory encounter (e.g., each prenatal visit and postnatal visit is an ambulatory encounter). Count the delivery as a single surgical case.
4. Administration of chemotherapy drugs.
5. Administration of immunizations.

Do not include:
1. Ambulatory encounters attributed to nonphysician providers. If your practice cannot break this out, report encounters and answer Y for "Yes" in column 17.
2. Encounters for the physician specialties of pathol- ogy or diagnostic radiology. (see #2 under "In- clude" above)
3. Encounters that include procedures from the surgery chapter (CPT codes 10040-69979) or anesthesia chapter (CPT codes 00100-01999). Report these as surgery/anesthesia cases in column 14.
4. Number of procedures, since a single encounter can generate multiple procedures.
5. Visits where there is not an identifiable contact between a patient and a physician or nonphysician provider (i.e., patient comes into the practice solely for an injection, vein puncture, EKGs, EEGs, etc. administered by an RN or technician).

Column 12 - Ambulatory encounters

Report total number of encounters (using the previ- ous definition) with the following Centers for Medicare and Medicaid Services (CMS) place of service codes:
11 Office
12 Home
22 Outpatient Hospital
23 Emergency Room
24 Ambulatory Surgical Center
31 Skilled Nursing Facility
32 Nursing Facility
33 Custodial Care Facility
34 Hospice

10

APPENDIX D:
COMPENSATION AND PRODUCTION SURVEY: 2003 GUIDE TO THE QUESTIONNAIRE BASED ON 2002 DATA

MEDICAL GROUP MANAGEMENT ASSOCIATION
Compensation and Production Survey: 2003 Guide to the Questionnaire Based on 2002 Data

50   Federally Qualified Health Center
52   Psychiatric Facility Partial Hospitalization
53   Community Mental Health Facility
54   Intermediate Care Facility for Mentally Retarded
55   Residential Substance Abuse Treatment Facility
56   Psychiatric Residential Treatment Center
62   Comprehensive Outpatient Rehabilitation Facility
65   End Stage Renal Disease Treatment Facility
71   State or Local Public Health Clinic
72   Rural Health Clinic
81   Independent Laboratory

Important: If ambulatory encounters in column 12 are reported, respondents must complete column 17.

Column 13 - Hospital encounters
Report the total number of encounters (using the previous definition) with the following CMS place of service codes:
21   Inpatient Hospital
25   Birthing Center
26   Military Treatment Facility
51   Inpatient Psychiatric Facility
61   Comprehensive Inpatient Rehabilitation Facility

Column 14 - Surgery/anesthesia cases
Report the total surgery/anesthesia cases performed annually by each provider. A surgery/anesthesia case is a case between a provider and a patient where at least one procedure performed is a procedure from the surgery chapter (CPT codes 10040-69979) or anesthesia chapter (CPT codes 00100-01999) of the Physicians' Current Procedural Terminology, Fourth Edition, copyrighted by the American Medical Association (AMA).

Please note that the number of cases, not procedures, should be counted since a case may consist of multiple procedures. Surgery/anesthesia cases include cases performed on an inpatient or outpatient basis, regardless of facility or site. For anesthesia care teams, anesthesiologist supervises one or more CRNAs, include total care team cases.

Columns 15 and 16 – RVUs
Report the relative value units, as measured by the Resource Based Relative Value Scale (RBRVS), not weighted by a conversion factor, attributed to all professional services. An RVU is a nonmonetary standard unit of measure that indicates the value of services provided by physicians, nonphysician providers, and other health care professionals. When answering this question, please note the following:

- The relative value units published in the November 1, 2001, *Federal Register*, effective for calendar year 2002, should be used.
- There are three components of RBRVS: Physician Work RVUs + Transitioned Practice Expense RVUs + Malpractice Expense RVUs. When answering, please report the sum total of Physician Work RVUs, Transitioned (Non-Facility) RVUs and malpractice expense RVUs.

In other words, if your practice is affiliated with a hospital and you utilize a split billing fee schedule for facility charges and professional charges, please report your total RVUs (specifically the transitioned practice expense component) as if you were a traditional freestanding medical practice that did not even utilize facility practice expense RVUs.
- *Transitioned* refers to the RVUs in effect for 2001.
- The *facility* total applies to services performed in a hospital, skilled nursing facility or ambulatory surgery. The *non-facility* total applies to services performed in a physician's office, patient home or facility or institution other than a hospital, skilled nursing facility or ambulatory surgery center.
- The Geographic Practice Cost Index (GPCI) should be set to 1.000 (neutral).

Column 15 - Total RVUs
Include RVUs for:
1. The physician work, malpractice and transitioned non-facility practice expense components of the RBRVS.
2. All professional services performed by provider.
3. The professional components of laboratory, radiology, medical diagnostic and surgical procedures.
4. For anesthesiology groups, provide the American Society of Anethesiologists (ASA) units. Use time measured in 15-minute increments.
5. All payers, not just Medicare.
6. Codes with a "0.00" value or no value by estimating RVUs. RVUs can be estimated by dividing the total gross charges for procedures without a published RVU by the average charge per RVU for procedures that have a published RVU.
7. Adjustments for modifiers (use percentage utilized by the CMS for Medicare reimbursement).

Do not include RVUs for:
1. Other scales, such as McGraw-Hill, California, etc.
2. The technical component (TC) associated with any medical diagnostic, laboratory, radiology, or surgical procedure. If your practice cannot break

11

APPENDIX D:
COMPENSATION AND PRODUCTION SURVEY: 2003 GUIDE TO THE QUESTIONNAIRE BASED ON 2002 DATA

MEDICAL GROUP MANAGEMENT ASSOCIATION
Compensation and Production Survey: 2003 Guide to the Questionnaire Based on 2002 Data

this out, please report RVUs and answer Y for "Yes" in column 15A.
3. RVUs attributed to nonphysician providers. If your practice cannot break this out, please report RVUs and answer Y for "Yes" in column 17.

Important: If Total RVUs in column 15 are reported, respondents must complete columns 15A and 16.

Column 15A - Technical component included in total RVUs

RVUs for laboratory, radiology, medical diagnostic, and surgical procedures may have two components: the physician's professional RVU (e.g., interpretation) and the technical RVU for the operation and use of the equipment. If total RVUs (column 15) do not include the technical component (indicated by the modifier -26 and referred to as a professional services only billing), circle N for "No." If total RVUs does include the technical component (indicated by no modifier code and referred to as a global fee billing), circle Y for "Yes."

Column 16 - Physician Work RVUs
Include RVUs for:
1. The physician work component of the RBRVS.
2. All professional services performed by the provider.
3. All payers, not just Medicare.
4. Codes with a "0.00" value or no value by estimating RVUs. RVUs can be estimated by dividing the total gross charges for procedures without a published RVU by the average charge per RVU for procedures that have a published RVU.
5. Adjustments for modifiers (use percentage utilized by the CMS for Medicare reimbursement).

Do not include RVUs for:
1. Anesthesiology groups. Instead, provide ASA units under total RVUs, column 15. Leave column 16 blank.
2. The transitioned facility or non-facility practice expense components or the malpractice component of the RBRVS.
3. Other scales, such as McGraw-Hill, California, etc.
4. Physician work RVUs attributed to nonphysician providers. If your practice cannot break this out, please report physician work RVUs and answer Y for "Yes" for column 17.

Important: If physician work RVUs in column 16 are reported, respondents must complete column 17.

Column 17 - Nonphysician provider productivity
For physicians, state if the productivity measures (columns 11 though 16) includes productivity attributed to a nonphysician provider working under a physician's supervision by circling Y for "Yes" or N for "No." For nonphysician providers, state whether the productivity measures includes productivity attributed to another (e.g., nonphysician provider) by circling Y for "Yes" or N for "No."

Management Compensation Matrix
The matrix requests information for Columns 1 through 13 on pages 6 and 7 of the questionnaire. Instructions for completing each column follows.

Column 1 - Employee tracking code
See page 8, column 1 for definition.

Column 2 - Position title
CHANGES HAVE BEEN MADE TO SOME POSITION DESCRIPTIONS. Select <u>one</u> position that best describes each individual's responsibilities from the list on pages 6 and 7 of the questionnaire and place the corresponding number in column 2. The numbers by the positions described below correspond to the positions listed on pages 6 and 7 of the questionnaire. If the position falls under "Other," write his/her position in column 2.

Physician Executive Positions
1. **Physician Chief Executive Officer (CEO)/President:**
   • Position requires candidate to be a licensed physician;
   • Usually found in larger practices or in some form of an integrated system or network, e.g., Physician Hospital Organization (PHO), MSO, etc.;
   • Since administrative duties are substantial, the delivery of health care services is minimal;
   • Develops and monitors organizational policy with other management personnel and board of directors;
   • Responsible for the overall operation of the organization, including patient care and contract relations;
   • Oversees activities related to the growth and expansion of the organization;
   • Plays a major role in the organization's strategic process;
   • Typically serves as the liaison between the organization, the community and the board of directors;

12

MEDICAL GROUP MANAGEMENT ASSOCIATION™

Appendix D:
Compensation and Production Survey: 2003 Guide to the Questionnaire Based on 2002 Data

MEDICAL GROUP MANAGEMENT ASSOCIATION

Compensation and Production Survey: 2003 Guide to the Questionnaire Based on 2002 Data

- Oversees a team of senior management personnel; and
- Usually reports to the governing body of the organization.

2. **Medical Director:**
   - Position requires candidate to be a licensed physician;
   - The senior medical administrative position within a medical group practice;
   - Physician's time is devoted to both administrative duties and the delivery of health care services;
   - In larger organizations there may be more than one Medical Director;
   - Responsible for all activities related to the delivery of medical care and clinical services e.g., cost management, utilization review, quality assurance and medical protocol development;
   - Typically oversees the activities of group physicians, including the recruiting and credentialing processes; and
   - Usually reports to the Physician CEO/President and/or to the governing body of the organization.

3. **Associate/Assistant Medical Director:**
   - Position requires candidate to be a licensed physician;
   - Time is devoted to both administrative duties and the delivery of health care services;
   - Typically assists the Medical Director in all respects, from the administration of medical care and clinical services to utilization review and medical protocol development. If there are multiple Associate/Assistant Medical Directors, the functional areas of medical administration are usually divided up among physicians with this position title; and
   - Usually reports to the Medical Director and/or Physician CEO/President.

Executive Management Positions
4. **Chief Executive Officer (CEO)/Executive Director:**
   - Highest nonphysician executive position in the organization;
   - Typically found in larger practices, or in some form of an integrated system, e.g., PHO, MSO;
   - Develops and monitors organizational policy in conjunction with other management personnel and board of directors;
   - Responsible for the overall operation of the organization, including patient care, contract relations and activities that relate to the future growth of the organization, e.g., strategic planning and marketing;
   - Oversees a team of senior management personnel who have direct responsibility for specific functional areas of the organization;
   - Typically serves as a liaison between the organization and staff members, businesses, individuals in the community and board of directors; and
   - Reports to the governing body of the organization.

5. **Administrator:**
   - The top nonphysician professional administrative position with less authority than a CEO;
   - Maintains broad responsibilities for all administrative functions of the medical group, including operations, marketing, finance, managed care/third party contracting, physician compensation and reimbursement, human resources, medical and business information systems and planning and development;
   - Typically oversees management personnel with direct responsibilities for the specific functional areas of the organization; and
   - Reports to the governing body of the organization.

6. **MSO Administrator/Executive Director:**
   - Oversees all activities of a hospital or investor-owned MSO, that provides practice management services to physician practices and clinics;
   - Responsibilities range from the daily operations of multiple sites to developing strategic plans;
   - Monitors the marketing of MSO services to physician clients;
   - Typically serves as a liaison between various organization levels, from the physicians to the governing entities of the organization, e.g., a hospital or health system, investors in the MSO or a board of directors;
   - Oversees the provision of management services to newly integrated practices; and
   - Usually reports to the governing body of the MSO.

7. **Chief Operating Officer (COO):**
   - Consults, advises and assists the CEO and/or Practice Administrator in providing leadership and direction in planning, directing and coordinating both patient and non-patient care activities;

13

APPENDIX D:
COMPENSATION AND PRODUCTION SURVEY: 2003 GUIDE TO THE QUESTIONNAIRE BASED ON 2002 DATA

MEDICAL GROUP MANAGEMENT ASSOCIATION
Compensation and Production Survey: 2003 Guide to the Questionnaire Based on 2002 Data

- May be the second senior administrative position, and assume the duties of the top administrator when necessary;
- Oversees the daily operations of the medical practice and/or other affiliated health care organizations;
- Responsibilities may include facilities management, business services, human resources management; and
- Usually reports to the senior administrative officer, or in some cases, to the governing body of the organization.

8. **Chief Financial Officer (CFO):**
   - Usually the organization's senior financial position;
   - Develops financial policies and oversees their implementation;
   - Typically monitors a variety of financial activities, including budgeting, analysis, accounting, billing, payer contracting, collections and the preparation of tax returns;
   - Usually prepares or oversees the preparation of annual reports and long-term projections to ensure that the organization's financial obligations are met;
   - May obtain funds for capital development;
   - May hold a designation as a Certified Public Accountant (CPA); and
   - Usually reports to the senior administrative officer, or to the governing body of the organization.

9. **Assistant Administrator:**
   - Provides assistance to the CEO and/or Practice Administrator with the management of one or more functional areas of the medical practice such as administration, managed care, human resources, marketing, patient accounting or operations;
   - Has a more limited scope of responsibility than a COO;
   - A medical group may have multiple assistant administrators;
   - Responsible for assisting the CEO and/or Practice Administrator in accomplishing organizational objectives; and
   - Usually reports to the senior administrative officer.

Senior Management Positions
(formerly General Managers)

10. **Ambulatory/Clinical Services Director: (formerly Director, Ambulatory/Clinical Services)**
    - A clinical operations position;
    - Monitors the daily operations of the organization's clinical function;
    - Develops, implements and monitors policies and procedures;
    - Monitors the activities of the nonphysician technical staff, e.g., radiology and laboratory technicians;
    - May oversee the medical records staff; and
    - Usually reports to CFO or senior administrative officer.

11. **Building and Grounds Director: (formerly Director, Facilities Management)**
    - Usually found in an organization with a facilities or building services department;
    - Develops and implements policies and procedures related to the organization's physical facilities, e.g., buildings;
    - Oversees related activities such as building maintenance, housekeeping, grounds preservation; and
    - Usually reports to COO.

12. **Business Services Director: (formerly Director, Business Services/Business Office Manager)**
    - Usually found in large organizations;
    - Directs and coordinates business office activities in an organization that has a top administrator;
    - Monitors the medical billing system;
    - Oversees areas of responsibility such as third party reimbursement, physician billing, collections, contract administration and management reporting; and
    - Usually reports to the senior administrative officer or to the organization's top financial position.

13. **Clinical Research Director: (formerly Director, Clinical Research)**
    - Analyzes and summarizes clinical data and outcomes, with responsibility for research design, methodology and data collection protocols;
    - Prepares grant proposals;
    - Participates in investigator meetings, seminars and regional or national research conferences;

14

APPENDIX D:

COMPENSATION AND PRODUCTION SURVEY: 2003 GUIDE TO THE QUESTIONNAIRE BASED ON 2002 DATA

MEDICAL GROUP MANAGEMENT ASSOCIATION

Compensation and Production Survey: 2003 Guide to the Questionnaire Based on 2002 Data

- Coordinates the activities of associates and investigators to ensure compliance with protocols and overall research objectives; and
- Usually reports to Medical Director or senior administrative officer.

14. Compliance Director: (formerly Compliance Officer)
- Develops, plans, organizes and administers programs to comply with applicable state and federal statues, regulations, policies and procedures within organization to ensure administrative and operational objectives are met;
- Identifies operational business risk issues;
- Develops a Corporate Compliance Plan, the Code of Conduct Handbook; and
- Usually reports to the CFO or COO.

15. Education and Training Director: (formerly Director, Education and Training/Training Manager)
- Only found in very large organizations with multiple locations;
- Supervises Training Managers;
- Develops and delivers education and training programs for the training needs of the organization's staff and patients;
- Evaluates programs to determine whether the training goals and objectives have been met;
- Monitors the delivery of on-going programs; and
- Usually reports to Human Resources Director or COO.

16. Finance Director: (New)
- Responsible for preparing financial statements and all general accounting functions;
- Develops, implements and monitors tax compliance, e.g., income, sales, use, etc., and has payroll oversight;
- Responsible for internal accounting policies and procedures;
- Supervises financial department;
- Directs all statistical analysis and reporting including monthly operating and medical management statistics; and
- Reports to CFO.

17. Human Resources Director: (formerly Director, Human Resources)
- Usually found in larger practices;
- Oversees all functions of an established human resources department within an organization;

- Using the organization's objectives and philosophy as a guide. Develops, implements and coordinates policies relating to all aspects of personnel administration, including recruitment, salary and benefits administration, EEO/AA and labor law compliance and employee relations; and
- Usually reports to the senior administrative officer.

18. Information Systems Director: (formerly Director, Management Information Services (MIS)/ Information Systems Manager)
- Implements and monitors all activities that relate to the organization's information system, including functions such as physician practice billing, scheduling, data processing, networking and system security;
- Oversees or resolves systems implementation and integration issues;
- Performs programming tasks when necessary; and
- Usually reports to the CFO or to the senior administrative officer.

19. Laboratory Services Director: (formerly Director, Laboratory Services/Laboratory Manager)
- Responsible for all activities related to the operations of a laboratory or several laboratories, from the initiation and implementation of test procedures to the oversight of laboratory personnel;
- May perform and monitor testing procedures in addition to administrative duties:
- Monitor budget activities that relate to the laboratory function; and
- Usually reports to the COO or to the senior administrative officer.

20. Managed Care Director: (formerly Director, Managed Care)
- Initiates and maintains relationships with managed care organizations as well as physician and ancillary providers;
- Develops and directs all managed care activities of the organization, including contract negotiations, product development and capitation payment procedures;
- May oversee risk and utilization management activities or claims administration for professional/medical purchased services; and
- Usually reports to the organization's Medical Director or the senior administrative officer.

15

Appendix D:
Compensation and Production Survey: 2003 Guide to the Questionnaire Based on 2002 Data

Medical Group Management Association
Compensation and Production Survey: 2003 Guide to the Questionnaire Based on 2002 Data

21. Marketing and Sales Director: (formerly Director, Marketing & Sales)
- The top marketing position in an organization with a distinct marketing and sales function;
- Typically found in larger organizations;
- May oversee the communications function;
- Develops marketing policies and programs that reflect the organization's goals and objectives;
- Oversees or conducts research designed to evaluate the organization's market position;
- Directs the implementation of policies and procedures that relate to the promotion of the organization;
- Performs administrative tasks such as department budgeting and supervises the Marketing/Communication specialist; and
- Usually reports to the senior administrative officer.

22. Medical Records Director: (formerly Director, Medical Records/Medical Records Manager)
- The individual in this position usually holds professional licensure in the area of medical records management;
- Usually found in large organizations and is considered part of the senior management team;
- Responsible for medical records library e.g., patient records;
- Oversees all medical records personnel;
- Monitors budget activities that relate to the medical records function; and
- Usually reports to the COO.

23. Nursing Services Director: (formerly Director, Nursing Services/Nursing Supervisor)
- Oversees all aspects of the organization's nursing practices;
- Typically found in large organizations;
- Is part of the senior management team;
- In most cases, requires certification as a Registered Nurse (RN);
- Oversees the nursing staff; and
- Usually reports to the COO.

24. Quality Improvement/Quality Assurance Director: (formerly Director, Quality Improvement/Quality Assurance)
- Develops and monitors programs designed to improve the quality of health care delivery e.g., outcome measurement;

- Develops policies and procedures designed to measure the quantitative and qualitative aspects of health care delivery;
- More likely to be found in larger organizations with some degree of integration with other health care organizations; and
- Usually reports to the CFO or to the senior administrative officer.

25. Radiology Services Director: (formerly Director, Radiology Services/Radiology Manager)
- Usually found in large organizations with several radiology departments;
- Responsible for all activities relating to the delivery of radiological services, including the development of policies and procedures;
- Oversees radiology personnel activities;
- Monitors the quality of all film products used;
- Monitors budget activities related to the radiology departments; and
- Usually reports to the COO or to the senior administrative officer.

26. Reimbursement Director: (formerly Director, Reimbursement)
- Oversees payment services for the practice, including establishing and maintaining the practice's fee schedules and fees that relate to managed care activities;
- Conducts regular analyses of reimbursement rates;
- Oversees coding activities; and
- Usually reports to the Managed Care Director, the CFO, or the senior administrative officer.

General Management Positions

27. Benefits Manager: (formerly Compensation/Benefits Manager)
- Oversees all aspects of the organization's salary/wage administration program as well as the benefits program;
- Determines eligibility for the benefits program;
- May provide assistance and information to employees with filing claims and the selection of benefits; and
- Usually assists and reports to the Human Resources Director.

16

APPENDIX D:
COMPENSATION AND PRODUCTION SURVEY: 2003 GUIDE TO THE QUESTIONNAIRE BASED ON 2002 DATA

MEDICAL GROUP MANAGEMENT ASSOCIATION
Compensation and Production Survey: 2003 Guide to the Questionnaire Based on 2002 Data

28. Branch/Satellite Clinic Manager:
- Oversees the daily administrative and operations activities of an assigned clinic in an organization with multiple clinics;
- Prepares the clinic's annual budget and supervises clinic staff;
- Oversees financial transactions, e.g., purchasing of supplies; and
- Usually reports to the COO or senior administrative position.

29. Business Office Manager: (formerly part of Director, Business Services/Business Office Manager)
- Not a Director or Senior Management level position;
- Responsible for directing and coordinating the overall functions of the Business Office;
- The top Business Office position in a mid-size or small organization without a Director of Business Services;
- Exercises general supervision over business office staff;
- Plans and directs registration, patient insurance, billing and collections and data processing to ensure accurate patient billing and efficient account collection; and
- Reports to the Finance Director or Business Services Director.

30. Clinical Department Manager:
- Manages operation of one or more medical/surgical departments, ancillary service departments or an ambulatory surgery facility;
- Usually found in larger practices;
- Assists with budget planning and approves department expenditures;
- May supervise department nonmedical staff; and
- Usually reports to the COO or the Nursing Services Director.

31. Clinic Research Manager: (New)
- Not a Director or Senior Management level position;
- Collects and analyzes clinical data and outcomes;
- The top Clinic Research position in a mid-size or small organization without a Clinical Research Director; and
- Usually reports to the Medical Director, the senior administrative officer or the Clinical Research Director.

32. General Accounting Manager: (formerly Controller)
- The second or third financial position in the organization;
- Assists the CFO or Finance Director with the financial responsibilities of the organization;
- Develops and oversees activities related to implementing and maintaining the integrity of the organization's financial reporting system;
- Assists with or oversees the budgeting process; and
- Usually reports to the CFO, Finance Director or in smaller organizations, to the senior administrative officer.

33. Laboratory Services Manager: (formerly part of Director, Laboratory Services/Laboratory Services Manager)
- Not a Director or Senior Management level position;
- The top laboratory position in a mid-size or small organization without a Laboratory Services Director;
- Responsible for the activities related to the delivery of laboratory services;
- Monitors the quality of services, products, supplies used;
- May monitor budget activities related to the laboratory department; and
- Reports to the COO, senior administrative officer or Laboratory Services Director.

34. Materials Management Manager: (formerly Director, Purchasing)
- Usually found in organizations with a separate purchasing department or function;
- Oversees all activities that involve the acquisition of equipment and supplies;
- May monitor budget activities, including the capital equipment budget; and
- Usually reports to the CFO.

35. Medical Records Manager: (formerly part of Director, Medical Records/Medical Records Manager)
- Not a Director or Senior Management level position;
- The top Medical Records position in a mid-size or small organization without a Medical Records Director;
- Oversees and coordinates all activities of the medical library, from maintenance tasks to the movement of patient records;

17

APPENDIX D:
COMPENSATION AND PRODUCTION SURVEY: 2003 GUIDE TO THE QUESTIONNAIRE BASED ON 2002 DATA

MEDICAL GROUP MANAGEMENT ASSOCIATION
Compensation and Production Survey: 2003 Guide to the Questionnaire Based on 2002 Data

• Oversees all medical records personnel;
• May monitor budget activities that relate to the medical records function; and
• Usually reports to the COO, Medical Records Director or Practice Administrator.

36. Nursing Manager: (New)
• Responsible for managing, supervising and administering the patient/nursing services in the clinic;
• In most cases, requires certification as a Registered Nurse (RN);
• Supervises nursing staff; and
• Reports to the Practice Administrator in smaller organization and the Nursing Services Director in larger organizations.

37. Office Manager:
• Manages the nonmedical activities of a larger medical practice;
• Typically found in a practice that does not have a Practice Administrator;
• The focus of this position usually rests on the daily operations of the organization;
• May oversee some financial activities, such as billing and collections; and
• Usually reports to the Practice Administrator, or the Business Services Director.

38. Operations Manager:
• Assists the top operations administrator;
• Coordinates and directs the overall operation of specific departments;
• Coordinates between departments to ensure that the organization meets internal and external regulatory requirements; and
• Usually reports to the COO or the senior administrative officer.

39. Patient Accounting Manager: (formerly Professional Fee Billing Coordinator/Billing Manager)
• Manages the billing process and billing staff for the practice;
• Manages insurance and other reimbursement functions; and
• Usually reports to the Reimbursement Director or the CFO.

40. Radiology Services Manager: (formerly part of Director, Radiology Services/Radiology Manager)
• Not a Director or Senior Management level position;
• The top Radiology position in a mid-size or small organization without a Radiology Director;
• Responsible for activities related to the delivery of radiological services;
• Monitors the quality of all film products used;
• May monitor budget activities related to the radiology departments; and
• Reports to the COO, the senior administrative officer or the Radiology Services Director.

41. Training/Education Manager: (formerly part of Director, Education and Training/Training Manager)
• Assists in delivering education and training programs for staff members and patients;
• Helps to identify the training needs;
• Evaluates programs to determine whether the goals and objectives have been met;
• Monitors the delivery of on-going programs; and
• Usually reports to the Training/Education Director or the COO.

Specialists
42. Benefits/Payroll Specialist: (New)
• Oversees all aspects of the organization's salary/wage administration program as well as the benefits program;
• Determines eligibility for the benefits program;
• May provide assistance and information to employees with filing claims and the selection of benefits; and
• Usually assists and reports to the Human Resources Director.

43. Marketing/Communication Specialist: (formerly Director, Public Relations/Communications)
• Usually found in organizations in which there is a separate publications/communications function;
• In some organizations, this person may be known as the "Public Relations Manager" and may report to the top marketing and sales position;
• Represents the organization at all media and other public relations events;
• May oversee the activities of public relations/communications staff; and
• Usually reports to the Marketing and Sales Director, the COO, or the senior administrative officer.

18

APPENDIX D:
COMPENSATION AND PRODUCTION SURVEY: 2003 GUIDE TO THE QUESTIONNAIRE BASED ON 2002 DATA

MEDICAL GROUP MANAGEMENT ASSOCIATION
Compensation and Production Survey: 2003 Guide to the Questionnaire Based on 2002 Data

Supervisors

44. Business Office Supervisor: (New)
- Responsible for supervising and coordinating activities of the business office;
- This position may be implemented in a multiple clinic setting;
- Supervises assigned business office staff; and
- Reports to the Business Office Manager or the Practice Administrator.

45. Clinic Supervisor: (New)
- Exercises supervision over assigned staff;
- Responsible for supervising and coordinating day to day activities of the clinic; and
- Reports to the Branch/Satellite Manager or the Practice Administrator.

46. Nursing Supervisor: (formerly part of Director, Nursing Services/Nursing Supervisor)
- Supervises a staff of nurses;
- In a large organization, may be one of several supervisors;
- Splits time between patient care and supervision of staff;
- Responsibilities are more limited than the Nursing Manager; and
- Reports to the Nursing Manager, the Nursing Services Director or the Practice Administrator.

47. Other: Please list the title and describe the position in column 2.

Column 3 - Total compensation
See page 8 in the Guide, column 3 for definition.

Column 4 - Bonus/incentive amount
Report the total dollar amount of any bonus or incentive payments received by each individual. The amount listed as a bonus/incentive should be included in total compensation, column 3.

Column 5 - Retirement benefits
See page 8 in the Guide, column 4 for definition.

Column 6 - Compensation method
From the options listed on page 7 of the questionnaire, select the choice that best describes the compensation method for each individual listed in column 2, and place the corresponding number in column 6. If the compensation method falls under "Other," write his/her compensation method in column 6.

Column 7 - Formal education
From the options listed on page 7 of the questionnaire, select the highest level of formal education attained by each individual listed in column 2, and place the corresponding number in column 7. If the education level falls under "Other," write his/her education level in column 7.

Column 8 - Years of management experience
Report the total years of management experience in health care delivery, health care administration and/or business administration for each individual listed in column 2.

Column 9 - Gender
Report gender for each individual listed in column 2 by circling M for "Male" or F for "Female."

Column 10 - ACMPE status
From the options listed on page 7 of the questionnaire, select the appropriate status designation in the American College of Medical Practice Executives (ACMPE), the professional credentialing arm of MGMA, for each individual listed in column 2 and place the corresponding number in column 10.

Column 11 - MGMA national member
Report whether each individual listed in column 2 is a national member of MGMA by circling Y for "Yes" or N for "No."

Complete column 12 for Physician Executive (position titles 1-3), Executive Management (position titles 4-9), and Senior Management (position titles 10-26) positions ONLY.

Column 12 - Professional organization fees
Report the dollar amount paid for professional organization dues and memberships, and educational conference fees and travel expenses related to those conferences over the fiscal year for each physician executive, executive management and senior management position listed in column 2. If your organization uses the MGMA *Chart of Accounts for Health Care Organizations*, please report the amounts by employee aggregated from: general ledger accounts 5845, 5855, and 5860, for Executive Management positions and Senior Management positions; and general ledger accounts 8245, 8255, and 8260 for Physician Executive positions.

19

APPENDIX D:
COMPENSATION AND PRODUCTION SURVEY: 2003 GUIDE TO THE QUESTIONNAIRE BASED ON 2002 DATA

MEDICAL GROUP MANAGEMENT ASSOCIATION
Compensation and Production Survey: 2003 Guide to the Questionnaire Based on 2002 Data

Complete column 13 for Physician Executive positions (position titles 1-3) ONLY.

Column 13 - Physician executive time percentage administrative/clinical

List the percentage of time spent performing administrative duties and clinical care responsibilities (e.g., a physician executive spending approximately 70% of their time in an administrative capacity and 30% of their time performing clinical functions should report 70% on the "Admin" line and 30% on the "Clinical" line).

Questionnaire Contact

25-30. If we need to clarify any responses, it would be helpful to have the name of the person who is most familiar with the completed questionnaire. Please provide complete information.

31. Please provide the Federal Tax ID # for the observed practice.

Please provide the Federal Tax ID # for the observed practice reported in the questionnaire. This information will be used for internal tracking purposes only, and will not be released under any circumstances.

32. Hours to complete

Add together the total number of hours for each individual who worked on this questionnaire.

Questions 33 through 43

Respondent Ranking Reports contain customized comparisons of an organization's self-reported data to median values compiled from the survey results. The individual identified on the questionnaire label will receive the Respondent Ranking Report and complimentary survey report for your organization. If this information is incorrect, please provide complete information on lines 33 through 45 for the appropriate recipient.

Parent Organization Information

The observed medical practice is the medical practice for which data has been reported. If you indicated in question 8 on page 2, ownership of the observed practice by a 'hospital/integrated delivery system', 'MSO', 'PPMC', 'University' or 'Other' type of organization, please provide the name and location of the parent organization (owner) in the spaces provided.

Medical Group Management Association
104 Inverness Terrace East
Englewood, Colorado 80112-5306
www.mgma.com
877.ASK.MGMA (275.6462)

20

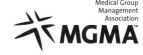

NOTES:

NOTES:

MEDICAL GROUP MANAGEMENT ASSOCIATION™

NOTES:

NOTES:

MEDICAL GROUP MANAGEMENT ASSOCIATION™

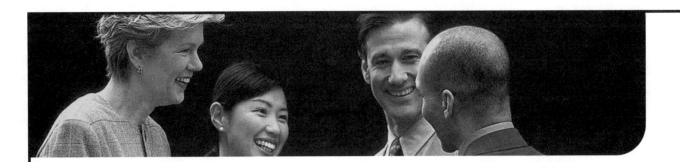

MGMA membership is great in theory.
It's *outstanding* in practice.

Vital resources. Valued results. That's why more than 19,000 of your peers and their practices depend on the benefits Medical Group Management Association (MGMA) membership provides. Whatever your professional needs, we're ready to help with:

INFORMATION. Fresh, relevant information gives you an advantage, whether you're making everyday decisions or planning long-term strategies. From industry-standard survey reports to the world-class MGMA Information Center, we keep you informed. The MGMA Health Care Consulting Group is also available to assist in improving finances, productivity and understanding benchmarking.

NETWORKING. Every professional knows the value of sharing ideas and advice with trusted colleagues. Online and in person, as an MGMA member you'll develop meaningful professional relationships that positively affect your career and your practice.

EDUCATION. We deliver varied opportunities to enhance your knowledge and skills. Online, in person, via audio and video — and special events — MGMA offers ongoing dynamic learning opportunities.

ADVOCACY. As the nation's principal voice for medical group practice, MGMA has been protecting your interests, keeping you abreast of crucial developments — and keeping you involved — for more than 75 years.

CERTIFICATION. If you want to be among the very best at the American College of Medical Practice Executives (ACMPE) can set you on the course toward respected professional board certification and Fellowship.

Want more information on membership?
Go to **www.mgma.com**, e-mail **membership@mgma.com** or call toll-free **877.275.6462**, ext. 889.

Medical Group
Management
Association

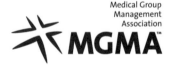

Survey Report CD-ROM Order Form

Improve your bottom line with the Medical Group Management Association's (MGMA's) survey reports on CD-ROM. These interactive tools allow you to benchmark your practice performance, run customized data comparisons and identify opportunities for improvement.

Gain analytical and graphing capabilities with the CD-ROM. Use it as a complement to your reports.

We put it together. You put it to use.

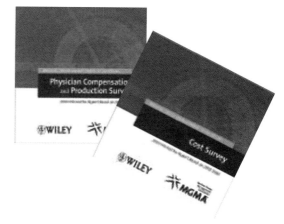

MGMA # _____

First name _____ MI _____ Last name _____

Title _____ Organization _____

Address _____ ☐ Work address ☐ Personal address

City _____ State _____ ZIP _____

Phone _____ Ext. _____ Fax_____ E-mail _____

☐ Male   Birth year _____   ☐ Please send me a **FREE** brochure about MGMA membership. (MAA)

☐ Female   Year started in health care _____   ☐ Please send me a **FREE** brochure about ACMPE® board certification in medical practice management. (AMD)

Item No.	Qty.	Description	Member	Affiliate	Other	Total Price
Cost Survey Report CD-ROM						
PMM-6041		Single user, single computer system	$415	$465	$515	
PMM-6042		Network license, single site, single access	$725	$810	$895	
PMM-6043		Network license, single site, unlimited simultaneous access	$1,200	$1,350	$1,495	
Physician Compensation and Production Survey Report CD-ROM						
PMM-6047		Single user, single computer system	$415	$465	$515	
PMM-6048		Network license, single site, single access	$725	$810	$895	
PMM-6049		Network license, single site, unlimited simultaneous access	$1,200	$1,350	$1,495	

Online
The Store at
www.mgma.com
Search by the four-digit item number.

Phone
For credit card orders: Call toll-free
877.ASK.MGMA

Mail   Mail this form with your check payable to:
Medical Group Management Association
P.O. Box 17603
Denver, CO 80217-0603

Fax
Fax this form for credit card orders to:
303.643.4439

Shipping and handling
Orders are shipped via UPS. Federal Express is also available.

Special mail	Add
UPS Priority (next day air)	$15.50
UPS 2nd day	$10.50

All orders must be prepaid

☐ Check enclosed

☐ VISA   ☐ MasterCard   ☐ AMEX

Card # _____ Exp. date _____

Cardholder's name _____

Authorized signature _____

Today's date _____

Subtotal	
Shipping/handling	$7.50
Sales tax*	
Special mail	
Total	

*Please add sales tax if a resident of Colorado: Denver metro area 3.7%; outside Denver metro area 2.9%; District of Columbia, 5.75%; Texas, 6.25%.

Medical Group
Management
Association
MGMA

MGMA Survey Report Order Form

MGMA # _____

First name _____ MI _____ Last name _____

Title _____ Organization _____

Address _____ ☐ Work address ☐ Personal address

City _____ State _____ ZIP _____

Phone _____ Ext. _____ Fax _____ E-mail _____

☐ Male   Birth year _____   ☐ Please send me a **FREE** brochure about MGMA membership. (MAA)

☐ Female   Year started in health care _____   ☐ Please send me a **FREE** brochure about ACMPE® board certification in medical practice management. (AMD)

Item No.	Qty.	Description	Member	Affiliate	Other	Total Price
		Academic survey report				
PMM-5978		Academic Practice Compensation and Production Survey for Faculty & Management: 2003 Report Based on 2002 Data	$295	$345	$495	
		Cost survey reports				
PMM-6053		Cost Survey: 2003 Report Based on 2002 Data	$250	$300	$460	
PMM-6041		Cost Survey CD-ROM (Single user, additional licenses available)	$415	$465	$515	
PMM-6057		Cost Survey for Cardiovascular/Thoracic Surgery & Cardiology Practices: 2003 Report Based on 2002 Data	$250	$300	$460	
PMM-6059		Cost Survey for Integrated Delivery System Practices: 2003 Report Based on 2002 Data	$250	$300	$460	
PMM-6058		Cost Survey for Orthopedic Practices: 2003 Report Based on 2002 Data	$250	$300	$460	
		Performance survey reports				
PMM-6067		Ambulatory Surgery Center Performance Survey: 2003 Report Based on 2002 Data	$185	$255	$340	
PMM-6066		Management Services Organization Performance Survey: 2003 Report Based on 2002 Data	$250	$300	$460	
PMM-6065		Performance and Practices of Successful Medical Groups: 2003 Report Based on 2002 Data (Members of both MGMA and ACMPE receive 10 percent off: $247.50)	$275	$325	$485	
		Production and compensation reports				
PMM-6064		Management Compensation Survey: 2003 Report Based on 2002 Data	$120	$150	$180	
PMM-6060		Physician Compensation and Production Survey: 2003 Report Based on 2002 Data	$265	$315	$475	
PMM-6047		Physician Compensation and Production Survey CD-ROM (Single user, additional licenses available)	$415	$465	$515	
		Special offers				
PMM-6044		Cost Survey CD-ROM (single user) and report	$565	$665	$875	
PMM-6050		Physician Compensation and Production Survey CD-ROM (single user) and report	$580	$680	$890	
PMM-6070		Essentials in Benchmarking, set of four survey reports: Cost Survey; Physician Compensation and Production Survey; Management Compensation Survey; Performance and Practices of Successful Medical Groups	$790	$940	$1,420	

Online
The Store at
www.mgma.com
Search by the four-digit item number.

Phone
For credit card orders: Call toll-free
877.ASK.MGMA

Mail
Mail this form with your check payable to:
Medical Group Management Association
P.O. Box 17603
Denver, CO 80217-0603

Fax
Fax this form for credit card orders to:
303.643.4439

Shipping and handling

Orders are shipped via UPS. Federal Express is also available by request.

Special mail	Add
UPS Priority (next day air)	$15.50
UPS 2nd Day	$10.50

All orders must be prepaid

☐ Check enclosed

☐ Please charge my: ☐ VISA   ☐ MasterCard   ☐ AMEX

Card # _____ Exp. date _____

Card holder's name _____

Authorized signature _____

Today's date _____

Subtotal	
Shipping/Handling	$7.50
Sales tax*	
Special mail	
Total	

*Please add sales tax if a resident of Colorado: Denver metro area 3.7%; outside Denver metro area 2.9%; District of Columbia 5.75%; Texas 6.25%

Medical Group Management Association

MGMA™